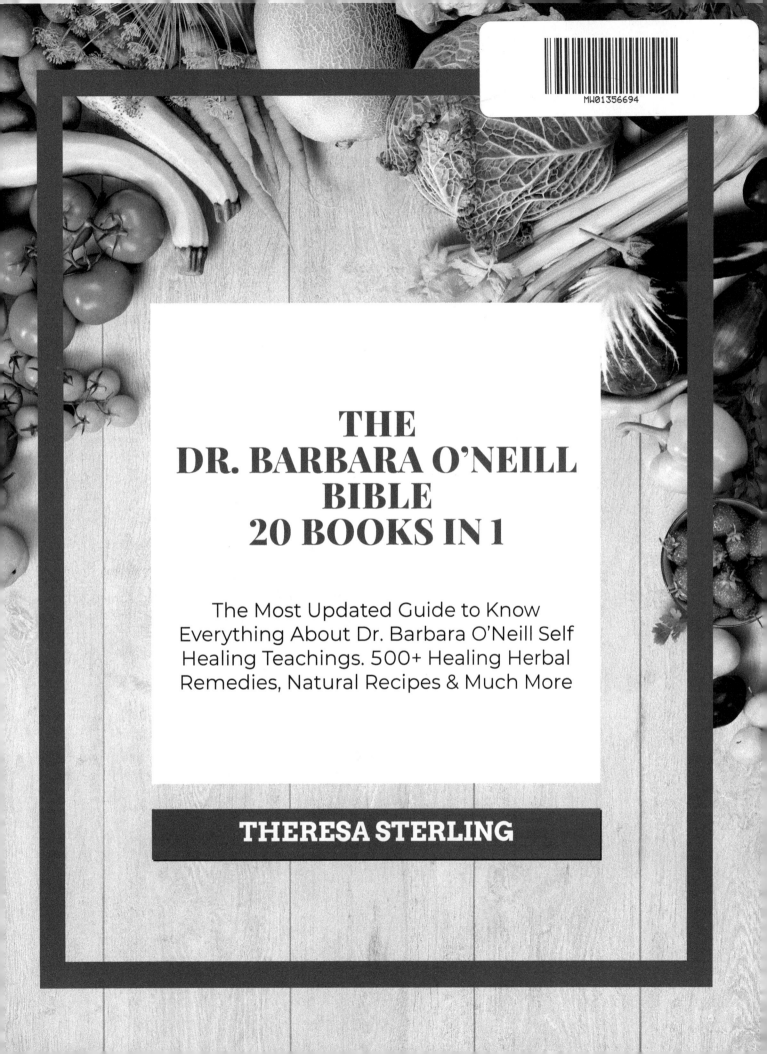

THE DR. BARBARA O'NEILL BIBLE 20 BOOKS IN 1

The Most Updated Guide to Know Everything About Dr. Barbara O'Neill Self Healing Teachings. 500+ Healing Herbal Remedies, Natural Recipes & Much More

THERESA STERLING

COPYRIGHT

© Copyright 2024 by Theresa Sterling - All rights reserved.

This document is intended to provide accurate and reliable information regarding the topic covered. The publication is sold with the understanding that the publisher is not required to render accounting, legal, or other professional services. If professional advice or other expert assistance is required, the services of a competent professional should be sought.

From a Declaration of Principles jointly adopted by a Committee of the American Bar Association and a Committee of Publishers and Associations.

No part of this document may be reproduced, duplicated, or transmitted in any form, electronic or printed, without the prior written permission of the publisher. Recording of this publication is strictly prohibited, and any storage of this document is not allowed without explicit consent from the publisher. All rights reserved.

The information contained herein is declared to be truthful and consistent, and any liability arising from negligence or otherwise, from the use or misuse of any policies, processes, or directions contained within, rests solely with the recipient reader. Under no circumstances will the publisher be held liable for any damages, reparations, or monetary loss due to the information herein, whether directly or indirectly.

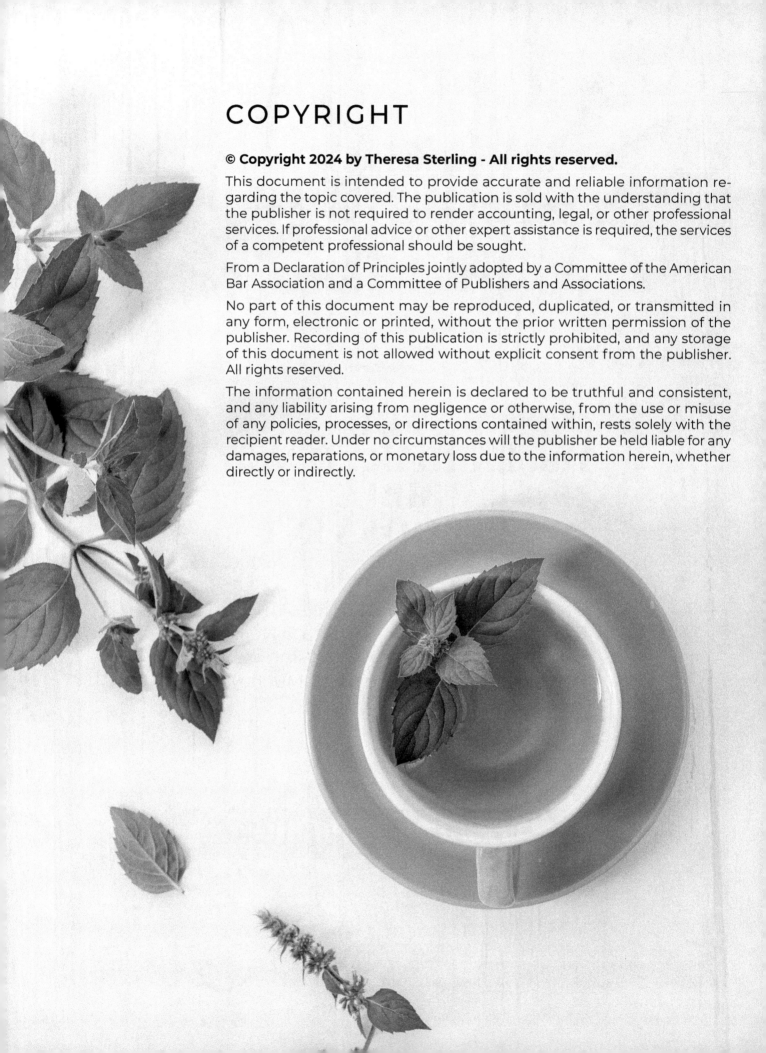

TABLE OF CONTENTS

BOOK 1
DR. BARBARA'S ENCYCLOPEDIA OF NATURAL REMEDIES

- ACKNOWLEDGMENT AND DISCLAIMER 13
- INTRODUCTION 13
- UNDERSTANDING NATURAL REMEDIES 14
- THE THERAPEUTIC BENEFITS OF HERBAL MEDICINE 15
- HOLISTIC APPROACH TO HEALING 15
- NATUROPATHIC USAGE OF HERBAL MEDICINE 16
- COMMONLY USED HERBS IN NATUROPATHIC MEDICINE 17
- INCORPORATING HERBAL MEDICINE INTO DAILY LIFE 18
- INTEGRATING NATURAL REMEDIES WITH MODERN MEDICINE 18

BOOK 2
THE SCIENCE OF HERBAL MEDICINE

- HOW KEY HERBS AFFECT THE BODY .. 22
- NATURAL REMEDY PROFILES FOR COMMON AILMENTS 23

BOOK 3
HERBS AND THEIR HEALING PROPERTIES

- INTRODUCTION 27
- DETAILED ESSENTIAL HERB PROFILES 27

BOOK 4
NATURAL REMEDIES FOR COMMON AILMENTS

- INTRODUCTION 39
- TREATMENTS FOR COLDS, FLU, INFLAMMATION, DIGESTIVE ISSUES, AND MORE 39

1. Common Cold and Flu 39
2. Inflammation 40
3. Digestive Issues 40
4. Stress and Anxiety 41
5. Nausea and Motion Sickness 41
6. Sore Throat 42
7. Herbal Immune-Boosting Tonic 42
8. Anti-inflammatory Turmeric Paste 43
9. Digestive Health Elixir 43
10. Stress-Relieving Lavender Bath 44

RECIPES OF COMMON REMEDIES 45

1. Elderberry Syrup 45
2. Elderberry Gummies 45
3. Elderberry Tea 46
4. Elderberry Tincture 46
5. Elderberry Lozenges 47
6. Marshmallow Root Tea 48
7. Marshmallow Root Cough Syrup 48
8. Marshmallow Root Infusion 49
9. Marshmallow Root Salve 49
10. Marshmallow Root Lozenges 50
11. Yarrow Tea 50
12. Yarrow Infused Oil 51
13. Yarrow Tincture 51
14. Yarrow Poultice 52
15. Yarrow Bath 52
16. Catnip Tea 53
17. Catnip Infused Oil 53
18. Catnip Tincture 54
19. Catnip Bath 54
20. Catnip Compress 55
21. Ginkgo Biloba Tea 55
22. Ginkgo Biloba Tincture 56
23. Ginkgo Biloba Infused Oil 56
24. Ginkgo Biloba Capsules 57
25. Ginkgo Biloba Lotion 57
26. Oregano Tea 58
27. Oregano Oil 58
28. Oregano Tincture 59
29. Oregano Infused Honey 59
30. Oregano Steam Inhalation 60
31. Tulsi Tea 60
32. Tulsi Infused Oil 61
33. Tulsi Tincture 61
34. Tulsi Honey 62
35. Tulsi Facial Steam 62
36. Licorice Root Tea 63
37. Licorice Root Decoction 63
38. Licorice Root Infused Oil 64
39. Licorice Root Honey Syrup 64
40. Licorice Root Steam Inhalation 65
41. Fenugreek Tea 66
42. Fenugreek Poultice 66
43. Fenugreek Seed Infusion 67
44. Fenugreek Seed Powder 67
45. Fenugreek Seed Capsules 68
46. Hawthorn Berry Tea 68
47. Hawthorn Tincture 69
48. Hawthorn Berry Syrup 69
49. Hawthorn Berry Jam 70
50. Hawthorn Berry Smoothie 70
51. Fennel Seed Tea 71
52. Fennel Infused Oil 71
53. Fennel Seed Mouthwash 72
54. Fennel Seed Steam Inhalation 72
55. Fennel Seed Poultice 73
56. Lemon Balm Tea 73
57. Lemon Balm Tincture 74
58. Lemon Balm Infused Oil 74
59. Lemon Balm Bath Soak 75
60. Lemon Balm Facial Steam 75
61. Basil Infused Water 76
62. Basil Essential Oil Massage Blend ... 76
63. Basil and Honey Cough Syrup 76
64. Basil Steam Inhalation 77
65. Basil Lemonade 77
66. Calendula Infused Oil 78
67. Calendula Salve 78
68. Calendula Tea 79
69. Calendula Bath Soak 79
70. Calendula Compress 80

BOOK 5
HERBAL REMEDIES IN DAILY LIFE

Practical advice 82
Tips for growing your herbs and preparing remedies at home 83

NUTRITION AND NATURAL REMEDIES 85

Investigating food, nutrition, and herbal remedy efficacy 85
Guidelines for a balanced diet 86

DETOXIFICATION AND BODY CLEANSING 88

Natural herbal detoxification and cleaning ...88
Foods and routines for periodic detoxification 89

BOOK 6
NATURAL REMEDIES FOR MENTAL AND EMOTIONAL WELL-BEING

NATURAL HERBS FOR MENTAL HEALTH AND EMOTIONAL HARMONY 93
HERBS FOR MENTAL AND EMOTIONAL SUPPORT 94
OTHER SUPPLEMENTS 96
NATURAL ANXIETY AND STRESS MANAGEMENT 96

BOOK 7
NATURAL REMEDIES FOR BEAUTY AND SKIN CARE

HERBAL SKIN CARE AND BEAUTY SOLUTIONS 100
TIPS FOR NATURAL ANTI-AGING AND SKIN HEALTH 101

BOOK 8
RECIPES FOR HEALTH AND WELLNESS

INTRODUCTION 104
DETAILED HERBAL REMEDY, TINCTURE, AND INFUSION RECIPES. 104
1. Lavender Relaxation Tea Infusion 104
2. Echinacea Immune-Boosting Tincture 105
3. Rosemary Scalp Stimulating Hair Rinse Infusion... 105
4. Lemon Balm Stress-Relief Tincture 106
5. Peppermint Digestive Tonic Infusion.......106
6. Calendula Healing Salve........................ 107
7. Chamomile Relaxing Bath Infusion 107
8. Ginger Digestive Tincture......................108
9. Elderberry Syrup Immune-Boosting Infusion 108
10. Turmeric Anti-Inflammatory Tincture ..109
How to properly store and administer these remedies 109

CASE STUDIES AND SUCCESS STORIES...110
Real-life success stories of natural remedy adopters...110
Lessons learned and tips from their experiences 111

BOOK 9
ADVANCED HERBAL MEDICINE

COMPLEX HERBAL FORMULATIONS AND THEIR THERAPEUTIC USES................................114
1. Immune Support Blend: 115
2. Stress Relief Formula: 115
3. Digestive Harmony Blend: 115
4. Hormonal Balance Formula: 116
5. Energy and Vitality Tonic: 116
6. Sleep Support Blend: 117
7. Joint and Muscle Comfort Formula: 117
8. Cognitive Function Enhancer: 117
9. Detoxification and Cleansing Blend: 118
10. Heart Health Support Formula: 118
Combining herbs for enhanced effects..........118

CONCLUSION..119

BOOK 10
PLANT-BASED NUTRITION BASICS

INTRODUCTION 122
UNDERSTANDING PLANT-BASED NUTRITION 123
WHAT IS A PLANT-BASED DIET? 123
Is Plant-Based Diet Beneficial for the Body? 124
Why it's Important to Reduce Consumption of Processed and Animal-

Based Foods.................................124
FOODS TO EAT AND AVOID 126
HEALTH BENEFITS OF
FOLLOWING A PLANT-BASED DIET 127
ENVIRONMENTAL BENEFITS OF
PLANT-BASED DIET 128
WHY YOU SHOULD ADOPT
PLANT-BASED EATING? 129
TIPS FOR FOLLOWING A PLANT-
BASED DIET 129

BOOK 11
THE SCIENCE OF WHOLE FOODS

INTRODUCTION 132
WHAT EXACTLY IS MEANT BY A
WHOLE FOODS DIET? 132
EXAMPLE OF WHOLE FOODS 133
WHY SHOULD YOU
INCORPORATE WHOLE FOODS
INTO YOUR DIET? 133
NUTRITIONAL BENEFITS OF
WHOLE FOODS 134
HOW WHOLE FOODS CAN HELP
NUMBER OF HEALTH ISSUES 135

BOOK 12
BUILDING A PLANT-BASED PANTRY

INTRODUCTION 138
WHY IS IT SO CRUCIAL TO HAVE
A WELL-STOCKED PANTRY? 138
ESSENTIAL INGREDIENTS TO
KEEP IN YOUR PLANT-BASED
PANTRY 139

ADDING FINAL ITEMS TO YOUR
GROCERY LIST 140
ORGANIZING YOUR PANTRY 141
TIPS FOR SOURCING
SUSTAINABLE AND ORGANIC
PRODUCTS..141

BOOK 13
DR. BARBARA COOKBOOK

INTRODUCTION 144
ESSENTIAL COOKING
TECHNIQUES EVERY PLANT-
BASED CHEF SHOULD MASTER..........144
FIVE EASY WAYS TO BEGIN
ENHANCING YOUR PLANT-
BASED COOKING ABILITIES................146
BREAKFAST RECIPES 147
Simple Avocado Toast 147
Raspberry and Chia Smoothie Bowl 148
Simple Breakfast Mix 149
Cheeky Cereal 149
Oatmeal-Free Breakfast 151
Plant-Powered Pancakes 152
Banana Nut Smoothie 153
Breakfast Scramble 154
Cinnamon Apple Toast 155
Chocolate Chia Pudding 156
Oat and Peanut Butter Breakfast Bar 156
Berry Blast Smoothie 157
Classic Tofu Scramble 157
Goji Breakfast Bowl 158
Fig Protein Smoothie.................................158
*Everyday Oats with Coconut and
Strawberries*..160
Peaches and Cream Oats 161
*Frosty Hemp and Blackberry Smoothie
Bowl*..162
Tropical Paradise Smoothie 164
Peach Crumble Shake 167
Banana Cream Pie Chia Pudding..............168
Oatmeal-Banana Pancakes 169
Pumpkin Spice Protein Oatmeal 170
Chocolate Quinoa Breakfast Bowl.............171

Baked Banana French Toast with Raspberry Syrup 172
Chocolate Peanut Butter Smoothie 173
Chickpea Scramble 174
Fruity Granola 175
Avocado Walnut Sandwich 176
Strawberry, Banana, and Coconut Shake 177
Spiced Orange Breakfast Couscous 177
Banana Bread 178
Pumpkin Pie Smoothie 179
Breakfast Parfaits 179

SOUPS AND SALADS 180
Loaded Kale Salad 180
Classic Lentil Soup with Swiss Chard 181
Roasted Fennel Salad 182
Cannellini Bean Soup with Kale 183
Quinoa and Black Bean Salad 184
Creamy Pumpkin and Toasted Walnut Soup 185
Classic Roasted Pepper Salad 186
Roasted Beet and Avocado Salad 187
Moroccan Aubergine Salad 188
Green Lentil Salad 189
Hearty Winter Quinoa Soup 190
Tomato Pumpkin Soup 191
Cauliflower Spinach Soup 194
Cherry Tomato Salad with Soy Chorizo 195
Creamy Squash Soup 196
Roasted Carrot Soup 197
Rocket Chickpeas Salad 198
Classic Cream of Broccoli Soup 199
Tarragon Cauli Salad 200
Old-Fashioned Green Bean Salad 201
Italian-Style Cremini Mushroom Soup 202
Creamy Avocado Salad with Herb Dressing 203
Quinoa and Avocado Salad 204
Red Bean and Corn Salad 205
Kidney Bean and Potato Soup 207
Creamy Golden Veggie Soup 208
Greek Orzo and Bean Salad 209

MAIN DISHES 210
Curried Mango Chickpea Wrap 210
Sushi Bowl 211
Sweet Potato Patties 212
Vietnamese Summer Rolls 213
Greek-Style Eggplant Skillet 214
Pesto and Sun-dried Tomato Quinoa 215
Olive and White Bean Pasta 216
Blackeyed Peas Burritos 217
Falafel Burgers 218
Savory Sweet Potato Casserole 219
Mango-Ginger Chickpea Curry 221
Rice with Asparagus and Cauliflower 222
Swiss Chard Skillet 223
Avocado Bread with Chickpeas 224
Chili Sin Carne 225
Brown Rice with Vegetables and Tofu 226
Veggie Curry 227
Barley Pilaf with Wild Mushrooms 228
Potage au Quinoa 229
Old-Fashioned Pilaf 230
Barley with Portobello Mushrooms and Chard 231
Traditional Tuscan Bean Stew 232
Beluga Lentil and Vegetable Mélange 233
Green Lentil Stew with Collard Greens 234
Classic Italian Minestrone 235
Mexican-Style Bean Bowl 236
Chickpea Garden Vegetable Medley 237
Old-Fashioned Lentil and Vegetable Stew ... 238
Brown Lentil Bowl 239

HEALTHY SIDES AND SNACKS 240
Roasted Carrots with Herbs 240
Easy Braised Green Beans 241
Braised Kale with Sesame Seeds 242
Sautéed Zucchini with Herbs 243
Sautéed Cauliflower with Sesame Seeds 244
Sautéed Turnip Greens 245
Yukon Gold Mashed Potatoes 246
Aromatic Sautéed Swiss Chard 247
Classic Sautéed Bell Peppers 248
Roasted Garden Vegetables 249
Herb Cauliflower Mash 250
Peppery Hummus Dip 254
Roasted Chickpeas 255
Traditional Baba Ganoush 256
Roasted Cauliflower Dip 257
Easy Zucchini Roll-Ups 258
Hummus Avocado Boats 260
Lettuce Wraps with Hummus and Avocado 261
Baked Zucchini Chips 262
Bell Pepper Boats with Mango Salsa 262
Stuffed Portobellos with Rice and Herbs 263

NATURAL SWEETS AND DESSERTS ... 264
Peanut Butter Date Bites 264
Chocolate N'ice Cream 264
Almond and Chocolate Chip Bars 265

Peanut Butter Oatmeal Bars 266
Raw Chocolate Mango Pie 267
Mini Lemon Tarts 268
Almond-Date Energy Bites 269
Easy Chocolate Squares 270
Zesty Orange-Cranberry Energy Bites 271
Funky Monkey Sorbet 272
Mango Coconut Cream Pie 273
Chocolate and Raisin Cookie Bars 274
Lime in the Coconut Chia Pudding 274
Almond Granola Bars 275
Chocolate Dream Balls 276
Chocolate Hazelnut Fudge 277
Decadent Hazelnut Halvah 278
Berry Compote with Red Wine 279
Coconut Cream Pie 280
Easy Chocolate Candy 281
Greek-Style Fruit Compote 282
Vanilla Ice Cream 283

GLOSSARY 284

MEASUREMENT CONVERSION
TABLE 285

30-DAY MEAL PLAN 286

CONCLUSION 288

BOOK 14
DR BARBARA 15-DAY
GUT CLEANSE PLAN

UNDERSTANDING GUT HEALTH:
THE FOUNDATION OF WELL-BEING .290

WHY A 15-DAY GUT CLEANSE?
THE SCIENCE BEHIND SHORT-
TERM INTERVENTIONS 291

WHAT DOES THE SCIENCE SAY
ABOUT GUT CLEANSES? 291

BOOK 15
PREPARING FOR YOUR
GUT CLEANSE

ASSESSING YOUR CURRENT
HEALTH 295
*How to Understand and Record Your
Baseline Gut Health* 295
Symptoms That Indicate Poor Gut Health ... 295

FUNDAMENTALS OF GUT
CLEANSING 297
*What is Detoxification? Separating Fact
from Fiction* 297
*The Role of Your Gut Microbiome in
Overall Health* 298

FOODS TO EMBRACE AND AVOID 301
*Comprehensive Lists of Beneficial and
Harmful Foods* 301
*The Importance of Organic and Whole
Foods* 304

BOOK 16
THE 15-DAY GUT CLEANSE PLAN

BREAKFAST RECIPES 307
Berry Chia Pudding 307
Turmeric Oatmeal 307
Spinach and Mushroom Egg Muffins 308
Coconut Yogurt Parfait 308
Avocado Breakfast Salad 309
Almond Butter Banana Toast 309
Veggie Breakfast Burrito 310
Blueberry Buckwheat Pancakes 310
Greek Yogurt Breakfast Bowl 311
Tofu Scramble 311

LUNCH RECIPES 312
Quinoa Salad with Lemon Herb Dressing ... 312
Zucchini Noodles with Pesto 314
Vegan Lentil Tacos 316

DINNER RECIPES 320
*Quinoa and Black Bean Stuffed Bell
Peppers* 320
Chicken and Vegetable Stir-Fry 321

Zucchini Noodles with Grilled Shrimp
And Pesto 321
Turkey and Vegetable Skillet 322
Vegetarian Lentil Curry 324
Miso Glazed Eggplant with Brown Rice 327

SNACK RECIPES 329
Avocado and Rice Cake 329
Cucumber and Hummus Bites 329
Energy Bites 330
Apple Slices with Almond Butter 330
Rice Cake with Cottage Cheese And
Sliced Strawberries 331
Carrot Sticks with Hummus 331
Trail Mix 332
Greek Yogurt with Berries 332
Edamame 333
Rice Cake with Smashed Avocado and
Cherry Tomatoes 333
Cottage Cheese with Pineapple 334
Almond Butter and Banana Rice Cake 334
Stuffed Bell Pepper Halves 335
Chia Seed Pudding 335
Turkey and Cheese Roll-Ups 336
Caprese Skewers 336
Seaweed Snack 337
Cucumber Slices with Tzatziki 337
Greek Yogurt Parfait 338
Coconut Yogurt with Mango 338

15-DAY MEAL PLAN 339

BOOK 17
SUPPLEMENTS FOR
ENHANCING GUT HEALTH

DIETARY SUPPLEMENTS 342
SAFE USAGE OF SUPPLEMENTS
DURING YOUR CLEANSE 345

BOOK 18
MIND-BODY PRACTICES TO
ENHANCE YOUR CLEANSE

INCORPORATING YOGA AND
MEDITATION 348
THE ROLE OF SLEEP AND HOW
TO IMPROVE IT 349
COMMON CHALLENGES AND
HOW TO OVERCOME THEM 351
Dealing with Detox Symptoms 351
Adjusting the Cleanse to Fit Your
Lifestyle and Needs 352
FAQS AND EXPERT ANSWERS 353
Responses to the Most Commonly
Asked Questions 353

BOOK 19
BEYOND THE CLEANSE

TRANSITIONING TO A
LONG-TERM GUT HEALTH PLAN 357
How to Safely Conclude Your Cleanse 357
STRATEGIES FOR MAINTAINING
GUT HEALTH POST-CLEANSE 357
BUILDING A HOLISTIC LIFESTYLE 359
Integrating Nutritional Changes into
Everyday Life 359
SUSTAINING MENTAL AND
PHYSICAL WELL-BEING 360
CONCLUSION 361

BOOK 20
430 EXTRA REMEDIES

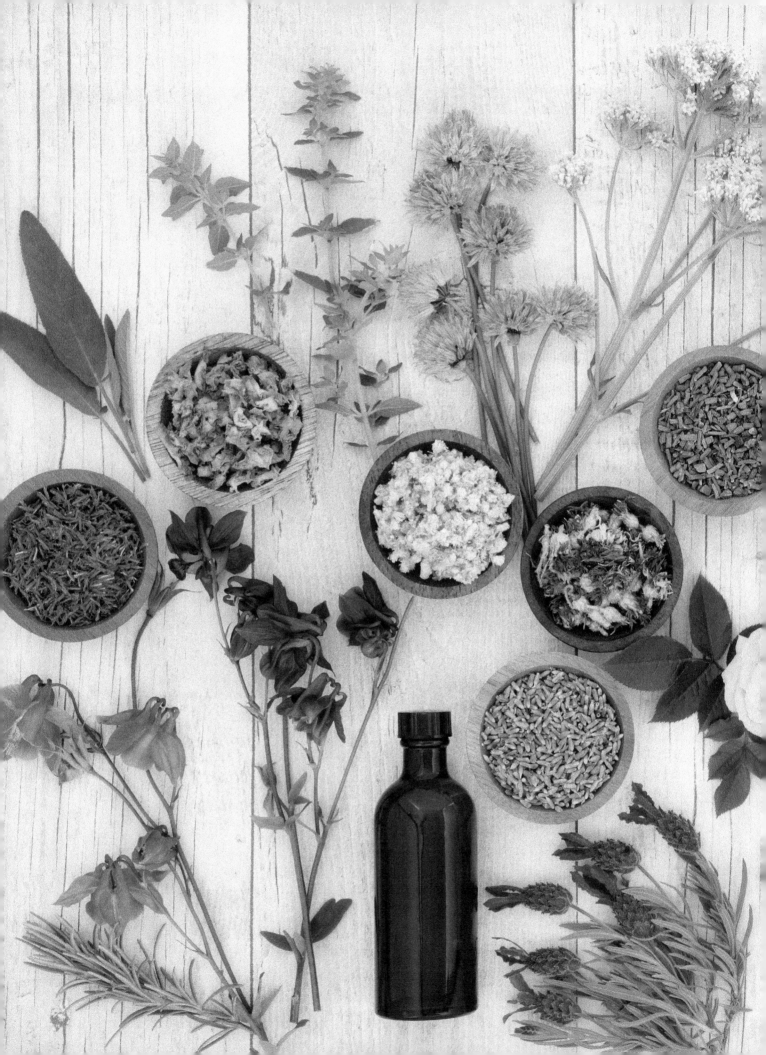

BOOK 1

DR. BARBARA'S ENCYCLOPEDIA OF NATURAL REMEDIES

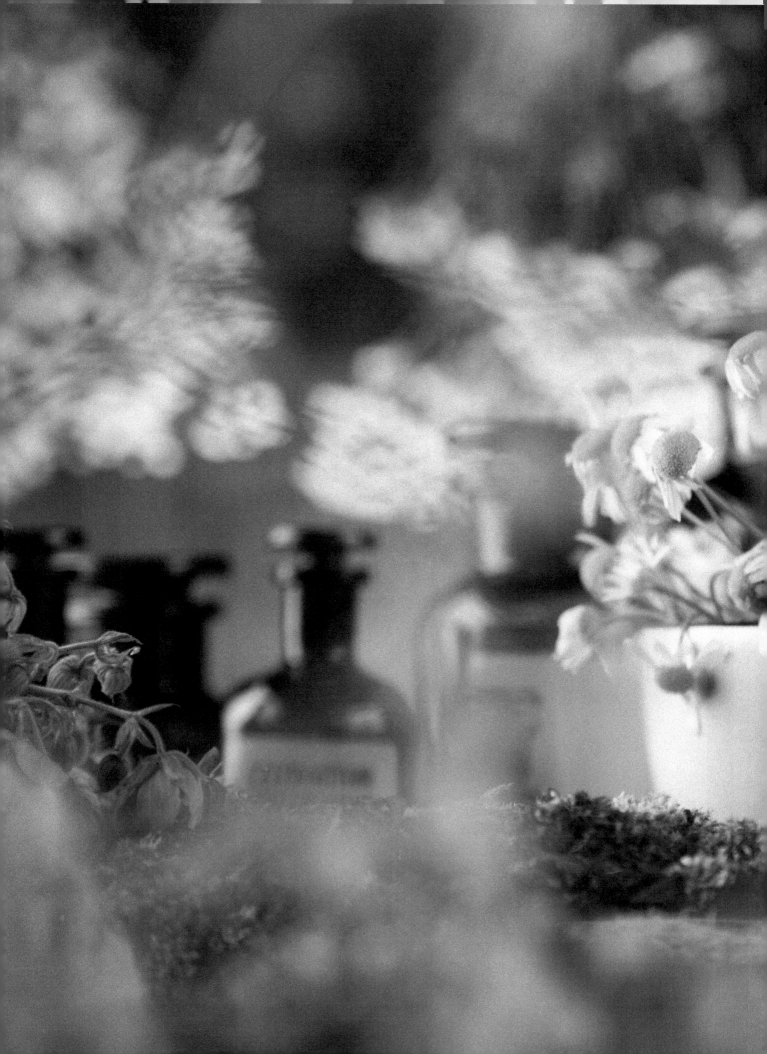

ACKNOWLEDGMENT AND DISCLAIMER

This book, although inspired by the teachings and philosophy of Barbara O'Neill, is an original work created and published in full adherence to copyright laws. It is important to clarify that while Barbara O'Neill's holistic approach to health and wellness has been a source of inspiration, the content within these pages is based on my own research, experiences, and interpretations.

The ideas, strategies, and recommendations in this book are not endorsed by, nor do they directly represent, the views or teachings of Barbara O'Neill. This work aims to honor her contributions to natural health and holistic living while presenting my personal perspective and understanding of these subjects.

The purpose of this book is to provide valuable information and insights to those seeking guidance on improving their health and well-being, with inspiration from Barbara O'Neill as a foundation. It should be considered an independent work, separate from Barbara O'Neill's publications and materials.

This book is not affiliated with, authorized by, sponsored by, or otherwise endorsed by Barbara O'Neill. All content is provided for informational purposes only and should not be taken as medical advice. Readers are encouraged to consult healthcare professionals for advice tailored to their individual health needs.

INTRODUCTION

Dr. Barbara's Encyclopedia of Natural Remedies is your go-to source for remedies and overall well-being. Many individuals in today's paced world are turning to healing methods to enhance their health and vitality. Within these pages, you'll discover a treasure trove of information and tips to help you achieve health and wellness. This comprehensive guide will lead you on a journey into the world of remedies.

Dr Barbara, a herbalist, doctor, and advocate for holistic living, will take you on an enlightening exploration of nature's healing powers. Drawing from her wealth of knowledge in plant medicine and holistic therapies acquired through years of experience, research and ancient wisdom, she empowers you to reclaim your vigor and manage your well-being.

At the core of this guidebook lies the belief that true healing occurs when the mind, body and spirit are in sync with each other. Driven by an approach that addresses mental, emotional and spiritual well-being, Dr Barbara's methods focus on restoring balance at every level while addressing the root causes of illness for lasting transformation and overall health.

The Encyclopedia of Natural Healing covers a range of topics, including remedies, nutritional therapy, lifestyle changes and mind-body techniques. Each element is careful. Chosen to offer information and practical tips for incorporating natural healing into your daily routine.

Within the herbal remedies section, you'll find a selection of botanicals and plants, each known for its medicinal properties. Dr Barbara's comprehensive guide introduces plant allies that can aid in support, digestion, stress relief and overall well-being. Whether you prefer herbs like chamomile and lavender or modern superfoods and adaptogenic herbs, there's something for everyone.

For insights on nourishing your body, enhancing health and preventing illness through nutrition therapy, look no further than Dr Barbara's exploration of superfoods, healing spices and rich foods. Her guidance on preparing meals that promote vitality and long-lasting wellness is invaluable.

In the lifestyle interventions section, the importance of establishing routines that contribute to your wellness is emphasized.

Dr Barbara provides tips on enhancing your health and well-being through avenues such as staying active, prioritizing good sleep habits, managing stress effectively and embracing mindfulness techniques. Additionally, the connection between your emotional and physical wellness is explored in detail within the mind-body practices section. Seek to boost your being, inner strength and resilience levels. Dr. Barbara can guide you in integrating mind-body activities like yoga, energy healing, controlled breathing exercises, and meditation practices into your daily regimen.

Empowering yourself to take control of your well-being journey, actively engaging in your healthcare decisions and acquiring knowledge are recurring themes emphasized throughout this encyclopedia authored by Dr. Barbara. This book serves as a companion and mentor as you navigate toward healing, whether you seek remedies for specific health issues or aim to prevent illnesses while enhancing your overall vitality.

May you discover the wisdom of nature within yourself, honor your body's ability to heal itself naturally and embark on a path towards health and vitality as you embark on this enlightening journey. Within the pages of Dr. Barbara's Encyclopedia of Natural Healing lies a wealth of health insights intertwined with the essence of nature.

UNDERSTANDING NATURAL REMEDIES

Phytotherapy, botanical medicine or herbal medicine all refer to the practice of improving health through the use of plants and their natural healing properties. It supports the body's healing abilities by harnessing the resources found in nature. Throughout history, civilizations such as the Greeks, Egyptians, and Chinese have utilized plants for culinary purposes. In today's healthcare landscape herbal medicine remains a component by offering approaches to conventional treatments. Naturopathic practitioners often blend healing methods with medical science to provide comprehensive care.

Importance of Herbal Medicine in Naturopathy

By supporting the body's natural healing mechanisms, medicine aims to tackle the root causes of illnesses. It emphasizes the healing properties found in nature. Herbal therapy aligns with this approach by utilizing ingredients to facilitate healing processes. In the realm of medicine, herbs are viewed as partners in restoring balance and well-being.

Herbal remedies play a role in medicine for treating various health conditions. Whether it's enhancing digestion or boosting immunity, herbs offer a range of benefits. Exploring the uses of plants is integral to understanding herbal medicine. Incorporating herbs into treatment plans can help individuals tap into nature's rejuvenating energies and feel revitalized.

Please note that this information is not advice, and it is important to consult with your healthcare provider before using any remedies.

THE THERAPEUTIC BENEFITS OF HERBAL MEDICINE

Exploring Nature's Pharmacy

A diverse array of plants, each possessing properties, thrives in the natural world. Natural environments ranging from grasslands to rainforests are rich with plants that offer a range of potential remedies.

The abundance and diversity of these plants enable therapy to address ailments effectively. It appears that there is a plant-based remedy for every illness. For instance, chamomile is beneficial for reducing inflammation, ginkgo biloba enhances memory, and hawthorn supports health.

The efficacy of therapy stems from the presence of chemical compounds within plants. These bioactive elements interact synergistically affecting processes to facilitate the healing process.

Active Compounds and Their Effects

The diverse array of compounds in medicinal plants offers a wide range of healing possibilities. Alkaloids and flavonoids are a couple of examples of these compounds that offer health benefits.

For example, apigenin, found in chamomile, is what gives it its calming properties. Curcumin, a component of turmeric, works by impacting signal pathways to reduce inflammation and discomfort.

In addition to these effects, many herbal ingredients also support antioxidants in the system and have properties. Herbal therapy is valued for its versatility in promoting health and preventing illness.

To improve being and overall quality of life, it's important to grasp the roles of these substances so we can harness nature's healing powers effectively.

HOLISTIC APPROACH TO HEALING

Balancing Body Systems with Herbs

To maintain health, as advocated by medicine, it is essential to nurture the well-being of one's mind, body and spirit in unity. Holistic practitioners delve into the causes of a person's health issues, looking beyond symptoms. Herbs play a role in regulating the body's hormones aiding in detoxification processes and enhancing resilience.

Traditional herbal remedies have confidence in the body's natural healing abilities. These remedies promote well-being and energy by aligning with the body's rhythms rather than simply masking symptoms.

By supporting functions and boosting immunity, herbs offer phytochemicals essential nutrients and bioactive compounds. They help regulate metabolism, facilitate tissue repair and bolster defenses.

Supporting the Body's Natural Process

The innate healing abilities of the body form the basis of medicine. Herbs support well-being and vitality by aligning with the body's rhythms of concealing them. The body's intrinsic functions and strength are enhanced by the minerals and compounds provided by herbs.

NATUROPATHIC USAGE OF HERBAL MEDICINE

Principles of Naturopathy

TREATING THE ROOT CAUSE

The main reason behind illnesses is the point of focus, in care. Naturopathic doctors aim to bring balance by pinpointing the core of the ailment. An essential aspect of these treatments involves using remedies that target the underlying issues affecting health. Maintaining health often involves utilizing herbs as solutions that tackle the root causes of health issues.

SUPPORTING THE HEALING POWER OF THE BODY

In the process of healing, naturopathic doctors work together with patients to remove agents and enhance the body's natural healing processes. The vital nutrients and compounds present in herbs help maintain functions and address any existing imbalances.

Integrating Herbal Medicine into Naturopathic Practices

CUSTOMIZED HERBAL FORMULAS

In medicine, it's crucial to take into account factors like a patient's well-being, lifestyle choices, diet and medical background when customizing treatment. Naturopathic doctors have the flexibility to personalize therapies using medicine based on needs and imbalances. They rely on a blend of wisdom, research and personal insights to ensure that herbal remedies are effective and safe for each patient.

HERBAL MEDICINE IN PREVENTIVE HEALTHCARE

When considering health, the use of herbs plays a role in both treating and preventing illnesses. Herbs offer health advantages, such as enhancing immunity, aiding in detoxification and managing stress effectively. Naturopathic doctors design health programs that focus on herbs, stress management, nutrition and lifestyle choices.

By incorporating herbs into their routine, individuals can take control of their well-being. This approach provides safe treatments that're essential components of naturopathic healthcare. Embracing remedies and following principles contribute positively to overall health.

COMMONLY USED HERBS IN NATUROPATHIC MEDICINE

A. Overview of Key Herbs and Their Properties

There are remedies derived from plants that offer various health benefits in herbal medicine. Naturopathic practitioners often use herbs to address a variety of symptoms and boost vitality. Let's explore some of the herbs utilized in medicine and the advantages they offer;

- **Echinacea (Echinacea purpurea):** Echinacea is well-liked for treating infections, the cold and flu due to its ability to boost the immune system. It aids in reducing symptoms and shortening their duration by enhancing immunity.
- **Ginger (Zingiber officinale):** Ginger is commonly utilized for its inflammatory and digestive properties, helping to ease symptoms of motion sickness, nausea and stomach discomfort. It also contributes to well-being by boosting the system and enhancing blood flow.
- **Turmeric (Curcuma longa):** Turmeric has become widely known for its antioxidant and anti-inflammatory properties. It can potentially help with health, inflammation and cardiovascular well-being. The active compound curcumin offers advantages for health conditions.
- **Holy Basil (Ocimum sanctum):** In medicine, basil, also known as tulsi, is greatly valued for its adaptogenic properties that support stress management and the development of resilience. Furthermore, holy basil is believed to enhance function, regulate blood sugar levels and improve focus and concentration.

B. Herbal Protocols for Common Health Concerns

To cater to health needs, naturopathic doctors create customized plans. Herbal treatments prove beneficial for health issues such as;

- **Immune Support:** Many individuals rely on herbs such as elderberry, echinacea and astragalus to boost their system and reduce the risk of getting sick.
- **Digestive Health:** Herbs such as peppermint, ginger and fennel are known for their ability to help with gas, nausea and indigestion due to their properties.
- **Stress Management:** Adaptogenic plants, like basil, Rhodiola and ashwagandha, support the body's response to stress while also promoting a sense of tranquillity, concentration and balance in both the mind and emotions.
- **Skin Conditions:** Calendula, aloe vera and chamomile are known for their soothing properties that can help reduce skin inflammation, heal wounds and promote the body's natural healing mechanisms.
- **Women's Health:** Supporting balance, easing cramps, and enhancing overall reproductive health are the objectives of herbal treatments like black cohosh, red raspberry leaf and dong quai.
- **Respiratory Wellness:** The licorice root, mullein, and thyme have properties for support the system, which can help with respiratory infections, congestion and coughs. Naturopathic doctors utilize approaches involving herbs to address imbalances and enhance health. Herbal remedies play a role in medicine by promoting well-being, easing various symptoms and boosting overall wellness. Please note that the statement above is shared for purposes only and should not be considered as advice.

INCORPORATING HERBAL MEDICINE INTO DAILY LIFE

A. Herbal Teas and Infusions

Creating your tea is an easy and delightful way to enjoy the goodness of herbs every day. You can brew an infusion that aids digestion, calms the senses or boosts your system.

- **Choosing Quality Herbs:** When preparing tea, opt for herbs of top-notch quality. To ensure you get the clean herbs, seek out trustworthy suppliers that follow sustainable harvesting methods.
- **Brewing Herbal Teas:** Brewing tea involves steeping the herbs in water for about 5 to 10 minutes. To retain the flavors and aroma, it's best to cover the tea while it steeps.
- **Popular Herbal Teas:** If you want a soothing tea, consider chamomile. Peppermint is good for digestion. Freshening breath and ginger might offer relief from inflammation and nausea. Experiment with herbs to discover your favorites.

B. Culinary Uses of Medicinal Herbs

Medicinal herbs not only have benefits but also add flavor and nutritional value to various dishes, like soups, sauces, salads and desserts.

- **Fresh vs. Dried Herbs:** Using dried herbs is preferable as they maintain their flavor and are easier to handle compared to ones. The ideal approach is to experiment with each option in your cooking endeavors.
- **Incorporating Herbs into Cooking:** To liven up salads, soups and pasta, you can sprinkle them with some parsley, cilantro or basil. For a boost in the taste of veggies, meats, and sauces, consider adding rosemary, dried thyme or oregano.
- **Herbal Infused Oils and Vinegar:** Enhance the taste of vinegar or olive oil by adding herbs, like rosemary or chili peppers, to make delicious dips, sauces and marinades. Integrate cooking herbs and herbal teas into your schedule for an environmentally friendly method to enjoy the rejuvenating effects of nature. To experience the benefits of remedies, try out plants and methods until you find one that suits your needs.

INTEGRATING NATURAL REMEDIES WITH MODERN MEDICINE

Blending remedies with healthcare has become a popular approach in the constantly evolving healthcare landscape to address the complex needs of patients. Care aims to consider the interconnectedness of the body, mind and spirit, striving for a method that merges ancient natural healing traditions with cutting-edge medical advancements. In this examination, we delve into how alternative medicines support medical practices by enhancing overall well-being, managing symptoms, improving treatment outcomes and preventing illnesses.

1. Understanding Natural Remedies and Modern Medicine

Understanding the principles and approaches of both these paradigms is essential before delving into their combination.

Natural Remedies: The phrase " remedy" encompasses a range of medical treatments that utilize natural substances, like herbs, minerals and traditional healing practices. Some examples include remedies, Ayurveda, Traditional Chinese Medicine (TCM) and indigenous healing methods that draw on wisdom. Practices like acupuncture, herbal supplements, plant-based extracts, therapeutic massages, dietary adjustments and mind-body activities such as meditation and yoga are commonly used in medicine. The underlying belief is that individuals possess an ability to heal themselves and that achieving wellness involves an approach to health.

Modern Medicine: On the side, modern medicine relies on concepts, evidence-driven practices and technological advancements. It encompasses interventions, such as advanced imaging techniques, prescription drugs, surgeries and medical devices. Guidelines and protocols are commonly utilized to guide treatment in contemporary healthcare, emphasizing the detection and management of illnesses.

2. The Integration of Natural Remedies with Modern Medicine

Preventive Care: On the side, modern medicine relies on concepts, evidence-driven practices and technological advancements. It encompasses interventions, such as advanced imaging techniques, prescription drugs, surgeries and medical devices. Guidelines and protocols are commonly utilized to guide treatment in contemporary healthcare, emphasizing the detection and management of illnesses.

Symptom Management: When it comes to term and end-of-life care natural remedies truly excel in managing symptoms and improving individuals well being. For example, many individuals dealing with conditions such as cancer, arthritis and persistent pain turn to acupuncture and massage therapies to address pain swelling and overall quality of life. Integrating supplements and herbal treatments alongside medicine can help reduce symptoms and minimize adverse effects. By blending these remedies with medical interventions, a more personalized and holistic approach to patient care is achievable, offering patients additional options for symptom relief.

Enhancing Treatment Efficacy: By addressing imbalances and enhancing the body's response to treatment, natural remedies could potentially enhance the effectiveness of medical approaches. Some plant extracts and herbal remedies, for instance, possess properties that might boost the efficiency of medications or reduce the required dosage for achieving therapeutic outcomes. Practices like meditation and other holistic activities could also contribute to better treatment outcomes by reducing stress levels, bolstering the system and enhancing well-being. Healthcare providers have the opportunity to enhance treatment outcomes while minimizing effects by integrating these methods into their care plans. Ultimately, this approach can lead to increased satisfaction and adherence to therapy regimens.

Personalized Healthcare: Every individual's healthcare needs, preferences and situations are unique. By blending remedies with medicine, we can offer a more personalized approach. Factors like a person's biology, cultural heritage and beliefs can play a role in choosing from the array of remedies. Understanding a person's traits, metabolism and nutritional deficiencies can guide the customization of treatments and supplements. Moreover, adjustments can be made to mind-body techniques to allow patients to incorporate their relaxation methods, mindfulness practices or spiritual rituals. By embracing this tailored approach, healthcare providers can enhance outcomes, boost involvement in their care and reinforce therapeutic relationships.

Supporting Overall Wellness: In contrast to medicine that targets treating symptoms, natural remedies aim to enhance overall health and well-being. The core principle of healing traditions such as Ayurveda, Traditional Chinese Medicine and Naturopathy revolves around achieving harmony and equilibrium among the mental and spiritual aspects. Integrating these approaches with medicine provides a more comprehensive view of wellness that extends beyond the mere absence of disease. Natural therapies play a role in addressing imbalances, strengthening the body's healing mechanisms and nurturing the mind and spirit to cope with stress and illness for optimal physical, mental and spiritual well-being.

Research and Collaboration: Through research and collaboration across fields, there is a growing effort to bridge the gap between natural remedies and modern medicine. An increasing number of individuals are delving into the study of treatments to explore their efficacy, safety and underlying mechanisms. These investigations aim to establish a foundation for integrating remedies into mainstream healthcare by bridging the knowledge from traditional practices with contemporary scientific insights. Professionals in conventional medicine stand to gain from cooperation as it fosters open dialogue, shared understanding and fresh perspectives. By blending elements from both approaches, healthcare providers have the opportunity to develop patient care strategies that leverage the benefits of traditional medicine alongside alternative therapies.

3. Challenges and Considerations

Blending remedies with healthcare could lead to enhanced patient treatment, yet various aspects and challenges need addressing beforehand;

Safety and Quality Control: There are concerns regarding the safety, purity and quality assurance of remedies as they do not undergo the same rigorous regulatory evaluation as pharmaceutical drugs. Healthcare providers need to exercise caution when recommending treatments to their patients. They must verify that these remedies come from sources and are free from contaminants, additives or potential allergens.

Evidence-Based Practice: The lack of evidence backing the safety and effectiveness of numerous treatments is concerning, especially with the rise in popularity of alternative remedies. It's crucial for healthcare providers to thoroughly evaluate the evidence supporting these treatments by examining research and sharing their findings with patients. Additionally, there is a necessity for data on how natural therapies work across different patient groups and medical settings, which calls for continued funding and development of research resources.

Integration into Clinical Practice: To incorporate therapies into healthcare, doctors need to have a good understanding of both conventional and alternative medicine along with being culturally aware. To guarantee the safe implementation of remedies in inpatient treatment, medical staff should have access to training programs and ongoing education opportunities that equip them with the required skills.

Patient Education and Informed Consent: To help patients make decisions about their treatment, they need to have an understanding of the potential side effects, benefits and constraints of natural therapies. Healthcare providers play a role in educating patients about evidence-based treatment options, empowering them to be involved in decision-making and honoring their preferences and independence.

Collaboration and Communication: Collaborations among professionals from different disciplines are vital for blending conventional treatments with modern healthcare. Ensuring consistent patient care involves fostering dialogue, sharing information and coordinating care plans within multidisciplinary teams.

There is a growing shift towards patient cantered care by blending therapies with modern medicine. Healthcare providers can better cater to their patient's needs by integrating the strengths of both approaches, considering how aspects like biology, psychology, social factors and environment influence health. Despite facing challenges like safety concerns and limited data and training, there are benefits to incorporating therapies alongside conventional treatment. By researching, educating and collaborating, we can leverage the potential of remedies to enhance global healthcare quality and improve patient outcomes.

BOOK 2
The Science of Herbal Medicine

HOW KEY HERBS AFFECT THE BODY

Here is an in-depth analysis detailing the ways important herbs impact the body physiologically.

1. Turmeric (Curcuma longa)

Turmeric, a spice, is widely used in both traditional medicine and cooking. It contains curcumin, a compound known for its anti-inflammatory properties.

Mechanism of Action: Curcumin operates in ways. It reduces the function of enzymes such as LOX and COX 2, leading to a decrease in the production of inflammatory substances like leukotrienes and prostaglandins. Additionally, curcumin affects pathways involved in inflammation signaling, such as mitogen-activated protein kinases (MAPKs) and nuclear factor kappa B (NF κB). Moreover, curcumin shields cells from harm by scavenging radicals and boosting the activity of antioxidant enzymes.

Effects: Inflammatory conditions like arthritis, IBD and heart disease could potentially benefit from turmeric and its active component, curcumin. Curcumin has been shown to reduce inflammation and oxidative stress offering relief for those dealing with disorders. Moreover, its ability to promote cell death in cancer cells and inhibit tumor growth highlights its potential as an anticancer agent due to its properties.

2. Ginger (Zingiber officinale)

Ginger is a plant, with applications in cooking and healthcare. It contains components like gingerol, shogaol and paradol, which offer antioxidant and anti-inflammatory properties.

Mechanism of Action: Ginger's bioactive elements operate through pathways. Gingerols and related compounds inhibit COX 2 and LOX enzymes, thereby blocking the production of mediators like prostaglandins and leukotrienes. Ginger can influence routes such as NF κB and MAPKs. Moreover, gingerols possess antioxidant qualities that combat radicals and enhance the effectiveness of the body's natural antioxidant enzymes.

Effects: When you're experiencing nausea due to factors such as undergoing chemotherapy, being pregnant or dealing with motion sickness, ginger could offer some relief. Conditions like osteoarthritis, rheumatoid arthritis and irritable bowel syndrome (IBS) are among the disorders that could potentially see improvements from gingers' inflammatory properties. By reducing stress and inflammation in the blood vessels, the antioxidant effects of ginger might also contribute to its cardiovascular advantages.

3. Garlic (Allium sativum)

Garlic has been utilized for its culinary purposes for centuries across cultures. Its unique aroma and health benefits are attributed to sulfur compounds such as allicin, diallyl sulfide and diallyl disulfide.

Mechanism of Action: Garlic sulfur compounds play a role in pharmacology. For instance, allicin, a component of garlic, has properties that can help prevent the growth of various microorganisms like bacteria, viruses, fungi and parasites. Additionally, garlic exhibits anti-inflammatory effects by reducing the production of enzymes and cytokines. Its impact on cholesterol metabolism, blood pressure regulation and prevention of platelet aggregation also contributes to lowering the risk of diseases. Diallyl sulfide is one of the chemicals in garlic that aids in these health benefits.

Effects: Garlic is believed to have effects on the system and can aid in combating illnesses like the flu, common cold and respiratory infections. Its anti-inflammatory properties may be beneficial for conditions involving inflammation, such as allergies, asthma and autoimmune diseases. Additionally, garlic is thought to help lower the risk of atherosclerosis and blood clots, improve blood circulation and reduce cholesterol levels, providing benefits.

4. Echinacea (Echinacea purpurea)

Echinacea, an American plant, is renowned for its capacity to boost the immune system. It contains alkamides, polysaccharides and variations of acid among its ingredients, all known for their anti-inflammatory properties.

Mechanism of Action: By enhancing the function of cells, like macrophages, natural killer cells and T lymphocytes, echinacea enhances the immune system. Moreover, it regulates responses by boosting production, including interleukins and interferons. Apart from its inflammatory effects, echinacea also adjusts inflammatory signaling pathways and reduces the release of inflammatory agents.

Effects: Catching the flu or respiratory infections, along with issues related to the upper respiratory tract, are common reasons why people turn to echinacea for prevention and treatment. Individuals dealing with conditions of ongoing infections or weakened immune systems might find value in its immune-boosting properties. Apart from its ability to reduce inflammation, echinacea is also beneficial in handling conditions such as psoriasis, eczema and arthritis.

5. Ginkgo Biloba (Ginkgo biloba)

Ginkgo biloba is well known for its ability to improve circulation and cognitive function. It is derived from the maidenhair tree. Contains compounds, like terpenoids and flavonoids, that have anti-inflammatory, vasodilatory and antioxidant effects.

Mechanism of Action: The bioactive elements found in Ginkgo biloba play a role in bodily functions. Flavonoids, known for their antioxidant properties, protect cells from damage by eliminating harmful free radicals. Moreover, Ginkgo enhances blood flow by dilating blood vessels and preventing clot formation, leading to improved circulation to tissues and the brain. The anti-inflammatory effects of Ginkgo could also be beneficial for conditions like atherosclerosis and peripheral artery disease by reducing inflammation in tissues and blood vessels.

Effects: Ginkgo biloba is commonly used to aid function and memory among older individuals facing dementia or age-related cognitive deterioration. Its effectiveness lies in enhancing blood flow to the brain, leading to nourishment and oxygen supply to brain cells. By reducing inflammation and oxidative stress in the brain, ginkgo may offer protection against conditions such as Parkinson's' and Alzheimer's.

NATURAL REMEDY PROFILES FOR COMMON AILMENTS

Many everyday health concerns, such as stomach issues, stress, trouble sleeping, the cold, breathing problems and joint discomfort, can be addressed with remedies that might ease symptoms and quicken recovery. These remedies offer an approach for individuals to take charge of their well-being alongside medical care. Your safety and health must consult healthcare before trying any remedies, especially if you have existing conditions or are taking medications.

1. Digestive Disorders

Description: Digestive issues, like indigestion, acid reflux, constipation, diarrhea, irritable bowel syndrome (IBS), and various other stomach problems, fall under the category of disorders. Signs such as feeling queasy, experiencing gas bloating, abdominal discomfort and alterations in bowel movements could be attributed to these conditions.

Natural Remedies: When faced with problems, a lot of individuals opt for solutions.

- **Peppermint:** If you experience bloating, indigestion, or irritable bowel syndrome (IBS), consider trying peppermint oil capsules or enjoying a cup of peppermint tea. These remedies may aid in soothing the muscles in your tract, reducing the occurrence and intensity of spasms.
- **Ginger:** Having ginger in tea or taking supplements could potentially aid in relieving issues, nausea, stomach discomfort and symptoms of motion sickness. This is believed to work by reducing inflammation and improving the movement of the stomach.
- **Probiotics:** Rebalancing the gut microbiota, improving digestion and alleviating issues such as IBS, constipation and diarrhea can be accomplished through the consumption of supplements containing bacteria such as Bifidobacterium and Lactobacillus.
- **Chamomile:** Chamomile tea's soothing properties and anti-inflammatory effects can help alleviate spasms, gas, bloating and indigestion.
- **Aloe Vera:** To alleviate symptoms of acid reflux, gastritis and inflammatory bowel disease (IBD), one may find relief by calming and healing tissues in the tract with the help of aloe vera juice or supplements.

2. Insomnia and Sleep Disorders

Description: Symptoms of insomnia and other sleep disorders include feeling sleepy during the day, impatience and decreased performance. These conditions are characterized by difficulties falling asleep, staying asleep, or achieving quality rest at night. Insomnia, sleep apnea, restless leg syndrome (RLS) and disruptions in rhythms are some of the sleep disorders.

Natural Remedies: You can improve the quality of your sleep, reduce stress and promote relaxation by using remedies.

- **Valerian Root:** Having some root tea or taking supplements could potentially assist in calming your mind, reducing anxiety and improving your sleep quality by boosting the levels of the neurotransmitter gamma-aminobutyric acid (GABA) in your body.
- **Lavender:** Using oil and aromatherapy can help relax you, reduce stress and anxiety, calm your nerves and improve your sleep quality.
- **Melatonin:** Using a melatonin supplement could assist in regulating your sleep patterns and improving the quality of your rest, particularly if you're dealing with jet lag or other disruptions to your body's rhythm.
- **Passionflower:** By boosting the levels of GABA and serotonin neurotransmitters that play a role in promoting a sense of calm and regulating mood, consuming passionflower tea or supplements could potentially reduce anxiety, improve sleep quality and induce relaxation.
- **Magnesium:** Taking magnesium supplements can help improve the quality of sleep, reduce muscle tension and promote relaxation by affecting neurotransmitter levels and boosting production.

3. Anxiety and Stress

Description: Feeling stressed and anxious is a concern, for feelings of worry, tension or discomfort often characterize well. Prolonged periods of stress and uneasiness can impact one's quality of life, mental health and physical well-being.

Natural Remedies: If you're dealing with anxiety or stress, some remedies could potentially help you unwind and improve your well-being.

- **Ashwagandha:** Ashwagandha supplements aid in supporting function and managing the body's stress response, leading to a reduction in cortisol levels, anxiety and overall stress.
- **Rhodiola Rosea:** Rhodiola supplements can help the body cope better with stress by reducing levels of stress hormones such as cortisol. This may result in stress levels, improved mood and enhanced resilience to situations.
- **Lemon Balm:** Adding some lemon balm supplements or enjoying a cup of lemon balm tea could potentially reduce feelings of anxiety, promote a sense of calmness and improve mood by increasing the levels of GABA, a neurotransmitter known for its soothing properties.

- **Kava Kava:** Kava supplements can help reduce anxiety, promote relaxation, and boost mood by enhancing neurotransmission and reducing activity in the amygdala, a brain region linked to processing emotions.
- **Holy Basil:** Drinking basil tea or taking supplements can help soothe the system and regulate the body's stress reactions, potentially reducing cortisol levels, anxiety and stress.

4. Common Cold and Respiratory Infections

Description: When a virus enters the tract, it can lead to various symptoms, like a scratchy throat, coughing, congestion, a runny nose, sneezing, fever and typically cold and respiratory issues. Even though these infections usually clear up by themselves, they can still be irritating and disrupt your activities.

Natural Remedies: Chilly weather can bring on symptoms like a stuffy nose. Using natural remedies might help with that as well as boost your immune system and speed up recovery time.

- **Echinacea:** You can potentially shorten the duration and severity of your symptoms, enhance your system, and accelerate your healing process from respiratory infections by consuming echinacea tea or supplements.
- **Vitamin C:** Vitamin C supplements can enhance the system, reduce the duration and severity of symptoms and speed up recovery from respiratory infections by boosting immune cell activity and reducing inflammation.
- **Zinc:** Taking zinc tablets or supplements can help boost the system by lessening the severity and duration of symptoms, speeding up recovery from respiratory infections and inhibiting virus replication while regulating immune responses.
- **Honey:** When you have a cold, honey can be beneficial in relieving your symptoms by calming your throat, suppressing coughing and decreasing inflammation in your system.
- **Garlic:** By enhancing the activity of cells and reducing inflammation, consuming garlic or garlic supplements could potentially speed up healing from respiratory infections, reduce the severity and duration of cold symptoms and boost immune system function.

5. Joint Pain and Arthritis

Description: Joint pain, inflammation, stiffness, and swelling are symptoms of arthritis and various musculoskeletal conditions. Arthritis presents itself in ways with each type having symptoms and underlying causes. Examples of arthritis types include gout, juvenile arthritis, osteoarthritis and rheumatoid arthritis.

Natural Remedies: There are ways found in nature that can help reduce discomfort in the joints, lower swelling, improve movement and slow down the beginning of arthritis.

- **Turmeric:** Curcumin extracts or turmeric supplements might help regulate responses, reduce inflammation, and alleviate pain and symptoms of arthritis.
- **Glucosamine and Chondroitin:** Taking glucosamine and chondroitin can assist individuals dealing with osteoarthritis in repairing cartilage, reducing inflammation, relieving joint discomfort and improving joint function by safeguarding joint structures from deterioration and providing essential components for cartilage formation.
- **Omega-3 Fatty Acids:** By inhibiting pathways that cause inflammation and boosting the production of substances that reduce inflammation, taking omega-3 acids as a supplement could potentially reduce inflammation, alleviate discomfort and help ease symptoms of arthritis.
- **Boswellia:** Boswellia supplements or extracts have the potential to alleviate pain, decrease inflammation and enhance symptoms by inhibiting inflammatory enzymes and regulating immune responses.
- **Capsaicin:** Topical capsaicin cream might be beneficial for pain, mobility and arthritis symptoms as it works by blocking pain signals, reducing inflammation and desensitizing pain receptors.

BOOK 3

Herbs and Their Healing Properties

INTRODUCTION

Studies in the field of science have demonstrated that essential herbs like echinacea, ginger, turmeric and garlic offer health benefits. Incorporating these herbs into your routine can enhance your system, reduce inflammation symptoms of different health conditions and promote overall well-being. By integrating these remedies into your diet and healthcare practices, you can discover ways to enhance your health and elevate your quality of life. It is crucial to consult with your healthcare provider before using herbs if you are currently taking medication or have existing health concerns. This step is important to ensure the safety and suitability of these herbs for your needs.

DETAILED ESSENTIAL HERB PROFILES

1. Aloe Vera

Benefits and Uses:

- **Skin Health:** Its soothing and anti-inflammatory properties make it beneficial for healing burns, injuries and various skin issues.
- **Digestive Health:** Offers assistance for stomach problems and digestive disorders, such as constipation and irritable bowel syndrome (IBS).
- **Immune Support:** It may enhance the system because of its antioxidants.

Scientific Backing:

In research, it has demonstrated potential in the fields of wound healing and skin conditions. Scientific studies have indicated its ability to improve health and reduce constipation.

2. Chamomile

Benefits and Uses:

- **Sleep Aid:** Helps with managing sleeplessness. Encourages a sense of calm.
- **Digestive Health:** Assists with stomach issues and baby colic.
- **Anti-Inflammatory:** Aids in reducing eczema and other skin conditions caused by inflammation.

Scientific Backing:

Through studies, chamomile has been shown to improve the quality of sleep. Its anti-inflammatory properties have been studied thoroughly. Confirmed in the realm of dermatology.

3. Peppermint

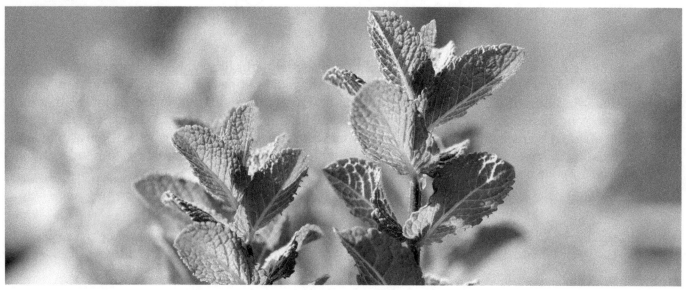

Benefits and Uses:
- **Digestive Aid:** Assists in managing bowel syndrome, bloating and digestive discomfort.
- **Respiratory Health:** It can assist in easing the effects of a cold and functions as a decongestant.
- **Pain Relief:** Helps ease discomfort in muscles and the mind.

Scientific Backing:

In studies peppermint oil has proven effective in relieving symptoms of bowel syndrome. Clinical research also backs its benefits in treating headaches and muscle pain.

4. Lavender

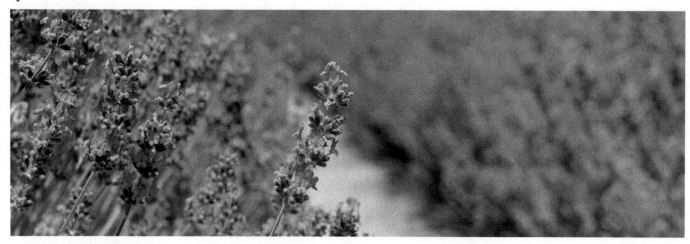

Benefits and Uses:
- **Anxiety and Stress Relief:** Promotes a sense of tranquility. Reduces feelings of tension.
- **Sleep Aid:** Assists in improving the quality of sleep.
- **Skin Health:** Ideal for calming skin and treating burns.

Scientific Backing:

Multiple studies have indicated that lavender has the potential to alleviate feelings of anxiety. Clinical trials have demonstrated its effectiveness in improving sleep quality and alleviating anxiety.

5. Milk Thistle

Benefits and Uses:

- **Liver Health:** It prevents elements from entering the liver and enhances the liver's functioning.
- **Antioxidant Properties:** Assists the body in handling stress.
- **Diabetes Management:** A helpful resource for controlling blood sugar levels.

Scientific Backing:

The active component found in milk thistle, known as silymarin, offers advantages for liver health. It could potentially shield the liver from harm. Research suggests it might also play a role in managing diabetes and reducing blood sugar levels.

6. St. John's Wort

Benefits and Uses:

- **Depression Treatment:** It is usually beneficial for individuals dealing with mild depression.
- **Anxiety Relief:** Affects issues with anxiety and mood.
- **Wound Healing:** Applied directly on cuts and burns.

Scientific Backing:

There is as much proof supporting its effectiveness in treating mild to severe depression as there is for traditional antidepressants. Additionally, there are indications that it could also help with reducing anxiety.

7. Rosemary

Benefits and Uses:

- **Cognitive Health:** Great for improving memory and maintaining concentration.
- **Digestive Health:** Aids in digestion. Relieves discomfort from gas.
- **Anti-Inflammatory:** Lessens swelling and discomfort.

Scientific Backing:

Reducing inflammation and easing discomfort are some of the benefits associated with rosemary. Studies have shown that rosemary can improve function and memory as well as aid in digestion.

8. Sage

Benefits and Uses:

- **Cognitive Health:** Improves brain function and enhances memory.
- **Menopausal Symptoms:** Alleviates heat wave. Night sweats.
- **Oral Health:** Its antibacterial properties make it perfect for mouthwash.

Scientific Backing:

Research suggests that sage can enhance memory and cognitive function. Studies also indicate its benefits in alleviating symptoms and promoting better dental health.

9. Thyme

Benefits and Uses:

- **Respiratory Health:** Treats bronchitis & coughs.
- **Antimicrobial Properties:** Treats infections caused by bacteria and fungi.
- **Digestive Aid:** Reduces gas and bloating.

Scientific Backing:

Research indicates that thyme could be beneficial for problems and combating microbes. Studies have also suggested its effectiveness in relieving issues.

10. Dandelion

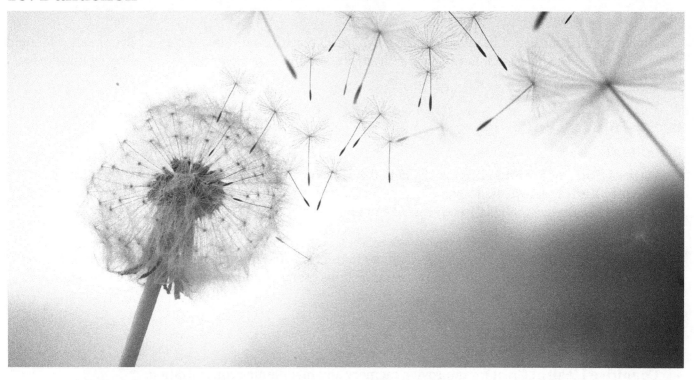

Benefits and Uses:

- **Liver Health:** Facilitates detoxification & liver function.
- **Digestive Health:** Assists with bowel regularity & digestion.
- **Diuretic:** Reduces water retention by acting as a natural diuretic.

Scientific Backing:

There is evidence to suggest that dandelion can contribute to the health of the liver and assist in its cleansing. It is widely believed to have effects on digestion. Acts as a diuretic too.

11. Valerian

Benefits and Uses:

- **Sleep Aid:** Contributes to better and longer sleep.
- **Anxiety Relief:** Lessens nervousness and encourages calmness.
- **Muscle Relaxant:** Relieves cramps & spasms in the muscles.

Scientific Backing:

Studies in the community support the use of valerian for improving sleep quality and reducing anxiety. Additionally, valerian is recognized for its muscle-relaxing properties.

12. Calendula

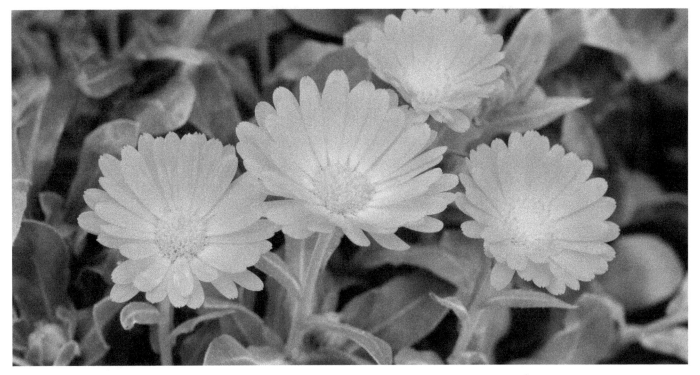

Benefits and Uses:
- **Skin Health:** Heals cuts, scrapes, and irritated skin.
- **Anti-Inflammatory:** Minimizes swelling and speeds up the healing process.
- **Oral Health:** An ingredient in mouthwashes that helps alleviate gingivitis & mouth ulcers.

Scientific Backing:

Calendula has been found to have healing properties for wounds and skin issues, with studies indicating its impact on oral health due to its anti-inflammatory properties.

13. Lemon Balm

Benefits and Uses:
- **Anxiety and Stress Relief:** Promotes serenity and alleviates nervousness.
- **Cognitive Health:** Improves mental acuity and memory.
- **Digestive Aid:** Reduces indigestion and associated pain.

Scientific Backing:

Studies indicate that lemon balm could be beneficial for managing anxiety and cognitive challenges. Additionally, research supports its effects on digestion.

14. Hawthorn

Benefits and Uses:
- **Heart Health:** Promotes heart health and alleviates symptoms of heart failure.
- **Antioxidant Properties:** Minimizes inflammation & oxidative stress.
- **Digestive Aid:** Comforts gastrointestinal problems, including gas.

Scientific Backing:

The positive impacts of hawthorn on heart health and overall well-being have been extensively recorded. Studies suggest that it supports digestion and functions as an antioxidant.

15. Fenugreek

Benefits and Uses:

- **Lactation Aid:** Aids nursing mothers in producing more milk.
- **Blood Sugar Control:** Lowers blood sugar levels and aids in diabetic management.
- **Digestive Health:** Relieves constipation and other gastrointestinal problems.

Scientific Backing:

Studies have demonstrated that fenugreek can aid in regulating blood sugar levels and improving lactation. There is evidence supporting its benefits for digestion, too.

16. Licorice Root

Benefits and Uses:

- **Digestive Health:** Comforts those suffering from acid reflux & gastritis.
- **Respiratory Health:** Assists with coughing & sore throats.
- **Anti-Inflammatory:** Lowers inflammatory levels and bolsters immune system performance.

Scientific Backing:

The healing benefits of licorice root have been widely recorded in aiding respiratory issues. Its capacity to decrease inflammation has also been thoroughly researched.

17. Oregano

Benefits and Uses:

- **Antimicrobial Properties:** Defeats infections caused by bacteria, fungi, and viruses.
- **Digestive Health:** Helps with gastrointestinal problems and promotes gut wellness.
- **Anti-Inflammatory:** Lessens swelling and discomfort.

Scientific Backing:

Research has proven the properties of oregano. Additionally, studies have indicated its impact on digestion and inflammation reduction.

18. Ginkgo Biloba

Benefits and Uses:

- **Cognitive Health:** Improves mental acuity and memory.
- **Circulatory Health:** Enhances blood circulation and alleviates signs of circulatory diseases.
- **Antioxidant Properties:** Attenuates free radical damage and shields cells from harm.

Scientific Backing:

The positive impacts of ginkgo biloba on heart health and brain function have been widely researched.

Moreover it has been thoroughly examined for its properties.

19. Catnip

Benefits and Uses:

- **Relaxation and Sleep:** Assists with restlessness and promotes relaxation.

- **Digestive Health:** Relieves gas and bloating as well as cramps.
- **Respiratory Health:** The cold and respiratory infection symptoms are alleviated.

Scientific Backing:

Catnip is known for its ability to relieve stress and digestive issues, with plenty of documented evidence supporting its effectiveness. Additionally, there are indications that it can also contribute to improving health.

20. Elderberry

Benefits and Uses:

- **Immune Support:** Improves immunity and lessens the severity of flu and cold symptoms.
- **Antioxidant Properties:** Decreases inflammation and oxidative stress.
- **Respiratory Health:** Relieves lung infection symptoms.

Scientific Backing:

Numerous research studies have demonstrated the effects of elderberry on boosting the system and relieving cold symptoms. Additionally, it is recognized for its properties and positive impact on health.

21. Marshmallow Root

Benefits and Uses:

- **Digestive Health:** Discomforts gastrointestinal problems such as gastritis and ulcers.
- **Respiratory Health:** Relieves coughs & sore throats.
- **Skin Health:** Assists in the recovery of skin irritations.

Scientific Backing:

Studies have demonstrated the effects of marshmallow root on digestive health. Moreover, research has indicated its efficacy in addressing skin conditions.

22. Fennel (Foeniculum vulgare)

Benefits and Uses:

- **Digestive Health:** Regulates gas, indigestion, & gas pain. Medicated to alleviate newborn colic.
- **Respiratory Health:** Assists in relieving coughs and clearing out congestion in the respiratory system.
- **Hormonal Balance:** This could potentially help with menopausal and period-related symptoms.

Scientific Backing:

Studies have indicated that fennel could help ease colic in babies and improve wellness in grown-ups. Research suggests that its expectorant properties have been utilized to address issues. While additional research is needed, there are hints that fennel might aid in managing symptoms of menopause and menstrual irregularities.

23. Holy Basil (Tulsi) (Ocimum sanctum)

Benefits and Uses:

- **Stress and Anxiety Relief:** Functions as an adaptogen, assisting the body in handling stress.
- **Immune Support:** Supports the immune system and aids in the battle against infections.
- **Anti-inflammatory and Antioxidant Properties:** Decreases oxidative stress & inflammation.

Scientific Backing:

Studies have indicated that Tulsi could potentially reduce stress and anxiety, showcasing its properties. Scientific studies suggest that it can enhance the system and aid in combating illnesses. The scientific literature is full of proof of its inflammatory characteristics.

24. Yarrow (Achillea millefolium)

Benefits and Uses:

- **Wound Healing:** Helps wounds and scrapes recover faster.
- **Digestive Health:** Puts an end to gas, bloating, and painful cramps.
- **Anti-inflammatory:** Lowers inflammatory levels and may help reduce arthritic symptoms.

Scientific Backing:

Research has revealed that yarrow has the potential to reduce inflammation and accelerate wound healing, supporting its use in this regard. Studies suggest that it can be beneficial in addressing issues like indigestion, gas and other gastrointestinal problems. Its anti-inflammatory properties have also been found effective in alleviating symptoms of arthritis.

25. Valerian Root (Valeriana officinalis)

Benefits and Uses:

- **Sleep Aid:** Encourages unwinding and enhances the quality of slumber.
- **Anxiety Relief:** Alleviates tension and anxious feelings.
- **Muscle Relaxant:** Relieves cramps & spasms in the muscles.

Scientific Backing:

Valerian root has been found to be effective in improving the quality and length of sleep in trials. Several research studies have demonstrated its ability to relieve anxiety symptoms, highlighting its properties. Additionally, research supports its use as a muscle relaxant, which can help ease cramps and spasms.

26. Nettle (Urtica dioica)

Benefits and Uses:

- **Anti-inflammatory:** Lowers inflammatory levels and may help reduce arthritic symptoms.
- **Allergy Relief:** Reduces the severity of allergic rhinitis & hay fever.
- **Nutrient-Rich:** Supports general well-being by supplying necessary nutrients.

Scientific Backing:

The anti-inflammatory properties of nettle are widely known, with evidence showing its effectiveness in easing arthritis and joint pain. Research supports its use in managing allergies and relieving symptoms of hay fever. Studies have extensively examined the benefits of nettle, highlighting its capacity to offer minerals and support overall health.

27. Slippery Elm (Ulmus rubra)

Benefits and Uses:

- **Digestive Health:** Those suffering from irritable bowel syndrome (IBS) or acid reflux may find relief by using this remedy.
- **Respiratory Health:** By creating a barrier, it alleviates coughs and sore throats.
- **Skin Health:** Aids in the recovery from skin irritations and wounds.

Scientific Backing:

Studies have indicated that slippery elm could be beneficial for managing bowel syndrome (IBS) and acid reflux, making it a potential treatment option for these conditions. Additionally, research suggests that it can help ease coughs and soothe sore throats, contributing to improved health. Scientific findings also support its effectiveness in addressing skin irritations and promoting wound healing.

28. Garlic (Allium sativum)

Benefits:

- **Antimicrobial Properties:** Garlic contains compounds, like allicin, that have properties that can inhibit the growth of bacteria, viruses, fungi and parasites. It has been traditionally used for both preventing and treating infections.
- **Cardiovascular Health:** Studies have indicated that consuming garlic supplements could reduce the chances of developing heart-related conditions, like heart disease and stroke, by lowering cholesterol levels, reducing blood pressure and preventing platelet clumping.
- **Anti-inflammatory Effects:** Garlic's anti-inflammatory properties can potentially ease symptoms of conditions like bowel disease and arthritis by reducing inflammation in the body.
- **Immune Support:** Garlic enhances the system by boosting production and activating immune cells.

Uses:

You can consume garlic in its form, cook it or opt for supplements. It is commonly utilized in cooking to enhance the flavor of dishes. Garlic is also available in forms like capsules, pills and liquid extracts.

Scientific Backing:

Many studies suggest that garlic possesses properties that benefit the heart and enhance the system.

Studies indicate that consuming garlic supplements could enhance heart health, reduce blood pressure and lower cholesterol levels.

Research also supports the use of garlic for strengthening the system and treating infections as a treatment.

29. Ginger (Zingiber officinale)

Benefits:

- **Anti-inflammatory Effects:** Ginger contains elements, like gingerols and shogaols, that have potent inflammatory properties. This enables them to diminish inflammation and ease symptoms linked to conditions such as bowel disease and arthritis.
- **Gastrointestinal Relief:** Ginger helps with digestion by speeding up stomach movement and reducing stomach spasms, leading to relief from nausea, indigestion, motion sickness and other related symptoms.
- **Immune Support:** Ginger shows its ability to enhance the system and reduce inflammation, indicating its role in modulating immunity.
- **Antioxidant Activity:** Ginger helps protect cells by getting rid of radicals, reducing the chances of developing long-term health issues.

Uses:

Ginger, whether fresh, dried or in form, can be used in dishes. It is an ingredient in teas, soups, stir-fries and desserts. The market offers a range of ginger supplements, like pills, liquid extracts and capsules.

Scientific Backing:

According to research, ginger is known to have properties that can reduce inflammation and aid digestion. Support the immune system. Clinical studies have demonstrated that taking ginger supplements can effectively relieve symptoms of nausea, indigestion and motion sickness. Additionally, research suggests that ginger may offer benefits for problems as well as conditions like rheumatoid arthritis and osteoarthritis.

30. Turmeric (Curcuma longa)

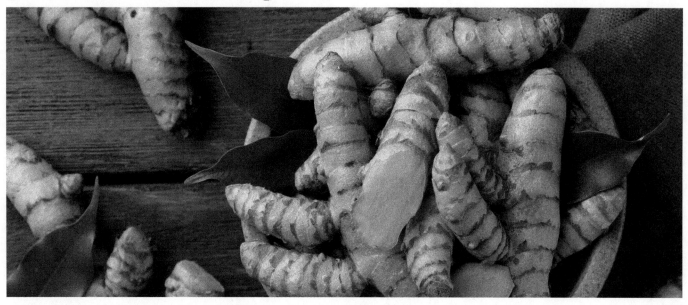

Benefits:

- **Anti-inflammatory Effects:** Curcumin, a compound found in turmeric, has been known to alleviate inflammation and pain, making it a useful remedy for conditions like arthritis, inflammatory bowel disease and heart issues.
- **Antioxidant Activity:** Curcumin helps by scavenging radicals and protecting cells from harm, showcasing its antioxidant properties that can reduce the chances of developing long-term health issues.
- **Pain Relief:** The pain-relieving properties of turmeric can ease the discomfort associated with conditions such as arthritis.
- **Brain Health:** Curcumin, with its inflammatory and antioxidant effects, has the potential to support brain health and protect against conditions like Alzheimer's and Parkinson's' disease.

Uses:

You can enjoy turmeric in ways such as using it fresh, dried or in form. It is an ingredient in curries, soups, sauces and beverages. Turmeric supplements come in forms, like capsules, pills and powdered extracts that you can choose from.

Scientific Backing:

Scientists have extensively. Documented the properties of curcumin, including its anti-inflammatory, antioxidant and neuroprotective effects. Studies have also demonstrated that curcumin has pain-relieving qualities and can improve symptoms. Furthermore, research has indicated that curcumin holds the potential to address health concerns such as cancer prevention, cardiovascular well-being and cognitive function.

31. Echinacea (Echinacea purpurea)

Benefits:

- **Immune Support:** Echinacea enhances the system by increasing the production of cytokines and boosting the activity of cells, which play crucial roles in regulating immune responses. It has been traditionally used for treating and preventing conditions such, as influenza and the common cold.
- **Anti-inflammatory Effects:** People with conditions, like arthritis and autoimmune diseases may experience relief from inflammation by using echinacea as it possesses inflammatory properties.
- **Antioxidant Activity:** Echinacea antioxidants protect cells from stress. Reduce the risk of chronic diseases.

- **Wound Healing:** Echinacea may help speed up wound healing and reduce the risk of infection by enhancing responses and promoting tissue repair.

Uses:

Echinacea supplements come in forms, like capsules, pills, and liquid extracts. They are commonly used to reduce inflammation, boost the system and manage infections. To enjoy echinaceas benefits, you can brew a soothing tea using dried plant components, like roots, leaves or flowers.

Scientific Backing:

Studies suggest that echinacea could enhance the system, decrease inflammation and shield cells from harm caused by radicals. Clinical research has demonstrated that taking echinacea can reduce symptoms and duration of illnesses such as the flu and common cold. Additionally, studies point to the benefits of echinacea in addressing health conditions like skin ailments, allergies, and arthritis.

BOOK 4
Natural Remedies for Common Ailments

INTRODUCTION

Natural remedies could potentially aid in addressing a range of health concerns and enhancing well-being. It's advisable to consult with your healthcare provider before trying out any remedies, especially if you are currently unwell, expecting a baby, breastfeeding or taking medications. If you experience any reactions discontinue the treatment away and seek medical advice if your symptoms persist beyond a few days.

TREATMENTS FOR COLDS, FLU, INFLAMMATION, DIGESTIVE ISSUES, AND MORE

Here are a few specific natural remedies for health issues, along with instructions on how to prepare and use them correctly

1. Common Cold and Flu

REMEDY: GINGER LEMON HONEY TEA

INGREDIENTS

- 1-inch piece of fresh ginger, sliced
- 1 tablespoon fresh lemon juice
- 1 tablespoon raw honey
- 1 cup hot water

PREPARATION

1. Place the ginger slices in a cup then add them to a pot of boiling water.
2. Let it steep for 5 to 10 minutes with the lid on.
3. Remove the ginger pieces, mix in some honey and lemon juice and savour the drink while it's still warm.

Safety and Effectiveness:
Ginger's antibacterial properties make it a helpful solution for combating flu symptoms. Lemons, known for their Vitamin C content, play a role in maintaining a robust immune system. Honey is renowned for its soothing effect on throats. Possesses antibacterial qualities. Although generally safe for the majority of individuals, with allergies are advised against using this medication. Those taking blood thinners or facing bleeding concerns should moderate their intake of ginger to avoid any complications.

2. Inflammation
REMEDY: TURMERIC MILK (GOLDEN MILK)

INGREDIENTS
- 1 cup milk (dairy or plant-based)
- 1/2 teaspoon turmeric powder
- 1/4 teaspoon ground cinnamon
- 1/4 teaspoon ground ginger
- Pinch of black pepper (to enhance turmeric absorption)
- Sweetener of choice (optional)

PREPARATION
1. Warm the milk in a saucepan on heat.
2. Season with pepper, ginger, cinnamon and turmeric.
3. Combine all ingredients while stirring continuously.
4. Sweeten with sugar to your preference.
5. Pour into a cup and savor while it is still warm.

Safety and Effectiveness:
Turmeric contains curcumin, which is known for its inflammatory properties. The absorption of curcumin is enhanced when paired with pepper. It's generally safe to use this remedy. It's advisable to consult your doctor if you are pregnant, nursing or taking any medications.

3. Digestive Issues
REMEDY: PEPPERMINT TEA

INGREDIENTS
- 1 teaspoon dried peppermint leaves or 1 peppermint tea bag
- 1 cup hot water

PREPARATION
1. Grab a cup. Put in some peppermint leaves or a tea bag.
2. Add the peppermint to the boiling water.
3. Let it steep for 5 to 10 minutes with the lid on.
4. Strain the tea. Remove the tea bag.
5. Add honey or lemon to your liking for sweetness.
6. Savour each sip.

Safety and Effectiveness:

If you're feeling a bit of stomach discomfort or swelling, peppermint could help. Avoid it if you have reflux or GERD. Generally, using this remedy shouldn't cause any problems.

4. Stress and Anxiety

REMEDY: LAVENDER ESSENTIAL OIL INHALATION

INGREDIENTS

- Lavender essential oil
- Diffuser or handkerchief

PREPARATION

1. Pour water into a diffuser and add a couple of drops of essential oil. Inhale the scent as you switch on the diffuser. Alternatively, take breaths while putting an amount of lavender oil on a tissue.

Safety and Effectiveness:
Using oil can help reduce stress and anxiety because of its calming properties. Avoid contact with the skin when using lavender oil. If it causes any irritation to your skin, discontinue use.

5. Nausea and Motion Sickness

REMEDY: GINGER CHEWS

INGREDIENTS

- Dried ginger chews or crystallized ginger

PREPARATION

1. If you start to feel nauseous or unwell due to motion sickness, simply chew on a piece of ginger. Enjoy some candied ginger.

Safety and Effectiveness:
Many individuals discover that ginger can alleviate feelings of nausea and vomiting. Ginger chews are a choice for relief. It's crucial for individuals dealing with gallbladder issues or taking blood thinning medication to moderate their ginger consumption.

6. Sore Throat
REMEDY: SALTWATER GARGLE

INGREDIENTS
- 1 teaspoon salt
- 1 cup warm water

PREPARATION
1. Boil some salt water.
2. Gargle with it for 30 seconds, then spit it out.
3. Repeat as needed during the day.

Safety and Effectiveness:
One method to reduce inflammation and eliminate bacteria in the throat involves gargling with saltwater. To avoid burns, ensure that the water is warm rather than hot. Even young children can safely adopt this remedy.

7. Herbal Immune-Boosting Tonic

INGREDIENTS
- 1 tablespoon dried echinacea root
- 1 tablespoon dried astragalus root
- 1 tablespoon dried elderberries
- 1 tablespoon dried rose hips
- 4 cups water
- **Optional:** honey or lemon for taste

PREPARATION
1. Place the water, elderberries, rose hips, astragalus root and echinacea root in a pot.
2. Allow the ingredients to boil first and then simmer for 30–45 minutes.
3. Remove it from the heat. Let it cool for a bit.
4. Strain the liquid into a container.
5. Add honey or lemon to your liking.
6. You can store the tonic in the refrigerator for up to a week.
7. **Usage**:
8. Boost your system. Ward off colds and flu by consuming half to one cup of the herbal tonic every day. If you're under the weather, consider increasing your intake to two or three cups until you start feeling better.

Safety and Effectiveness:
The herbal tonic contains herbs like echinacea, astragalus, elderberries and rose hips to boost your

system. Make sure to check with your healthcare provider before using it if you're pregnant, nursing or taking any medications. Avoid consuming it if you have allergies to any of the ingredients.

8. Anti-inflammatory Turmeric Paste

INGREDIENTS

- 1/2 cup turmeric powder
- 1 cup water
- 1/4 cup coconut oil
- 1-2 teaspoons freshly ground black pepper

PREPARATION

1. Combine the powder with water in a saucepan.
2. Stir constantly as you cook it over heat until it thickens into a paste.
3. Remove the pan from the heat. Add coconut oil and black pepper.
4. Once the mixture has cooled, transfer it to a jar.
5. Seal it tightly. Store the paste in the refrigerator for up to two weeks.
6. **Usage**:
7. Enhance your well-being and combat inflammation by consuming half to one teaspoon of turmeric paste daily. Incorporate the paste as a topping on crackers or toast. Blend it into milk or tea for a soothing beverage.

Safety and Effectiveness:
Turmeric contains curcumin, which is known for its inflammatory properties. Curcumin is effectively absorbed when taken with pepper. If you experience gallbladder issues or have allergies to any ingredients, it's advisable to avoid using this supplement. Before starting any regimen, pregnant or nursing individuals and those taking medications should seek advice from their healthcare provider.

9. Digestive Health Elixir

INGREDIENTS

- 1 tablespoon apple cider vinegar
- 1 tablespoon fresh lemon juice
- 1 teaspoon raw honey
- 1/2 teaspoon grated ginger
- 1/2 teaspoon ground cinnamon
- 1 cup warm water

PREPARATION

1. Blend the apple cider vinegar, honey, lemon juice, cinnamon, ginger and grated ginger in a cup.

Stir thoroughly as you mix with water. Allow the elixir to sit for a while to let the flavors meld for results. Take it easy on the elixir.
2. **Usage**:
3. For health, its recommended to consume the digestive health elixir once a day to support digestion, reduce gas and ease bloating. For effectiveness, consider drinking it after meals.

Safety and Effectiveness:
Improving your health and maintaining the acid balance can be achieved by incorporating apple cider vinegar into your routine. Lemon juice, known for its vitamin C content, supports the liver's functioning. Both cinnamon and ginger are helpful for digestion and reducing inflammation. If you experience issues like acid reflux ulcers or have sensitivities to ingredients, it's advisable to steer off using these remedies. Before starting any regimen, especially if you're nursing or taking medications, it's wise to seek advice from your healthcare provider.

10. Stress-Relieving Lavender Bath

INGREDIENTS

- 1/2 cup Epsom salt
- 10-15 drops of lavender essential oil

PREPARATION

1. Fill up a bathtub with water. Add some Epsom salt and a few drops of oil to the water. Stir the mixture until the salt and oil dissolve. Relax in the tub for twenty to thirty minutes, allowing the calming fragrance of lavender to envelop you.
2. **Usage**:
3. If you find it hard to unwind, soothe yourself, or sleep well, consider having a lavender-infused bath. To maximize the calming benefits opt for a bath, before bedtime, in the evening.

Safety and Effectiveness:
Epsom salt contains plenty of magnesium, a mineral that can help relax and rejuvenate the body.
Lavender essential oil is known for its calming properties that can ease tension and anxiety.
If you have allergies to any of the ingredients, it's best to avoid consumption.
Stop using it if it causes any skin irritation to prevent discomfort.
Before using it, make sure to consult your healthcare provider if you're pregnant, nursing or taking any medications.

RECIPES OF COMMON REMEDIES

1. Elderberry Syrup

INGREDIENTS

- 1 cup dried elderberries (or 2 cups fresh elderberries)
- 4 cups water
- 1 cup raw honey
- 1 cinnamon stick
- 1 teaspoon dried ginger root
- 5 whole cloves

PREPARATION

1. First, bring a pot filled with elderberries, water, ginger, a cinnamon stick and cloves to a boil. Let the mixture simmer for 45 minutes to an hour until the liquid reduces by half. Remove it from the heat. Allow it to cool slightly. To extract juice from the berries, mash them using a spoon or potato masher. Strain the mixture through cheesecloth or a fine mesh strainer into a glass jar. Once strained, add honey. Mix thoroughly. Seal the syrup in a glass jar before storing it in the refrigerator.

Safety and Effectiveness:
When elderberry syrup is ingested, it has the potential to relieve flu symptoms and reduce their duration, all while boosting the system. Consuming raw elderberries might cause stomach discomfort due to the presence of glycosides. However, cooking the berries removes these chemicals. It's important to note that honey should not be fed to infants under one year old due to the risk of botulism.

2. Elderberry Gummies

INGREDIENTS

- 1 cup elderberry syrup (see above recipe)
- 1/4 cup hot water
- 1/4 cup cold water
- 1/4 cup gelatin powder

PREPARATION

1. Mix the gelatin powder and cold water in a bowl. Let it sit for a few minutes to thicken. In a saucepan gently warm the elderberry syrup and hot water until just heated. Once warm, combine the

mixture with the gelatin, stirring until fully dissolved. Pour the mixture into silicone molds or onto a parchment-lined baking sheet. Chill the gummies in the refrigerator for two hours to set. Remove them from the molds. Cut them into squares if using a baking dish. Store in an airtight jar, in the fridge.

Safety and Effectiveness:
A convenient way to give children elderberry syrup is through these candies.
It's best to store the gummies in the refrigerator for freshness. Remember to do that.
By cooking the elderberries they become safe for consumption to the syrup.

3. Elderberry Tea

INGREDIENTS

- 2 tablespoons dried elderberries (or 1/4 cup fresh elderberries)
- 2 cups water
- 1 teaspoon dried ginger root
- 1 cinnamon stick
- Honey or lemon to taste (optional)

PREPARATION

1. In a saucepan, gently melt the ginger root and cinnamon stick along with the elderberries in water. Allow it to simmer, covered, for fifteen to twenty minutes once it reaches a boil. After letting it steep for 5 minutes, remove it from the heat. Before serving, strain the tea into a teapot or individual cups using a fine mesh sieve. If you prefer a taste, feel free to add some honey or lemon.

Safety and Effectiveness:
Elderberry tea is known for its soothing effects helping to strengthen the system and alleviate symptoms of the flu and cold. To ensure safety, boiling the berries is a practice when preparing elderberry-based remedies.

4. Elderberry Tincture

INGREDIENTS

- 1 cup dried elderberries (or 2 cups fresh elderberries)
- 2 cups vodka or other high-proof alcohol

PREPARATION

1. Grab a glass jar. Place the elderberries inside.
2. Coat the berries with vodka by shaking them until covered.
3. Seal the jar tightly. Give it a shake.

4. Occasionally shake the jar. Store it in a dark area for four to six weeks.
5. After four to six weeks, strain the tincture through cheesecloth or a fine mesh strainer into a glass container.
6. Remember to keep the tincture stored in a location.

Safety and Effectiveness:
Just a small amount of tincture can deliver the benefits of elderberry. The alcohol content in the tincture helps preserve it. Draw out components from the elderberries. It's best for those aiming to reduce their alcohol intake to avoid consuming this tincture.

5. Elderberry Lozenges

INGREDIENTS

- 1/2 cup elderberry syrup (see syrup recipe above)
- 1/2 cup honey
- 2 tablespoons lemon juice
- 2 cups powdered sugar (for dusting)

PREPARATION

1. To prepare elderberry syrup, combine honey, lemon juice and elderberries in a saucepan. Stir the mixture constantly overheat until it reaches 300°F on a candy thermometer, indicating the hard crack stage.
2. Quickly spread the mixture thinly onto a parchment paper-lined baking sheet or into silicone candy molds.
3. Once the tablets have cooled completely, they should be solid. If you don't have molds break the mixture into pieces and dust with powdered sugar to prevent sticking. Seal them promptly.
4. Store in a place.

Safety and Effectiveness:
Elderberry lozenges are known for their effectiveness in soothing coughs and sore throats. The elderberries undergo a cooking process at heat to ensure safety. To maintain their effectiveness and prevent sticking it is recommended to store the tablets in a place.

6. Marshmallow Root Tea

INGREDIENTS

- 1 tablespoon dried marshmallow root
- 1 cup hot water
- Honey or lemon (optional)

PREPARATION

1. Put the dried marshmallow root in a teapot or infuser.
2. Make sure the marshmallow root is fully covered in boiling water.
3. Allow it to steep for around ten to fifteen minutes or longer if desired.
4. Strain the mixture to pour yourself a soothing cup of tea.
5. For added flavor, consider mixing in some honey and a squeeze of lemon juice based on your taste preferences.

Safety and Effectiveness:
When dealing with issues like throats, coughs and digestive troubles, drinking marshmallow root tea could be beneficial due to its soothing effect on membranes. It's generally safe for most people to consume. Individuals who are nursing or taking medications should consult with their healthcare provider beforehand.

7. Marshmallow Root Cough Syrup

INGREDIENTS

- 1/4 cup dried marshmallow root
- 1 cup water
- 1/2 cup raw honey
- 1 teaspoon ground ginger (optional)

PREPARATION

1. In a saucepan, combine the water and marshmallow root.
2. Simmer for 20 to 30 minutes once it reaches a boil.
3. Strain out the root. Pour the liquid into a dish.
4. Add honey to the liquid. Stir until it dissolves.
5. If using ground ginger mix it in now thoroughly.
6. Pour the syrup into a glass container and refrigerate.

Safety and Effectiveness:
Marshmallow root acts as a soothing agent, aiding in the relief of coughs and throat discomfort. Additionally, honey possesses qualities that further assist in soothing the throat.

8. Marshmallow Root Infusion

INGREDIENTS

- 1/4 cup dried marshmallow root
- 1-quart cold water

PREPARATION

1. Place the dried marshmallow root in a glass jar.
2. Add water to the jar until it is half full, then pour it over the marshmallow root.
3. Let it sit at room temperature, covered for 4 to 8 hours or overnight.
4. Transfer the infused liquid into a container lined with vaseline.

Safety and Effectiveness:
If you experience irritation in the membranes of your urinary tract, you could consider trying a cold infusion made from marshmallow root. This remedy is generally safe for people. Individuals with existing health conditions should consult a doctor before using it.

9. Marshmallow Root Salve

INGREDIENTS

- 1/4 cup dried marshmallow root
- 1/2 cup olive oil or coconut oil
- 1/4 cup beeswax
- 10 drops lavender essential oil (optional)

PREPARATION

1. In a boiler mix together the olive oil and marshmallow root. Be cautious not to overheat the oil while gently warming the blend for one to two hours. Strain out the marshmallow root from the oil. Use a boiler to melt the beeswax; once the beeswax is melted blend in your infused oil thoroughly. If you opt for oil stir it in after removing from heat. Once the mixture has fully cooled, transfer it into glass or tin containers.

Safety and Effectiveness:
The soothing and healing properties of marshmallow root make this ointment perfect for addressing skin, minor cuts and skin issues. Remember to do a patch test to check for any reactions; if not it's safe to apply on the skin.

10. Marshmallow Root Lozenges

INGREDIENTS

- 1/4 cup dried marshmallow root
- 1 cup water
- 1 cup honey
- 1/4 cup powdered sugar (optional for dusting)

PREPARATION

1. Heat the water. Marshmallow root in a saucepan until it comes to a boil. Let it simmer with the lid on for twenty to thirty minutes. Once strained, return the liquid to the pot. When the mixture reaches 300°F (hard crack stage), as indicated by a candy thermometer, stir in the honey and continue heating. Pour the mixture evenly into silicone molds and a lined baking sheet. Allow the lozenges time to cool and set. Cut them into pieces and dust them with sugar if you plan to bake them on a lined baking sheet. Store them in a place out of sight.

Safety and Effectiveness:
If you have a cough or sore throat, consider using a marshmallow root lozenge. The process is ensured to be safe because of the cooking heat involved. Store them in a place to maintain their efficacy and prevent them from becoming sticky.

11. Yarrow Tea

INGREDIENTS

- 1 tablespoon dried yarrow flowers and leaves
- 1 cup boiling water
- Honey or lemon (optional)

PREPARATION

1. Brew a cup of tea by steeping yarrow in water for about ten to fifteen minutes. Strain the mixture to enjoy your tea. If you like, you can enhance it with a touch of honey and a squeeze of lemon juice based on your taste preferences.

Safety and Effectiveness:
Yarrow tea can be beneficial for addressing problems, reducing fever, and easing symptoms of flu and colds due to its inflammatory and fever-reducing properties. It is advisable to refrain from consuming yarrow tea during pregnancy. If you have an allergy to plants in the Asteraceae family. However, for the majority of people, it is typically safe to consume.

12. Yarrow Infused Oil

INGREDIENTS

- 1 cup dried yarrow flowers and leaves
- 2 cups olive oil or almond oil

PREPARATION

1. Place the dried yarrow in a dry glass container.
2. Ensure that the yarrow is completely submerged in oil before pouring it over.
3. Seal the jar tightly. Place it in a warm spot for two to four weeks, gently shaking it each day.
4. Transfer the oil into a jar after filtering it through cheesecloth or a fine strainer.

Safety and Effectiveness:
Yarrow-infused oil is known for its inflammatory properties, which can accelerate wound healing and reduce inflammation. While applying it topically is generally safe, it's an idea to conduct a patch test to check for any potential allergies.

13. Yarrow Tincture

INGREDIENTS

- 1 cup dried yarrow flowers and leaves
- 2 cups vodka or other high-proof alcohol

PREPARATION

1. Please begin by obtaining a glass jar and placing the dried yarrow inside it. Ensure that the yarrow is fully immersed in the alcohol before you pour it in. Seal the jar tightly. Store it in a cool location for a period of four to six weeks, remembering to gently shake it every few days. Once strained using cheesecloth or a fine mesh strainer transfer the tincture into a glass container.

Safety and Effectiveness:
If you're experiencing indigestion, a low fever, or the flu, consider using a yarrow tincture. The tincture. Extracts the properties of yarrow with the help of alcohol concentration. It's not recommended for individuals looking to reduce their alcohol intake.

14. Yarrow Poultice

INGREDIENTS

- Fresh yarrow leaves and flowers (enough to cover the affected area)
- A small amount of water (if needed)

PREPARATION

1. To get the juices out of picked yarrow flowers and leaves you can. Chop them.
2. If the plant material is too dry, you can add some water to create a paste.
3. Yarrow paste could be beneficial for treating wounds, scrapes or insect bites when applied topically.
4. Cover it with a bandage or cloth. Leave it on for at least an hour.
5. After removing the poultice, rinse the area with water.

Safety and Effectiveness:
Yarrow poultices can be beneficial in treating wounds and reducing inflammation due to their anti-inflammatory properties. They are generally safe for people. Individuals with allergies to Asteraceae plants should avoid using them.

15. Yarrow Bath

INGREDIENTS

- 1 cup dried yarrow flowers and leaves
- 2 quarts boiling water

PREPARATION

1. Throw the dried yarrow into a pot or bowl.
2. Let the yarrow steep in water for twenty to thirty minutes.
3. Strain the infusion into a tub of water.

Safety and Effectiveness:
Yarrow is a herb to include in a bath to alleviate muscle pain and inflammation due to its inflammatory and pain relieving properties. It is generally safe to use. Its recommended to perform a patch test. Avoid using it if you are pregnant or allergic to Asteraceae plants.

16. Catnip Tea

INGREDIENTS

- 2 teaspoons dried catnip leaves
- 1 cup boiling water
- Honey or lemon (optional)

PREPARATION

1. Grab your teapot or strainer and place the dried catnip leaves inside.
2. Heat some water. Pour it over the catnip leaves.
3. Let it steep for around ten to fifteen minutes.
4. Pour yourself a cup of tea after straining it.
5. If you like you can sweeten it with a bit of honey and a squeeze of lemon juice.

Safety and Effectiveness:
Catnip tea's mild calming properties can help nerves, aid digestion, and relieve tension. It is generally safe for use. Pregnant or nursing women should avoid it due to its soothing effects.

17. Catnip Infused Oil

INGREDIENTS

- 1 cup dried catnip leaves and flowers
- 2 cups olive oil or coconut oil

PREPARATION

1. Grab a spotless glass jar. Place the dried catnip inside.
2. Coat the catnip thoroughly in the oil.
3. Seal the jar tightly. Position it in a warm spot for two to four weeks, remembering to give it a gentle shake every day.
4. Transfer the oil into a jar after straining it using cheesecloth or a fine mesh strainer.

Safety and Effectiveness:
Infused with catnip oil possesses inflammatory properties that can help reduce inflammation and soothe minor skin irritations. It's generally safe to apply. Its recommended to perform a patch test first to check for any potential allergies.

18. Catnip Tincture

INGREDIENTS

- 1 cup dried catnip leaves and flowers
- 2 cups vodka or other high-proof alcohol

PREPARATION

1. Move the dried catnip into a glass jar. Ensure that the catnip is completely immersed in alcohol before pouring it on top. Seal the jar tightly. Place it in a dark area for four to six weeks, giving it a gentle shake every few days. Once strained through cheesecloth or a fine mesh strainer, transfer the tincture to a sterilized glass container.

Safety and Effectiveness:
Catnip extract, known for its muscle-relaxing properties, can help reduce anxiety, aid digestion, and promote sleep. It's advisable to avoid it if you don't drink alcohol or if you're pregnant or nursing.

19. Catnip Bath

INGREDIENTS

- 1 cup dried catnip leaves and flowers
- 2 quarts boiling water

PREPARATION

1. Throw the dried catnip into a pot or bowl. Let it soak in water for about 20 to 30 minutes. Strain the mixture. Pour it into a tub of water.

Safety and Effectiveness:
Catnip is often added to baths for its soothing and anti-inflammatory properties, which can help alleviate stress, reduce muscle tension and promote relaxation. While generally considered safe, pregnant or nursing women should avoid using it. To ensure no negative reactions occur it's advisable to conduct a patch test.

20. Catnip Compress

INGREDIENTS

- 1/2 cup dried catnip leaves and flowers
- 2 cups boiling water
- Clean cloth or bandage

PREPARATION

1. Place the dried catnip in a bowl.
2. Let the catnip steep in water for around fifteen to twenty minutes.
3. Once strained, allow the herbal infusion to cool to a temperature.
4. You can use the catnip infusion to moisten a bandage or cloth for application.
5. Apply the cloth on the affected area (like a sprain, cut or insect bite) for about fifteen to twenty minutes.

Safety and Effectiveness:
Catnip compresses can be helpful in relieving insect stings, minor wounds and inflammation due to their inflammatory and pain-relieving properties. While applying them topically is generally safe, it's advisable to perform a patch test to check for any allergic reactions.

21. Ginkgo Biloba Tea

INGREDIENTS

- 1 teaspoon dried ginkgo biloba leaves
- 1 cup boiling water
- Honey or lemon (optional)

PREPARATION

1. Place the dried ginkgo leaves in a teapot or infuser.
2. Pour boiling water over the ginkgo leaves in a pot.
3. Allow it to steep for ten to fifteen minutes.
4. Pour the tea through a strainer into a cup.
5. If desired, sweeten with honey. A squeeze of lemon juice.

Safety and Effectiveness:
Ginkgo biloba tea enhances blood circulation and cognitive function due to its properties. While generally safe for consumption, without oversight, individuals who are pregnant, nursing, taking blood thinners or experiencing bleeding problems should consult their healthcare provider before incorporating this product into their routine.

22. Ginkgo Biloba Tincture

INGREDIENTS

- 1 cup dried ginkgo biloba leaves
- 2 cups vodka or other high-proof alcohol

PREPARATION

1. Place the dried ginkgo leaves in a glass container. Ensure that the leaves are fully submerged in alcohol before pouring it over them. Seal the jar tightly. Store it in a cool place for four to six weeks, giving it a gentle shake every few days. Strain the tincture through cheesecloth or a fine mesh strainer. Transfer it to a glass container.

Safety and Effectiveness:
Apart from its ability to act as an antioxidant, ginkgo biloba tincture also enhances blood flow, leading to function. It's advised to avoid it if you don't drink alcohol. If you're pregnant, nursing or taking blood thinners, it's crucial to consult a healthcare provider.

23. Ginkgo Biloba Infused Oil

INGREDIENTS

- 1 cup dried ginkgo biloba leaves
- 2 cups olive oil or almond oil

PREPARATION

1. Place the dried ginkgo leaves in a glass container. Ensure that the leaves are fully immersed in oil before pouring it on them. Seal the jar tightly. Keep it in a warm spot for two to four weeks, giving it a gentle shake each day. Transfer the oil into a jar after straining it through cheesecloth or a fine sieve.

Safety and Effectiveness:
Using ginkgo biloba-infused oil can improve blood circulation to the scalp, promoting the growth of hair. It's generally safe to apply. It's wise to conduct a patch test first to check for any allergies.

24. Ginkgo Biloba Capsules

INGREDIENTS

- 1/2 cup dried ginkgo biloba leaves, finely ground
- Empty gelatin or vegetable capsules

PREPARATION

1. Grind the dried ginkgo biloba branches into a powder. Use a coffee grinder for this task.
2. Carefully fill the capsules with the ginkgo powder using a spoon or a capsule-filling machine.
3. Store the pills in a sealed container.

Safety and Effectiveness:
Enhancing blood flow and brain function can be achieved by taking ginkgo biloba supplements. While generally considered safe for the majority of people, individuals who are pregnant, breastfeeding or taking blood thinners should consult their healthcare provider before incorporating this supplement into their routine.

25. Ginkgo Biloba Lotion

INGREDIENTS

- 1/4 cup ginkgo biloba-infused oil (see infused oil recipe)
- 1/4 cup shea butter
- 1/4 cup coconut oil
- 10 drops essential oil (optional, such as lavender or chamomile)

PREPARATION

1. Mix the coconut oil and shea butter then gently heat them using a boiler. Once the ginkgo biloba oil has melted, remove it from the heat. Blend it in. If you choose to include oil mix it in thoroughly. Allow the mixture to cool to room temperature before transferring it into a jar and letting it solidify.

Safety and Effectiveness:
Ginkgo biloba lotion's anti-inflammatory and antioxidant properties can help reduce inflammation and improve circulation. It is generally safe to apply. It's important to conduct a patch test first to check for any allergies.

26. Oregano Tea

INGREDIENTS

- 1-2 teaspoons dried oregano leaves
- 1 cup boiling water
- Honey or lemon (optional)

PREPARATION

1. Prepare your teapot or infuser. Put in the dried oregano leaves. Place the oregano leaves into a pot of boiling water. Allow it to steep for around ten to fifteen minutes. Pour the tea into a cup. For a taste, consider adding some honey and lemon.

Safety and Effectiveness:
Oregano tea is known for its antiviral and antiinflammatory properties, which can help with respiratory issues, aid digestion and boost the immune system. It's generally safe to consume. Pregnant or nursing women should avoid it. Overindulging may lead to bloating.

27. Oregano Oil

INGREDIENTS

- 1 cup fresh oregano leaves
- 1 cup olive oil

PREPARATION

1. Thoroughly. Dry the oregano leaves. Gently crush them to release the oils. Place the leaves in a glass container. Ensure they are fully covered with olive oil before pouring it in. Seal the jar tightly. Place it in a spot for two weeks, giving it a gentle shake every few days. Transfer the infused oil into a jar after straining it through cheesecloth and a fine sieve.

Safety and Effectiveness:
Oregano oil's antibacterial and anti-inflammatory properties are beneficial for treating wounds, insect bites and skin irritations. It is generally safe to apply. It's important to conduct a patch test first to check for any allergies. Avoid using oils directly on the skin.

28. Oregano Tincture

INGREDIENTS

- 1 cup fresh oregano leaves
- 2 cups vodka or other high-proof alcohol

PREPARATION

1. Wash the oregano leaves thoroughly and gently dry them.
2. Chop the leaves into pieces. Put them in a clean glass jar.
3. Ensure that the leaves are fully immersed in alcohol before pouring it over them.
4. Seal the jar tightly. Store it in a dark place for around four to six weeks, giving it a gentle shake every few days.
5. Once ready, strain the tincture through cheesecloth or a fine mesh strainer into another glass container.

Safety and Effectiveness:

Due to its properties, oregano extract can be beneficial in fighting infections. Boosting the immune system. It is advisable to avoid oregano tincture if you do not consume alcohol. If you are pregnant, nursing or taking any medications, it is crucial to seek advice from a healthcare provider.

29. Oregano Infused Honey

INGREDIENTS

- 1 cup fresh oregano leaves
- 1 cup raw honey

PREPARATION

1. Thoroughly. Dry the oregano leaves.
2. Gently crush the leaves to release the oils.
3. Place the leaves in a glass container.
4. Mix the leaves with honey, ensuring they are fully coated.
5. Store the sealed jar in a spot for one to two weeks.
6. After straining through cheesecloth or a fine mesh strainer, transfer the honey to a container.

Safety and Effectiveness:

Honey mixed with oregano possesses properties and soothing qualities that can help alleviate throat discomfort and boost immunity. It's best to steer if you're allergic to honey or oregano; otherwise, it typically poses no harm for the majority of people. It's advisable not to give honey to infants under one year of age.

30. Oregano Steam Inhalation

INGREDIENTS

- 1/4 cup dried oregano leaves
- 4 cups boiling water

PREPARATION

1. Place the dried oregano leaves in a bowl.
2. Drop the oregano leaves into the water.
3. Cover your head with a towel. Lean over the bowl to trap the steam inside.
4. Inhale the steam for ten to fifteen minutes.

Safety and Effectiveness:
Oregano's antibacterial and anti-inflammatory properties make it a great choice for steam inhalation to alleviate congestion and respiratory issues. While generally safe for people, it's important to be cautious with the water to avoid injury. If you are pregnant or nursing, it's best to consult with your doctor before using oregano for steam inhalation.

31. Tulsi Tea

INGREDIENTS

- 1 teaspoon dried tulsi leaves
- 1 cup boiling water
- Honey or lemon (optional)

PREPARATION

1. Place the dried tulsi leaves in a teapot or infuser.
2. Put the tulsi leaves into a pot of boiling water.
3. Allow them to steep for five to ten minutes.
4. Strain the tea to pour into a cup.
5. For added flavor consider sweetening with honey or a squeeze of lemon juice based on your taste preferences.

Safety and Effectiveness:
Tulsi tea is known for its antioxidant properties, which can help reduce stress, boost the system and enhance overall well-being. It is generally considered safe to consume. It's advisable to consult with your doctor before using it if you are pregnant, breastfeeding or taking any blood thinning medications.

32. Tulsi Infused Oil

INGREDIENTS

- 1 cup fresh tulsi leaves
- 1 cup carrier oil (such as olive oil or coconut oil)

PREPARATION

1. Thoroughly dry the tulsi leaves. Gently crush them to release their oils. Place the leaves in a glass container. Ensure the leaves are fully submerged in the carrier oil before pouring it over them. Seal the jar tightly. Place it in a spot for two weeks, remembering to give it a gentle shake every few days. Once ready, strain the oil through cheesecloth or a fine mesh strainer into a jar.

Safety and Effectiveness:
The anti-inflammatory and antibacterial properties of oil infused with tulsi have benefits in reducing inflammation, treating acne and promoting skin health. It's generally safe to apply. It's advisable to conduct a patch test first to check for any potential allergies.

33. Tulsi Tincture

INGREDIENTS

- 1 cup fresh tulsi leaves
- 2 cups vodka or other high-proof alcohol

PREPARATION

1. Make sure to wash and dry the tulsi leaves.
2. Next, finely chop the leaves. Place them in a glass container.
3. Ensure that the leaves are fully immersed in alcohol before pouring it over them.
4. Seal the jar tightly. Store it in a dark place for four to six weeks remembering to gently shake it every few days.
5. After straining the tincture using cheesecloth or a fine mesh strainer transfer it into another glass container.

Safety and Effectiveness:
Tulsi tincture is known for its ability to help reduce stress, boost the system and improve health due to its adaptogenic and antioxidant properties. It's best to avoid if you don't drink alcohol. If you are pregnant, nursing or taking medication, it's essential to seek advice from a healthcare provider.

34. Tulsi Honey

INGREDIENTS

- 1 cup fresh tulsi leaves
- 1 cup raw honey

PREPARATION

1. First, Dry the tulsi leaves thoroughly. Next, finely chop the leaves. Put them in a glass jar. Coat the leaves with honey, ensuring they are fully covered. Store the sealed jar in a spot for one to two weeks. Finally, strain the honey through cheesecloth or a fine mesh strainer. Transfer it to a container.

Safety and Effectiveness:
Tulsi-infused honey is known for its antioxidant properties, which can help reduce stress, boost the system and promote overall health. It is generally considered safe to consume. Individuals with allergies to tulsi or honey should avoid it.

35. Tulsi Facial Steam

INGREDIENTS

- Handful of fresh tulsi leaves
- 4 cups boiling water

PREPARATION

1. Place the tulsi leaves in a bowl. Gently drop them into the pot of water. Lean over the bowl. Cover your head with a towel to trap the steam. Inhale the steam for five to ten minutes.

Safety and Effectiveness:
Tulsi facial steam possesses inflammatory properties, which can help cleanse pores, decrease inflammation and promote skin health. It's important to handle water with care to avoid burns. Generally, it's safe for people if you're pregnant or nursing, its advisable to consult your doctor before using this product.

36. Licorice Root Tea

INGREDIENTS

- 1 tablespoon dried licorice root slices
- 1 cup water

PREPARATION

1. Boil some water in a saucepan.
2. Add the dried licorice root slices to the boiling water.
3. Simmer gently for 5 to 10 minutes.
4. Remove from heat. Let it steep for five minutes.
5. Strain the tea before pouring it into a cup.

Safety and Effectiveness:
Licorice root tea is known for its soothing properties that can help alleviate coughs, sore throats and respiratory problems. However, it's important to be cautious if you have blood pressure kidney issues or are taking medications that may interact with licorice root.

37. Licorice Root Decoction

INGREDIENTS

- 2 tablespoons dried licorice root powder
- 2 cups water

PREPARATION

1. Combine the water and powdered dry licorice root in a saucepan. Heat over heat until it boils. Stir occasionally. Let it simmer for 15 to 20 minutes on heat; after the liquid has cooled down, strain it into a cup.

Safety and Effectiveness:
Licorice root is known for its inflammatory and soothing properties, which can help with digestive issues like gastritis, upset stomach and acid reflux. However, prolonged or excessive use of licorice root may lead to loss of potassium, retention of salt and fluid retention. This is especially important to consider for individuals with high blood pressure, kidney problems or heart conditions.

38. Licorice Root Infused Oil

INGREDIENTS

- 1/2 cup dried licorice root slices
- 1 cup carrier oil (such as olive oil or coconut oil)

PREPARATION

1. Place the dried licorice root slices neatly in a dry and clean glass jar. Ensure that the licorice root is fully immersed in the carrier oil before pouring it over. Seal the jar tightly. Position it in a well-lit area for a period of two to four weeks, gently shaking it every day. Filter the infused oil into a container using cheesecloth or a fine mesh strainer.

Safety and Effectiveness:
Licorice root-infused oil is known for its soothing and hydrating properties, which can be beneficial for managing conditions like eczema, skin irritations and psoriasis. Its recommended to test a patch of skin to observe how your skin responds and discontinue use if any irritation occurs.

39. Licorice Root Honey Syrup

INGREDIENTS

- 2 tablespoons dried licorice root powder
- 1 cup honey
- 1/2 cup water

PREPARATION

1. In a saucepan stir the water and powdered licorice root together. Heat it on medium until it boils. Let it simmer, covered, over heat for 15 to 20 minutes. Then switch off the stove. Strain the mixture into a bowl. Mix the liquid with honey thoroughly.

Safety and Effectiveness:
Licorice root honey syrup is great for easing coughs, sore throats and respiratory congestion due to its soothing properties. It's important to note that honey can potentially lead to botulism, so it's not recommended for infants under one year old. Additionally, individuals with conditions like high blood pressure, kidney problems or heart issues should use caution when consuming honey.

40. Licorice Root Steam Inhalation

INGREDIENTS

- 2 tablespoons dried licorice root slices
- 4 cups boiling water

PREPARATION

1. Transfer the chopped, dried licorice root to a basin.
2. Boil enough water to cover the licorice root.
3. Hang over the basin. Put a towel over your head to keep the steam in.
4. Take a deep breath of the steam for 10–15 minutes.

Safety and Effectiveness:
Inhaling steam from licorice root can help ease sinusitis, nasal congestion and respiratory infections due to its antibacterial properties. Remember to exercise caution, as hot steam and water can cause burns. If you experience any irritation, discontinue use.

41. Fenugreek Tea

INGREDIENTS

- 1 teaspoon fenugreek seeds
- 1 cup water
- Honey (optional)

PREPARATION

1. To enhance the flavor, softly crush the fenugreek seeds.
2. Warm a pot of water until it reaches a boiling point.
3. Bring water to a boil and mix in the fenugreek seeds.
4. Simmer, with a lid on over heat, for 5 to 10 minutes.
5. Pour yourself a cup of tea after straining it.
6. If you prefer it sweeter consider adding some honey.

Safety and Effectiveness:
Fenugreek tea is beneficial for digestion, inflammation and managing blood sugar levels due to its fiber and antioxidant content. It's advisable to limit consumption during pregnancy as it can trigger contractions.

42. Fenugreek Poultice

INGREDIENTS

- 2 tablespoons fenugreek seeds
- 1/2 cup water
- Clean cloth or gauze

PREPARATION

1. Grind the fenugreek seeds finely using a spice grinder or mortar and pestle.
2. Mix the fenugreek powder with water to create a paste.
3. Spread the paste evenly on a piece of gauze or fabric.

Safety and Effectiveness:
Fenugreek poultices are known for their ability to speed up the healing process of wounds, reduce inflammation and provide relief for skin irritations due to their inflammatory and antibacterial properties. It's important to conduct a patch test before applying it to areas of the skin. If you experience any irritation, discontinue use immediately.

43. Fenugreek Seed Infusion

INGREDIENTS
- 2 tablespoons fenugreek seeds
- 2 cups water

PREPARATION
1. In a saucepan mix together the fenugreek seeds and the water.
2. Heat over heat until it boils.
3. Reduce heat. Let it simmer gently for 10 to 15 minutes.
4. Remove from the stove. Allow it to cool down to room temperature.
5. Strain the mixture. Pour it into a glass container.

Safety and Effectiveness:
The protein and nicotinic acid in fenugreek seeds can help improve scalp health, lessen dandruff and promote hair growth. Before applying it to areas of your scalp, be sure to test it on a patch first. If it causes any irritation, discontinue use immediately.

44. Fenugreek Seed Powder

INGREDIENTS
- 2 tablespoons fenugreek seeds

PREPARATION
1. Crush the fenugreek seeds into a powder using a spice grinder or mortar and pestle.

Safety and Effectiveness:
Fenugreek seed powder is beneficial for nourishing hair follicles, promoting hair growth and preventing dandruff due to its protein, iron and nicotinic acid content. Before applying it to areas of the scalp, be sure to conduct a patch test. If any irritation occurs, discontinue use.

45. Fenugreek Seed Capsules

INGREDIENTS

- Fenugreek seed powder
- Empty gelatin or vegetable capsules

PREPARATION

1. You can put ground fenugreek seeds into capsules using either a spoon or a capsule-filling device.

Safety and Effectiveness:
Fenugreek seed capsules are beneficial for regulating blood sugar, enhancing digestion, and boosting milk production in breastfeeding mothers due to their phytoestrogens and rich fiber content. If you are expecting a baby, nursing or taking any medications, it's advisable to consult your healthcare provider before using fenugreek supplements.

46. Hawthorn Berry Tea

INGREDIENTS

- 1 tablespoon dried hawthorn berries
- 1 cup water
- Honey (optional)

PREPARATION

1. In a saucepan, heat the water until it boils.
2. Add the dried berries to the boiling water.
3. Let it simmer with a lid on for about 10 to 15 minutes over heat.
4. Remove it from the heat. Let it steep for five minutes.
5. Strain it to serve yourself a cup of tea.
6. If you prefer a taste, feel free to mix in some honey.

Safety and Effectiveness:
Hawthorn berry tea is known for its vasodilatory properties, which can help support heart health, improve circulation and lower blood pressure. While generally considered safe, it's advisable for nursing individuals well as those taking medication for heart conditions, to consult their healthcare provider before consuming this product.

47. Hawthorn Tincture

INGREDIENTS

- 1/4 cup dried hawthorn berries
- 1 cup vodka or other high-proof alcohol

PREPARATION

1. Grab a glass jar. Place the dried hawthorn berries inside. Mix the berries with the alcohol, ensuring they are fully submerged. Seal the jar tightly. Store it in a dark place for about four to six weeks, giving it a gentle shake every few days. Once ready, strain the tincture using cheesecloth or a fine mesh strainer. Transfer it to a glass container.

Safety and Effectiveness:
The tincture's antioxidant and vasodilatory properties are beneficial for supporting heart wellness, improving blood flow and easing symptoms of heart failure. It's best to avoid if you don't consume alcohol. Pregnant women, nursing mothers and individuals taking medication for heart conditions should consult their healthcare providers before using this product.

48. Hawthorn Berry Syrup

INGREDIENTS

- 1 cup dried hawthorn berries
- 2 cups water
- 1 cup honey

PREPARATION

1. Heat some water. Toss in the dried berries.
2. Let it come to a boil while simmering over heat.
3. Cover it up. Let it simmer for about 20 to 30 minutes or until the liquid is reduced by half.
4. Take it off the heat. Allow it to cool down a bit.
5. Strain out any solids using cheesecloth or a fine mesh strainer.
6. Mix the liquid with honey. Give it a good stir.
7. Transfer the syrup to a sealed glass container and refrigerate.

Safety and Effectiveness:
Hawthorn berry syrups antioxidant and vasodilatory properties are beneficial for supporting heart health, improving blood circulation and lowering blood pressure. While generally considered safe for use, individuals who are pregnant, nursing or taking medication for a heart condition should consult with their healthcare provider before incorporating this product.

49. Hawthorn Berry Jam

INGREDIENTS

- 2 cups fresh hawthorn berries
- 1 cup water
- 1 cup sugar
- 1 tablespoon lemon juice

PREPARATION

1. After you've removed the stems and leaves make sure to wash the berries. Place the berries and water in a pot. Let them boil until they burst. Let it simmer for about 20 to 30 minutes or until the berries become soft. Crush the berries using a fork or potato masher. Once the berries are mashed, mix in the sugar and lemon juice thoroughly; remember, as you cook, the jam will thicken, so stir it occasionally. Remove from heat. Allow it to cool before transferring it into clean glass containers.

Safety and Effectiveness:
The health benefits of berries can now be enjoyed in a jam that is convenient to use. The sugar content makes it generally safe for consumption, by people. It's important to consume it in moderation.

50. Hawthorn Berry Smoothie

INGREDIENTS

- 1/2 cup fresh hawthorn berries
- 1/2 cup plain yogurt or almond milk
- 1/2 banana
- 1/2 cup mixed berries (such as strawberries, blueberries, or raspberries)
- 1 tablespoon honey or maple syrup (optional)
- Ice cubes (optional)

PREPARATION

1. After you've taken off the stems and leaves give the hawthorn berries a rinse. Next, put all the ingredients together in a blender and blend until it becomes light and fluffy. If you'd like it colder, add some ice cubes before blending everything.

Safety and Effectiveness:
If you want to add berries to your diet in a straightforward manner that could potentially benefit your heart and blood vessels, consider blending them into a smoothie. As long as you don't have an allergic reaction to any of the ingredients, it should be safe to enjoy.

51. Fennel Seed Tea

INGREDIENTS
- 1 teaspoon fennel seeds
- 1 cup water
- Honey (optional)

PREPARATION
1. For a fennel flavor, lightly crush the seeds.
2. Heat the water in a saucepan until it boils.
3. Drop the fennel seeds into the boiling water.
4. Simmer over heat for 5 to 10 minutes.
5. Remove from heat. Let it steep for five minutes.
6. Strain to pour yourself a cup of tea.
7. Sweeten with honey if desired.

Safety and Effectiveness:
Fennel seed tea is known for its ability to ease indigestion due to its properties. While it is generally safe, for people nursing individuals should moderate their consumption. It's important to note that some individuals may have allergies to fennel.

52. Fennel Infused Oil

INGREDIENTS
- 1 cup fennel seeds
- 1 cup carrier oil (such as olive oil or coconut oil)

PREPARATION
1. Carefully grind the fennel seeds.
2. Once the fennel seeds are crushed, place them in a spotless glass container.
3. Coat the fennel seeds with the carrier oil until they are fully coated.
4. Position the jar in a lit area. Gently shake it every few days for two to four weeks once sealed.
5. Transfer the oil through cheesecloth or a fine mesh strainer into a jar.

Safety and Effectiveness:
Fennel-infused oil's soothing properties can help with stomach discomfort. Remember to test a patch of skin before using it widely. Only ingest infused oil under supervision.

53. Fennel Seed Mouthwash

INGREDIENTS

- 1 tablespoon fennel seeds
- 1 cup water

PREPARATION

1. Carefully grind the fennel seeds.
2. Heat the water in a saucepan until it boils.
3. Add the ground fennel seeds to the boiling water.
4. Simmer, covered, on heat for 5 to 10 minutes.
5. Let it cool down to room temperature once taken off the heat.
6. Strain out the seeds from the mixture.

Safety and Effectiveness:
Fennel seed mouthwash is known for its inflammatory properties, making it a good choice for freshening breath and soothing mouth discomfort. It is generally safe to use. Individuals with fennel allergies should avoid it.

54. Fennel Seed Steam Inhalation

INGREDIENTS

- 2 tablespoons fennel seeds
- 4 cups boiling water

PREPARATION

1. Crush the fennel seeds
2. Take the fennel seeds. Crush them in a bowl.
3. Put the fennel seeds into a pot of boiling water.
4. To trap the steam, bend over the pot. Cover your head with a towel.
5. Inhale from the steam for around ten to fifteen minutes.

Safety and Effectiveness:
The soothing properties of fennel seed steam can help ease coughs and congestion in the system. Remember to be careful to avoid getting burnt by the steam and hot water.

55. Fennel Seed Poultice

INGREDIENTS

- 2 tablespoons fennel seeds
- Hot water
- Clean cloth or gauze

PREPARATION

1. Gently grind the fennel seeds.
2. Mix the fennel seeds in a bowl.
3. Add water gradually until a paste forms.
4. Spread the paste using a cloth or gauze.

Safety and Effectiveness:
A fennel seed poultice can help ease bloating and menstrual pains due to its properties. Remember, hot water and steam can lead to burns, so use caution. If you experience any irritation, discontinue use.

56. Lemon Balm Tea

INGREDIENTS

- 1 tablespoon fresh lemon balm leaves (or 1 teaspoon dried leaves)
- 1 cup boiling water
- Honey (optional)

PREPARATION

1. Place the lemon balm leaves in a heat teapot or cup.
2. Pour boiling water over the leaves.
3. Let it steep for 5 to 10 minutes.
4. Strain the tea to serve in a cup.
5. For a taste, consider adding honey.

Safety and Effectiveness:
Due to its soothing properties, lemon balm tea is fantastic for aiding in relaxation, easing tension and improving sleep quality. While it is generally safe for most people to enjoy, pregnant or nursing individuals should moderate their consumption.

57. Lemon Balm Tincture

INGREDIENTS

- Fresh lemon balm leaves
- High-proof alcohol (such as vodka or brandy)

PREPARATION

1. Place fresh lemon balm leaves, in a glass container in a manner.
2. Make sure the leaves are fully covered with alcohol.
3. Seal the jar tightly. Keep it in a dark place for four to six weeks giving it a gentle shake every few days.
4. After four to six weeks, strain the liquid using cheesecloth or a fine mesh strainer.
5. Transfer the tincture into a clean glass container. Seal it securely.

Safety and Effectiveness:
Lemon balm tincture is known for its soothing properties, which can help with reducing stress promoting relaxation and improving digestion. If you are pregnant, breastfeeding or taking any medications, it's advisable to consult your healthcare provider before using this product.

58. Lemon Balm Infused Oil

INGREDIENTS

- Fresh lemon balm leaves
- Carrier oil (such as olive oil or coconut oil)

PREPARATION

1. Remember to wash and dry the lemon balm leaves. Place them gently into a glass jar, ensuring they are fully immersed in the carrier oil. Keep the jar in a lit area. Give it a gentle shake every few days for two to four weeks once sealed. After this period, strain the oil through cheesecloth or a fine mesh strainer into a glass container.

Safety and Effectiveness:
Lemon balm-infused oil is known for its inflammatory properties, making it a helpful solution for skin issues, inflammation and stress. Remember to conduct a patch test before using it on skin areas and avoid it if you're allergic, to lemon balm.

59. Lemon Balm Bath Soak

INGREDIENTS

- Handful of fresh lemon balm leaves
- 1 cup Epsom salt
- Hot bathwater

PREPARATION

1. Place the Epsom salt and lemon balm leaves in a cloth bag or towel and tie it securely.
2. As the water in the bathtub warms up, hang the bag on the faucet.
3. Allow the bag to steep in the bathwater for ten to fifteen minutes.
4. Discard the bag afterward.
5. Enjoy a soak in the tub for twenty to thirty minutes.

Safety and Effectiveness:
Taking a bath with lemon balm can help ease muscle tension, promote relaxation and prevent any slips or falls when getting in and out of the tub.

60. Lemon Balm Facial Steam

INGREDIENTS

- Handful of fresh lemon balm leaves
- 4 cups boiling water

PREPARATION

1. Collect the lemon balm leaves. Place them in a heat-resistant bowl.
2. Cover the leaves with boiling water.
3. Lean over the bowl to trap the steam, and cover your head with a towel.
4. Take slow breaths for a couple of minutes.

Safety and Effectiveness:
The calming and germ-fighting properties of lemon balm make it a perfect choice for steam, as it can unclog pores, purify the skin and promote a sense of tranquility. Just remember to avoid getting burned by the steam and water.

61. Basil Infused Water

INGREDIENTS

- Fresh basil leaves
- Water

PREPARATION

1. Wash the fresh basil leaves under water. Pat them dry with a paper towel. Next, finely chop the basil leaves using a food processor. Fill up a pitcher with water and mix in the chopped basil leaves. Refrigerate the mixture for an hour to allow the flavors to blend.

Safety and Effectiveness:
Adding basil to water is a way to satisfy your thirst and could potentially assist with reducing inflammation and providing antioxidants. For the part, it should be harmless. However, individuals who have a sensitivity, to basil should avoid it.

62. Basil Essential Oil Massage Blend

INGREDIENTS

- 5-7 drops of basil essential oil
- 1 tablespoon carrier oil (such as coconut oil or almond oil)

PREPARATION

1. Mix the carrier oil and basil oil in a bowl.

Safety and Effectiveness:
If you're feeling muscle pain or a headache, consider applying basil oil. It has pain-relieving and inflammatory properties. To avoid skin irritation, make sure to blend oils with a carrier oil before applying them. Begin by testing a patch on your skin.

63. Basil and Honey Cough Syrup

INGREDIENTS

- Handful of fresh basil leaves
- 1 cup honey

PREPARATION

1. Wash the basil leaves in water. Pat them dry with a paper towel to clean them.

2. Heat the honey in a saucepan over heat until it turns into a thin syrup by bringing it to a gentle boil.
3. Let the basil leaves soak in the honey for 10 to 15 minutes.
4. Remove the pan from the stove. Allow the mixture to cool down.
5. After straining out the basil leaves, transfer the syrup into a container.

Safety and Effectiveness:
This syrup works well for soothing coughs and sore throats, as basil contains antitussive properties. Although it's generally safe for people, it's important to avoid giving honey-based remedies to children under one year old due to the risk of botulism.

64. Basil Steam Inhalation

INGREDIENTS
- Handful of fresh basil leaves
- 4 cups boiling water

PREPARATION
1. After washing the basil leaves in water, pat them dry with a paper towel.
2. Arrange the basil leaves in a heatproof bowl.
3. Dip the basil leaves into the boiling water.
4. Cover your head with a towel. Lean over the bowl to retain the steam.
5. Inhale deeply for five to ten minutes.

Safety and Effectiveness:
Inhaling basil steam could be beneficial for clearing nasal passages and easing congestion due to its decongestant properties. Remember to watch out for the steam and hot water to avoid getting burned.

65. Basil Lemonade

INGREDIENTS
- Handful of fresh basil leaves
- 4 cups water
- 1/2 cup fresh lemon juice
- 1/4 cup honey or maple syrup (adjust to taste)

PREPARATION
1. Rinse the fresh basil leaves with water. Pat them dry using a paper towel. In a pot, gently heat the maple syrup or honey with water until the sweetener is completely dissolved. Let it cool down to room temperature after removing from heat. Combine the basil leaves, lemon juice and sweetened water in a pitcher and mix thoroughly. Chill the mixture in the refrigerator after stirring it.

Safety and Effectiveness:
Enjoy the refreshing experience of reaping the anti-inflammatory advantages of basil by savoring a glass of basil-infused lemonade. Although generally beneficial, for people individuals who are expecting a baby or breastfeeding should moderate their consumption.

66. Calendula Infused Oil

INGREDIENTS

- 1 cup dried calendula flowers
- 1 cup carrier oil (such as olive oil or almond oil)

PREPARATION

1. Move the dried calendula flowers into a sealed glass jar.
2. Mix the flowers with the carrier oil, ensuring they are fully immersed.
3. Place the jar in a spot. Gently shake it every few days for four to six weeks after sealing.
4. After four to six weeks, strain the oil through cheesecloth or a fine mesh strainer into a glass container.

Safety and Effectiveness:
Calendula-infused oil's inflammatory and antibacterial properties can help soothe skin irritations, reduce inflammation and promote tissue healing. It's advisable to test an area before using the product on your body, and if any skin irritation arises, discontinue use.

67. Calendula Salve

INGREDIENTS

- 1/2 cup calendula infused oil
- 2 tablespoons beeswax pellets
- **Optional:** a few drops of essential oils such as lavender or tea tree oil (for added fragrance and antimicrobial properties)

PREPARATION

1. Mix the beeswax pellets with the calendula-infused oil and heat gently in a boiler until melted.
2. Remove from the heat source. Add the oils if desired.
3. Pour the mixture into containers, like small jars or tins.
4. Seal the containers once the salve has hardened and cooled.

Safety and Effectiveness:
Calendula salve's antibacterial and anti-inflammatory properties are beneficial for soothing skin

irritations, promoting healing and reducing inflammation. Prior to applying it on areas of the skin, perform a patch test. Cease usage if any irritation occurs.

68. Calendula Tea

INGREDIENTS

- 1 tablespoon dried calendula flowers
- 1 cup boiling water
- Honey (optional)

PREPARATION

1. Place the dried calendula blossoms in a heat cup. Pour water over the flowers. Cover them to steep for ten to fifteen minutes. Once steeped, strain the tea into another cup. If you prefer it sweeter you can stir in some honey.

Safety and Effectiveness:
Calendula tea is beneficial for your system, inflammation levels and overall health due to its inflammatory and antibacterial properties. While most people can enjoy it safely, pregnant or nursing individuals should moderate their consumption.

69. Calendula Bath Soak

INGREDIENTS

- Handful of dried calendula flowers
- 1 cup Epsom salt
- Warm bathwater

PREPARATION

1. Once the calendula flowers are dry, put them together with the Epsom salt in a muslin bag or clean cloth. Tie it securely.
2. As you fill the tub with water, hang the bag on the faucet.
3. Allow the bag to soak in the bathwater for ten to fifteen minutes.
4. Discard the bag.
5. Relax in the tub for twenty to thirty minutes and unwind.

Safety and Effectiveness:
Calendula's soothing and anti-inflammatory properties make it a perfect addition to your bath for easing discomfort, reducing swelling and promoting a sense of calm. Be careful not to slip when getting in or out of the tub.

70. Calendula Compress

INGREDIENTS

- Handful of fresh or dried calendula flowers
- Hot water
- Clean cloth or gauze

PREPARATION

1. Place the calendula blooms in a heat bowl, whether they're fresh or dried.
2. Pour water over the flowers to cover them entirely.
3. Let the blooms steep for around ten to fifteen minutes.
4. Soak a cloth or gauze in some of the calendula-infused water.
5. Before placing the compress on the area, wring out any excess liquid.

Safety and Effectiveness:

The anti-inflammatory and antibacterial qualities of calendula make it a useful compress for decreasing inflammation and encouraging healing.

To prevent burns, be careful while handling hot water. Stop using it immediately if it irritates your skin.

BOOK 5

Herbal Remedies in Daily Life

Practical advice

Enhance your well-being. Deepen your bond with nature by integrating remedies into your daily routine. This can help you on your path to health and a stronger connection, with your body and surroundings.

1. Start with Education and Research

Before you start using any herbs as a remedy, it's important to get to know them. Understand their benefits, potential risks and the right doses. Books, research, trusted herbalists, and doctors can provide information. By learning about the qualities and functions of herbs, you can make informed decisions to safely incorporate them into your routine for results.

2. Identify Your Wellness Goals

When selecting remedies, it's crucial to consider your health concerns and wellness goals. Certain herbs can address issues such as enhancing digestion, reducing stress, improving abilities and strengthening immunity. By understanding your life goals, you can tailor your routine to incorporate herbs that align with your desired outcomes.

3. Incorporate Herbs into Daily Rituals

Using remedies regularly and smoothly in your life can enhance their benefits. You can easily integrate herbs into your tasks by following these tips;

- **Morning Routine:** Starting your day with smoothies or teas infused with healing herbs is an idea. If you're looking to reduce inflammation in the morning, consider blending ginger and turmeric into your beverage. Additionally, incorporating herbs like Ashwagandha and Rhodiola could potentially assist in managing stress effectively.
- **Meal Preparation:** For a nutritious meal, consider incorporating culinary herbs and spices. Ingredients like cinnamon, cumin and oregano do not enhance the flavor of dishes. Also offers various health benefits. Additionally, you can elevate the taste of salads, soups and main dishes by using herbs like parsley, cilantro and basil as garnishes.
- **Afternoon Pick-Me-Up:** Indulge in a snack or a soothing infusion while taking a break for lunch. For a pick me up and aid consider sipping on some peppermint tea. If you fancy almonds, opt for a handful dusted with turmeric and honey; they'll satisfy your cravings. It can also aid in reducing inflammation.
- **Evening Wind-Down:** Unwind before bedtime with a calming ritual. If you're finding it hard to relax at night consider sipping on chamomile tea or incorporating a couple of drops of oil into a cozy bath or a soothing massage.

4. Keep Supplies Handy

Make sure to have your supplies to stay consistent with your herbal routine. Have a selection of your herbs, teas, tinctures and essential oils available by keeping them well stocked. To seamlessly incorporate herbs and herbal products into your habits without any disruptions, designate an area in your kitchen or pantry for storing them.

5. Listen to Your Body

Monitor the shifts in your body as you incorporate remedies into your routine. Since each individual's body reacts uniquely, there isn't a one-size-fits-all solution for maintaining health. Be mindful of how your body responds and adapt your regimen accordingly. If you experience any discomfort or adverse reactions discontinue the usage. Consult with your healthcare provider promptly.

6. Maintain Balance and Moderation

Using remedies, in moderation and balance is key for reaping their health benefits. It's essential to be mindful of side effects and interactions with medications, so it's advisable to consume herbs and herbal products in moderation. To prevent tolerance and ensure an intake of nutrients and compounds, consider changing the rotation of herbs you use from time to time.

7. Seek Professional Guidance

Seek advice from a certified herbalist, naturopathic physician or healthcare professional if you are not well-versed in remedies or if you are facing health concerns. They can evaluate your situation, offer tailored recommendations following the assessment, monitor your development and adjust your herbal therapy regimen accordingly.

8. Practice Patience and Consistency

Remember, herbal remedies usually require patience to show results. Must be used regularly for benefits. Using supplements is a commitment to your well-being that yields long-term rewards rather than quick fixes. By following your regimen, you may experience increased energy, strength and overall health over time.

Tips for growing your herbs and preparing remedies at home

If you want to grow your herbs and create your remedies at home, here are some tips to keep in mind;

1. Choose the Right Location

For a herb garden, opt for a spot with sunlight. To prevent root rot caused by moisture, ensure the area has drainage. Indoor herb gardens require around six to eight hours of sunlight daily, so planting them near a window is essential.

2. Start with Easy-to-Grow Herbs

For beginners in gardening, it's best to begin with low-maintenance herbs. Mint, basil, thyme, rosemary and chives are options for newcomers. These herbs are perfect for those to garden, as they require care and can thrive in various conditions.

3. Provide Adequate Watering

Remember to water your herbs to keep the soil moist but not overly wet. Check the moisture levels by touching the soil with your finger; if it feels dry it's time to give your plants a watering. Herbs prefer an environment to flourish but be cautious not to overwater them as this could lead to root rot.

4. Incorporate Organic Practices

Minimize your exposure, to pesticides and chemicals by tending to your garden in a manner. To cultivate herbs in your garden it's essential to enrich the soil with elements such as compost and matured manure. Embrace companion. Attracting insects is two eco-friendly methods for pest control in order to maintain a pest-free environment.

5. Harvest Herbs Correctly

To ensure your herbs grow robust and lush with yields, it's essential to harvest them. Trim the inches of the stems meticulously using sharp scissors or pruning shears, making sure not to take more than one-third of the plant at once. The morning is ideal for herb harvesting as this is when their essential oils are most potent and flavourful.

6. Preserve Excess Herbs

When you have fresh herbs, consider creating an herb preserve. Popular methods for preserving herbs include making infusions and extracts, drying them and freezing them. To dry herbs, you can hang them down in a fridge them into ice cube dishes with a small amount of water or olive oil.

7. Research Herbal Remedies

Discover the range of uses and healing properties that plants offer, allowing you to create your natural remedies in the comfort of your home. Explore solutions for managing stress, alleviating headaches, easing indigestion and treating cold symptoms. Experiment with treatments, like tea tinctures, infused oils, balms and compresses, to find the application method that suits you best.

8. Invest in Quality Tools and Equipment

To keep your remedies effective and safe, it's crucial to use sterile gardening gloves, shears, drying racks and storage glass jars. These items are vital for gardening and preparing herbs.

9. Consult Reliable Sources

To expand your knowledge of herbalism and natural remedies, it's essential to seek information from sources. To enhance your understanding of herbs, consider exploring resources such as books, websites and classes conducted by experts in the field. Engage with communities and forums dedicated to herbalism to connect with minded individuals and exchange insights and experiences.

10. Practice Patience and Persistence

Growing your herbs and creating remedies requires determination, patience and a willingness to learn from both successes and setbacks. Embrace new plants, techniques and recipes with a heart and mind. Herbalism is a craft that demands ongoing exploration. As you refine your gardening skills. Deepen your knowledge of herbs, trust your instincts, and sharpen your skills.

By following these guidelines, you'll be on the path to cultivating a herb garden and utilizing its healing properties for yourself and your loved ones. Engaging in herbalism and tending to a garden are fulfilling ways to enhance your well-being while strengthening your bond with the world.

NUTRITION AND NATURAL REMEDIES

Investigating food, nutrition, and herbal remedy efficacy

The connection between diet, nutrition and the effectiveness of remedies is complex. Plays a significant role in maintaining good health and well-being. Let's delve deeper into how these factors interact with each other.

1. Nutrient Absorption and Bioavailability

The way our bodies take in and utilize nutrients and herbal substances is heavily impacted by the food we eat. Herbal substances are best absorbed when included in a diet, in phytonutrients, minerals and vitamins. Vitamin C and other nutrients can enhance the body's absorption of antioxidants, while dietary fats aid in absorbing soluble herbal compounds.

2. Synergistic Effects

The combined effects of nutrients in meals and the healing qualities of herbs can potentially boost the effectiveness of the nutrients. For instance, the presence of piperine in pepper can improve the body's ability to absorb curcumin, which is the key element in turmeric, especially when paired with black pepper. Additionally, herbal teas have been shown to increase the intake of phytochemicals and antioxidants in herbs when consumed alongside meals, in vitamin C.

3. Gut Microbiota

The trillions of organisms residing in the tract form the gut microbiota, playing a crucial role in supporting functions such as immunity and nutrient processing. The effectiveness of remedies could be influenced by elements that impact the diversity and makeup of the gut microbiota. Consuming fruits, vegetables, and whole grains provides prebiotics that nourish bacteria in the gut, enhancing the potency and absorption of herbal treatments.

4. Inflammatory Balance

Several health concerns, like conditions, heart disease and metabolic issues, are linked to long-term inflammation. Some minerals and food items possess inflammatory qualities, with diet playing a crucial role in controlling inflammation pathways. Adding inflammatory herbs to your meals could potentially decrease inflammation levels. Turmeric, ginger and green tea are known for their inflammatory properties.

5. Metabolic Health

Diet plays a role in influencing metabolic health, affecting aspects like insulin sensitivity, lipid metabolism and blood sugar control. For individuals dealing with diabetes and metabolic syndrome, incorporating remedies such as melon, cinnamon and fenugreek can offer benefits in lowering blood sugar levels and improving lipid profiles. By combining these treatments with a diet and regular exercise routine, one can enhance both metabolic outcomes and overall well-being.

6. Nutrient Deficiencies and Herbal Supplementation

Natural remedies might not be as effective if your body lacks nutrients, potentially affecting your metabolism and overall health. For example, immune-boosting herbs, like echinacea and elderberry, may not work optimally if you're deficient in magnesium, zinc and vitamin D. This could impact your system's function and how your body responds to stress. To enhance the healing properties of treatments and address nutritional needs herbal supplements could be beneficial.

7. Individual Variability and Personalized Nutrition

The effectiveness of treatments and dietary adjustments can differ from person to person based on factors such as diet, genetics, lifestyle and overall health. Personalized nutrition strategies aim to optimize the benefits of changes and herbal treatments by tailoring them to each individual's nutritional requirements, metabolic processes and health goals. Integrative healthcare professionals consider their patient's preferences, sensitivities and genetic backgrounds when creating customized plans for their needs and herbal therapies.

8. Adverse Food-Herb Interactions

Some foods and herbal remedies can interact with each other, affecting how they are absorbed and used in the body. For instance, grapefruit juice has been found to slow down the breakdown of herbs and medications, leading to levels in the bloodstream and potential side effects. It's important to consult your doctor before introducing any remedy into your diet and be aware of possible interactions between food and herbs.

The relationship between diet, nutrition and the effectiveness of medicines is complex. Influences various aspects of health. To achieve health outcomes, it is advisable to consume a rounded diet rich in minerals, phytonutrients and prebiotics. This supports the absorption and utilization of components along with their combined benefits. Individuals can enhance the impact of medicine on health by integrating herbal therapies with a nutritious diet tailored to their specific needs.

Guidelines for a balanced diet

To enhance the effectiveness of remedies in improving health and wellness, it is essential to establish a foundation by adhering to these guidelines for a well-rounded diet; for outcomes, prioritize consuming plant-based foods, staying adequately hydrated and listening to your body's cues. Additionally aim to minimize the intake of processed foods whenever feasible.

1. Eat a Variety of Whole Foods

Include a number of fruits, vegetables, legumes, nuts, seeds, lean meats and whole grains in your meals. For a rounded intake of vitamins, minerals, antioxidants, and phytonutrients, aim for a selection of colorful fruits and veggies.

2. Emphasize Plant-Based Foods

Ensure that the majority of your diet includes plant-based foods. To maintain a diet high in phytochemicals, fiber, and essential nutrients, make sure to consume plenty of fruits, vegetables, herbs and spices. A nutrient-packed plant-based diet supports well-being. It could potentially enhance the effectiveness of homemade remedies.

3. Include Healthy Fats

Fatty fish, like mackerel and salmon, along with avocados, nuts, seeds and olive oil, are sources of fats. The body requires these fats to absorb nutrients producing hormones and performing tasks efficiently. Moreover, they enhance the absorption of components that dissolve in fat, making them more accessible to the body.

4. Limit Processed Foods and Sugars

Minimize intake of carbohydrates, sugary treats and sweet beverages. Opt for foods to support natural treatments by reducing inflammation, maintaining stable blood sugar levels and preventing nutrient deficiencies. Prioritize consuming foods in their state, for health benefits.

5. Prioritize Nutrient-Dense Foods

For the value, without exceeding your calorie intake, opt for foods packed with essential vitamins, minerals and plant-based nutrients. Examples include grains, legumes, nuts, seeds, cruciferous vegetables, berries and leafy greens. Consuming rich meals supports health and provides your body with the necessary fuel for optimal performance.

6. Stay Hydrated

Ensuring you stay hydrated is essential for supporting function, digestion and detoxification. It's important to drink an amount of water throughout the day to maintain hydration levels. There are ways to enhance hydration with added health benefits, like enjoying tea-flavored water or coconut water. For nutrients and herbal remedies to work effectively, the body needs to be hydrated for absorption and distribution.

7. Include Herbal Teas and Infusions

To enhance your being and health make it a habit to enjoy herbal teas and infusions daily. Opt for teas made from herbs like echinacea, ginger, chamomile and peppermint for their medicinal properties. Not only do these herbal brews help in hydrating you, calming your senses and aiding digestion. They also offer various other health benefits.

8. Listen to Your Body

Monitor how your body responds to remedies and the impacts of diets. Each individual has needs and responses to herbs and other natural elements. To support your health and well-being, listen to your body's cues. Adjust your diet and herbal routine as needed.

9. Consider Individual Needs and Preferences

When deciding on your routine and diet, consider your health goals, food preferences and medical history. Personalize your nutrition and herbal practices to suit your needs and tastes. For guidance, consult with a healthcare provider or nutrition specialist who's a certified dietitian.

10. Practice Moderation and Balance

To maintain a balance, incorporate herbs into your diet. Follow a moderate eating plan. Avoid overly restrictive diets that may lead to deficiencies or imbalances. For well-being and energy, include a variety of nutrient-packed foods in your meals. Use herbal remedies in moderation.

Top of Form

DETOXIFICATION AND BODY CLEANSING

Natural herbal detoxification and cleaning

It's an idea to set a couple of days to get organized, declutter and prepare for the upcoming abundance of the new year. Making space for creativity, revisiting goals and adopting habits that support both the mind and body are all ways to approach this period. The terms "cleansing" and "detoxifying" hold significance during this season.

Our ancestors have long incorporated roots and herbs into their diets, even though "detoxing" appears to be a modern response to what is perceived as a more toxic environment today. Recent studies have revealed that certain herbs like dandelion, burdock, nettle, Schisandra and red clover possess properties that aid our body's natural detoxification processes. Herbalists continue to use these plants to support and enhance these functions, honoring wisdom rather than promoting extreme detox regimes.

The lymphatic system, system, skin, liver and kidneys all play roles in maintaining the body's fluid balance. Nature has provided us with an array of plants that cater specifically to each of these organs' needs. Whether it's protecting the skin or supporting liver function, there is a plant remedy for every requirement.

Best Herbs to Support Your Natural Detoxification Systems

- **Schisandra:** In the realm of Traditional Chinese Medicine (TCM), the Schisandra berry goes by the name wǔ wèi zi, which translates to the «five-taste fruit.» What sets it apart from fruits is its ability to encompass all five flavors: sour, bitter, savory and sweet. Each taste signifies aspects of nature, bodily systems and healing properties. According to healing practices, this exceptional fruit rejuvenates the body›s life force, known as ch›i or qi, with research supporting its beneficial effects on liver health.
- **Red Clover:** Farmers often choose to sow cover crops that can fix nitrogen, like the rejuvenating clover, a plant belonging to the pea family. Red clover is popular for its ability to support skin health, making it a favorable choice for a daily detox routine.
- **Dandelion:** Dandelion, a loved herb known for its bitterness, contains properties that support the body›s natural detoxification process and gently activate the liver. The bitter elements in dandelion root excite the taste buds, prompting a series of reactions that promote bile production and enhance digestion. Widely valued in medicine, dandelion serves as an effective tonic for aiding fat digestion and facilitating waste elimination.
- **Burdock:** For quite some time, people have praised this plant›s ability to balance the body supporting the elimination processes and enhancing the absorption of nutrients. Burdock root is commonly utilized to support kidney health and maintain skin, thanks to its content of inulin and prebiotic starch.
- **Nettle:** One of the respected spring remedies is nettle, a wild green, in the spring. While nettle was initially known for its skin benefits, it is now recognized for enhancing health and supporting well-being. Following a winter or holiday period when your body might feel sluggish, this plant could assist.

Simple Ways to Incorporate These Herbs into Your Life

Herbal teas and tinctures offer ways to incorporate these plants into your routine if you're looking for some inspiration. Whether you aim to support your skin, liver or kidneys in their natural detoxification processes, our wide range of cleansing teas can be a companion. While herbs play a role, they are one piece of the puzzle when it comes to leading a healthy lifestyle and restoring balance in your life. It's important to acknowledge the complexity of your body's ecosystem and treat it with the care it deserves. Have you considered ways to enhance cleansing" in your life? Your dietary choices, the organization of your living and work spaces, the ingredients, the products you use and even the quality of your relationships all contribute to this process.

Foods and routines for periodic detoxification

Our two-week cleanse regimen aims to rejuvenate your body. This plan is designed to assist you in eliminating toxins while savoring meals that are both purifying and invigorating. Cleanse your system naturally with these nourishing options. Experience a renewed sense of vitality afterward.

Foods to eat

- **Hydrating Foods:** Cucumber, celery, watermelon, and other water-rich veggies and fruits should be part of your daily diet.
- **Leafy Greens:** The chlorophyll and nutritional richness of kale, spinach, & Swiss chard will be enhanced.
- **Citrus Fruits:** Vitamin C & natural detoxification help may be found in citrus fruits, including limes, lemons, and oranges.
- **Cruciferous Vegetables:** For the benefit of your liver, include broccoli, cauliflower, & Brussels sprouts in your diet.
- **Herbal Teas:** Dandelion, green, & ginger teas are great detoxifiers, and you may drink them all day long.
- **Lean Proteins:** For well-rounded diets, choose skinless chicken, tofu, fish, and beans.
- **Healthy Fats:** Avocados, almonds, & olive oil are great sources of healthy fats.
- **Whole Grains:** To get fiber and sustained energy, brown rice, quinoa, & oats are good choices.
- **Nuts and Seeds:** For extra nutrition, add chia seeds, almonds, and flaxseeds.
- **Detox Smoothies:** Incorporate cleansing herbs into a fruit and vegetable smoothie for a healthy and revitalizing beverage.

Consume cruciferous vegetables such as kale and broccoli to aid the liver's detoxification processes.

Foods not to eat

- **Processed Foods:** Cut down on processed sweets, snacks, and fast meals as much as possible.
- **Added Sugars:** In order to aid in the detoxification process, stay away from sugary beverages, sweets, and snacks.
- **Artificial Additives:** If you want to eat clean, you should cut out items that include colors, artificial flavors, and preservatives.
- **Caffeine:** To aid in detoxifying and encourage hydration, cut down or cut out coffee.
- **Alcohol:** To get the most out of your detoxification process, cut down or quit drinking altogether.
- **Individual Dietary Needs:** Make changes to the diet plan according to personal tastes and dietary requirements.
- **Regular Hydration:** Stay hydrated for optimal detoxification and health by drinking plenty of water.
- **Regular Physical Activity:** You may boost the detox process by doing modest activity, such as walking or yoga.
- **Consult a Healthcare Professional:** Talk to your doctor if you need specific recommendations for detoxing.

Main benefits

The detox program lasts for two weeks. Aims to cleanse the body of toxins while boosting energy levels. It includes meals, antioxidants and beverages to help rehydrate and support health.

How to budget for this meal plan?

Make sure you keep tea and lemon water available. You can save money by buying a variety of fruits and vegetables, like kale, spinach, cucumbers and berries, in bulk. Purchasing broccoli, celery and avocados in quantities can also help you cut costs. Consider buying chia seeds, quinoa and flaxseeds in amounts to save money well.

14-Day Detox Meal Plan

This diet plan focuses on incorporating nourishing foods that support the body's natural detoxification processes. By including a variety of foods high in minerals, fiber and antioxidants, you can help your body rejuvenate and reset.

Day 1
- **Breakfast:** Smoothies made with strawberries, spinach, blueberries, & chia seeds, accompanied with a glass of lemon water
- **Lunch:** Salad made of quinoa, celery, avocado, cucumber, & a dressing made of lemon and turmeric.
- **Dinner:** Quinoa cooked with garlic and served with steamed broccoli baked salmon.

Day 2
- **Breakfast:** Smoothie made with green tea, almonds, flaxseeds, overnight oats, and sliced strawberries
- **Lunch:** A salad with cucumber, avocado, grilled chicken, & leafy greens (spinach, kale).
- **Dinner:** Vegetables (bell peppers, broccoli, etc.) and tofu stir-fried in a ginger-turmeric sauce.

Day 3
- **Breakfast:** Smoothie made with pineapple, ginger, chia seeds, and kale for digestion.
- **Lunch:** A salad of lentils and beets tossed with mixed greens, cucumber, and a dressing made with apple cider vinegar.
- **Dinner:** Quinoa pilaf, roasted Brussels sprouts, & baked chicken breast

Day 4
- **Breakfast:** Toasted green tea, avocado, & sliced tomatoes on healthy grain bread.
- **Lunch:** Veggie sticks dipped in hummus and cucumbers
- **Dinner:** Fish tacos cooked on the grill with a slaw made of cabbage, avocado, & lime dressing.

Day 5
- **Breakfast:** A dish of berry smoothies garnished with flaxseeds and chopped almonds served with lemon water
- **Lunch:** Grilled shrimp, spinach salad and avocado dressed with a lemon-turmeric vinaigrette
- **Dinner:** Quinoa cooked with garlic, greens, and roasted chickpeas

Day 6
- **Breakfast:** Prosciutto, chia seeds, green tea, a variety of fruit, and honey drizzled on top.
- **Lunch:** A salad of quinoa tabbouleh tossed with cucumber, olive oil, tomatoes, and parsley
- **Dinner:** lemon-garlic sauce, Grilled asparagus, and baked fish

Day 7

- **Breakfast:** Smoothie made with spinach, banana, flaxseeds, and ginger for a detox.
- **Lunch:** A salad of greens tossed with almonds, grilled chicken, and a dressing made with apple cider vinegar.
- **Dinner:** Quinoa, corn, broccoli, & tofu stir-fried in a ginger-turmeric sauce with chopped bell peppers and garlic

Day 8

- **Breakfast:** Oatmeal with chopped strawberries & almonds on top, served with lemon water
- **Lunch:** A salad of kale, grilled shrimp, avocado, and a vinaigrette made with lemon & turmeric.
- **Dinner:** Quinoa cooked with garlic and topped with baked chicken breast, roasted Brussels sprouts,

Day 9

- **Breakfast:** green tea, Toasted avocado, & sliced tomatoes on healthy grain bread.
- **Lunch:** Veggie sticks dipped in hummus and cucumbers
- **Dinner:** Fish tacos cooked on the grill with a slaw made of cabbage, avocado, & lime dressing.

Day 10

- **Breakfast:** A dish of berry smoothies garnished with flaxseeds and chopped almonds served with lemon water.
- **Lunch:** Grilled shrimp, spinach salad & avocado dressed with a lemon-turmeric vinaigrette
- **Dinner:** Quinoa cooked with garlic, greens, & roasted chickpeas

Day 11

- **Breakfast:** Prosciutto, chia seeds, green tea, a variety of fruit, and honey drizzled on top.
- **Lunch:** A salad of quinoa tabbouleh tossed with olive oil, cucumber, tomatoes, & parsley
- **Dinner:** Grilled asparagus, baked fish, lemon-garlic sauce

Day 12

- **Breakfast:** Detox smoothie with spinach, banana, ginger, and flaxseeds
- **Lunch:** A salad of greens tossed with grilled almonds, chicken, and a dressing made with apple cider vinegar.
- **Dinner:** Quinoa, corn, broccoli, and tofu stir-fried in a ginger-turmeric sauce with chopped bell peppers and garlic

Day 13

- **Breakfast:** Oatmeal with chopped strawberries & almonds on top, served with lemon water
- **Lunch:** A salad of kale, grilled shrimp, avocado, and a vinaigrette made with lemon & turmeric.
- **Dinner:** garlic-infused quinoa, Roasted Brussels sprouts, & baked chicken breast

Day 14

- **Breakfast:** Toasted avocado, green tea, & sliced tomatoes on healthy grain bread.
- **Lunch:** Veggie sticks dipped in hummus and cucumbers
- **Dinner:** Fish tacos cooked on the grill with a slaw made of cabbage, avocado, & lime dressing.

BOOK 6
Natural Remedies for Mental and Emotional Well-Being

NATURAL HERBS FOR MENTAL HEALTH AND EMOTIONAL HARMONY

Maintaining a sense of harmony is crucial for both mental well-being and, over the years individuals have sought solace in herbs as a comforting and supportive remedy during times. Whether incorporated into aromatherapy, taken as a supplement, or brewed into a calming tea, herbs enable us to connect with the healing properties of nature. Integrating herbs into our self-care routine can serve as a beneficial method to enhance emotional and mental wellness, especially in conjunction with professional therapy when needed.

How Herbal Traditions Use Herbs To Support Mental And Emotional Health

Traditional Chinese Medicine

In Chinese Medicine (TCM), it is believed that the mind and body are closely connected and that emotional well-being can affect health. TCM views health conditions as imbalances, in qi, which can be addressed through practices like acupuncture, herbal remedies and dietary adjustments. Herbal medicines, like St. Johns wort, valerian root and ginseng, are commonly used in TCM to address issues.

Ayurveda

In Ayurveda the vata, pitta and kapha doshas are. An imbalance among them could result in health challenges. Ayurvedic philosophy views well-being as a state influenced by internal and external factors. The holistic approach to medicine involves adjustments, lifestyle changes and therapies incorporating herbs, meditation and other mind-body practices to address mental health concerns. Herbs like bacopa brahmi) Withania somnifera (Ashwagandha) and Convolvulus pluricaulis (shankhapushpi) are commonly used in Ayurvedic practices to enhance wellness by harmonizing doshas and supporting the nervous system. Additionally, Ayurveda emphasizes the importance of maintaining a lifestyle through nutrition, sufficient sleep, regular exercise and stress relief techniques such as yoga and meditation.

Western Herbalism

In herbalism, the connection between soul, body and mind is recognized. Various factors, like stress, poor diet, sleep deprivation, hormonal issues and environmental toxins, can cause mental disturbances, a concern that herbalists address.

Besides easing stress and anxiety while promoting balance, herbal remedies target the causes of mental imbalances to support mental well-being.

HERBS FOR MENTAL AND EMOTIONAL SUPPORT

St. John's Wort (H. perforatum, Hypericum spp.)

Throughout history, individuals have relied on St. John wort, a plant known for supporting emotional well-being by reducing anxiety and boosting mood. Studies indicate that St. John's wort can be beneficial in easing levels of depression. The neurotransmitters serotonin, dopamine and norepinephrine play roles in regulating mood stability. Here's how they interact with this herb. Thanks to its calming properties, St. John wort may help alleviate anxiety symptoms. Additionally, it has the potential to improve sleep quality, making falling asleep easier and enhancing comfort during rest.

Withania somnifera (Ashwagandha)

Ashwagandha, known for its properties, can help the body cope with stress and anxiety effectively. Its primary functions involve reducing stress levels and enhancing the body's resilience. Being an adaptogen, ashwagandha contributes to well-being by maintaining a balance in systems.

One key benefit is its ability to decrease cortisol levels, a hormone released during situations. Elevated cortisol levels are associated with anxiety and stress. Studies suggest that ashwagandha can lower cortisol levels, thereby reducing anxiety and promoting a sense of calmness.

Moreover, research indicates that ashwagandha can improve mood by alleviating feelings of sadness and anxiety. By regulating mood and enhancing neurotransmitter levels like dopamine and serotonin in the brain, it enhances well-being.

The adaptogenic nature of ashwagandha enables the body to better handle stressors and build resistance against them. This quality can be particularly helpful for individuals experiencing worry and stress.

Additionally, promising results have been observed regarding ashwagandhas impact on sleep quality for those facing sleep disturbances due to stress and anxiety.

Passiflora incarnata (Passionflower)

For ages, traditional healers have acknowledged the healing properties of passionflower, scientifically termed Passiflora incarnata. It's a suggestion for those feeling anxious and seeking improved sleep quality.

Addressing anxiety: Studies suggest that passionflower could potentially ease anxiety and promote a sense of tranquillity through its calming effects. One way in which this natural remedy aids in managing anxiety is by enhancing the levels of the neurotransmitter GABA.

Due to its attributes, passionflower serves as a solution for achieving a peaceful night's sleep. Individuals struggling with falling asleep or staying asleep may find it particularly beneficial, especially if they experience "monkey mind", a condition characterized by racing thoughts. Passionflowers' sedative properties can aid in relaxation. Promoting sleep.

Matricaria recutita (Chamomile)

If you're feeling anxious about something, having a cup of chamomile tea can help you unwind. Chamomile acts as an agent that soothes and stabilizes the system during times of worry or restlessness. The natural compound apigenin present in chamomile interacts with receptors to those targeted by anti-anxiety medications. Some studies suggest that chamomile could potentially uplift mood by boosting dopamine and noradrenaline levels;

this is in addition to the plant's ability to modulate signals in the brain for relaxation purposes. Moreover, the bitter flavor of chamomile aids in digestion, leading to an effect on the system by triggering the parasympathetic nervous system's "rest and digest" response, promoting a sense of relaxation.

Piper methysticum (Kava)

Herbalists have a deal of respect for kava, also known scientifically as Piper methysticum, due to its soothing properties. This plant's ability to interact with the brain's GABA receptors is responsible for its effects. Moreover, kava has been historically used to alleviate pain, promote sleep and enhance emotional well-being.

Kava may offer benefits in managing panic attacks by leveraging its anxiety-reducing qualities. Theoretically, it aids in anxiety control by increasing GABA levels in the brain.

In terms of depression, kava shows promise in alleviating symptoms like mood, fatigue and hopelessness. One way it could be beneficial is by reducing anxiety levels that are often associated with depression. Another possible mechanism is promoting relaxation.

Lavandula angustifolia (Lavender)

Lavender serves purposes that promote emotional wellness, whether enjoyed as a fragrant tea, a refreshing essential oil or a soothing addition to a bath. Its calming effects help combat feelings of anxiety and promote relaxation. Research suggests that inhaling lavender oil can reduce anxiety levels and enhance mood. For those seeking sleep, lavender's tranquil and soothing qualities make it a popular choice for addressing sleep troubles. Consider incorporating oil, tea or bath salts into your routine to improve your sleep quality.

Leonurus cardiaca (Motherwort)

"No plant can ease feelings of sadness like this one. It can lift your mood, strengthen your heart and bring a smile to your face.". Nicholas Culpeper, an astrologer, physician, herbalist and botanist from England.

Improving well being and reducing stress and anxiety are benefits of motherworts calming effects on the nervous system.

By reducing stress levels and promoting relaxation, motherwort might help alleviate symptoms of depression.

Motherwort could improve sleep quality, which could positively impact health. Its soothing properties make it a useful aid for achieving sleep.

Enhancing memory and focus are functions that motherwort shows promise in boosting.

Tilia spp. (Linden)

Feeling anxious, stressed or just not at ease? Linden, a remedy, could help by regulating the release of those feel neurotransmitters in your brain.

A study back in 2015 looked into how linden flower extract can ease symptoms of depression and anxiety during menopause. The research showed that menopausal women who took linden flower extract had milder feelings of anxiety and hopelessness compared to those who took a placebo. These findings suggest that linden flower juice might offer a solution for women dealing with feelings of sadness and anxiety during menopause.

Albizia julibrissin (Albizia)

The mimosa tree, also known as Albizzia julibrissin, is renowned in Chinese Traditional Medicine (TCM) for its ability to soothe the spirit and promote well-being. Throughout history, individuals have sought solace in its bark and flowers to address feelings of unease, sorrow, tension and agitation.

Components such as saponins, flavonoids and alkaloids are present in mimosa trees, with studies indicating their potential to mitigate feelings of anxiety and depression. These substances may impact the levels of mood-regulating neurotransmitters like dopamine, serotonin and gamma-aminobutyric acid (GABA).

OTHER SUPPLEMENTS

Omega 3's

Numerous research studies have explored the impact of omega-3 acids on conditions like depression and various mental health concerns. Omega 3s influence neurotransmitters, which are crucial brain molecules regulating emotions and behavior. These fatty acids play a role in managing the activity of neurotransmitters such as serotonin and dopamine, which are associated with moods and could potentially elevate their levels. The anti-inflammatory properties of omega-3 fatty acids have prompted researchers to consider the role of inflammation in symptoms. By reducing brain inflammation omega 3 fatty acids might be beneficial in alleviating depression symptoms. The incorporation of omega-3 acids into brain cell membranes shows promise in improving transmission and overall brain functionality.

Magnesium

The nervous system, along with bodily processes, depends on magnesium. Like omega-3 fatty acids, magnesium plays a role in balancing neurotransmitters in the brain. It's been noted that serotonin levels could increase as a result. Research has indicated that inflammation might play a part in health problems such as anxiety and depression; magnesium possesses inflammatory properties. Due to its soothing impact on the system, magnesium could be beneficial for reducing anxiety and improving sleep quality.

NATURAL ANXIETY AND STRESS MANAGEMENT

Using remedies alongside medical treatments is generally considered safe. Before making any adjustments or trying out natural supplements, it's important to consult with a healthcare provider, as they could potentially impact the effectiveness of anti-anxiety medications. Additionally, your doctor may recommend therapies worth exploring.

1. Exercise

Engaging in activity has been proven by studies to help ease certain anxiety symptoms. Some research indicates that rigorous exercise regimes might yield outcomes compared to less intense ones, as, per a reputable source. If you experience anxiety stemming from circumstances, incorporating exercise into your routine could be beneficial. A 2016 study suggests that exercise may be advantageous for individuals dealing with anxiety related to smoking.

2. Meditation

Managing stress and anxiety could potentially see improvement through practicing meditation as it helps calm down racing thoughts. Different types of meditation, such as insight meditation, yoga-based meditation and mindfulness-based meditation, might offer some benefits.

3. Relaxation exercises

When feeling anxious, certain people unconsciously tense their muscles. Progressive relaxation methods can help alleviate feelings of anxiety and stress.

4. Journaling

When feeling anxious, discussing your feelings with someone could be beneficial. Research suggests that engaging in activities, like journaling, can assist individuals in managing anxiety. For instance, emotion-driven journaling has been shown in a 2018 study to reduce distress and improve one's state of mind.

5. Time management strategies

When juggling responsibilities simultaneously, some people might start feeling overwhelmed. These could include family matters, work-related tasks and health commitments. Knowing your steps can help in handling anxieties

To ease their worries, individuals can employ efficient time management strategies. Moreover, breaking down projects into more achievable tasks can help in completing them with reduced stress levels.

6. Aromatherapy

Breathing in the soothing scent of plant oils could help ease stress and anxiety. Experiment with fragrances to discover which ones suit you best; different people may react differently to scents.

There is some encouraging research on the benefits of lavender in managing anxiety disorders based on several studies.

7. Cannabidiol oil

The oil derived from the cannabis plant, often referred to as cannabidiol or CBD, does not contain the psychoactive component THC found in cannabis products. Research on the effectiveness of CBD oil for purposes is ongoing, with results in addressing anxiety. Some health stores and online pharmacies offer CBD oil without requiring a doctor's prescription in regions where legal, medical cannabis physicians may also suggest using this oil for conditions.

8. Herbal teas

Many people appreciate the calming effects of teas, which can help reduce anxiety and promote sleep. Some teas are known to have an impact on relaxing the mind, making the experience of brewing and savoring a cup of tea even more soothing. In a study conducted in 2018, it was suggested that chamomile tea might influence cortisol levels, a stress hormone related to anxiety.

9. Herbal supplements

Many herbal remedies, like teas, claim to alleviate anxiety. However, these claims lack evidence to support them. It is essential to consult with a physician about herbal supplements and potential interactions with medications.

10. Time with animals

Pets offer more than affection and companionship; they can also provide support. Recent studies from 2018 suggest that individuals dealing with health issues, such as anxiety, could find solace in having a pet. While cats and dogs are choices for animal lovers, those with allergies can take comfort in knowing that a furry companion is not essential for emotional well-being.

Other treatment options

Seeking therapy for anxiety that interferes with life is recommended for individuals assuming there are no underlying medical conditions like thyroid issues. Therapy can provide an understanding of anxiety. Prove benefits in addressing areas such as making healthy lifestyle choices and overcoming trauma.

Studies have demonstrated that therapy (CBT) is an effective treatment for anxiety by helping individuals recognize the impact of negative thinking on their emotions and behaviors. It aims to replace responses with constructive ones.

Whether it's work-related anxieties, traumatic experiences, or generalized anxiety disorder, CBT has been shown to provide relief. Additionally, medication can be used to manage anxiety under the guidance of a doctor.

Prescribed medications may include anxiety drugs like Xanax and Valium, selective serotonin reuptake inhibitors (SSRIs) for depression prevention or sedatives for improved sleep quality. It's essential to follow the dosage due to potential serious side effects associated with these medications. Natural remedies for anxiety could. Even replace therapy.

Book 7

Natural Remedies for Beauty and Skin Care

HERBAL SKIN CARE AND BEAUTY SOLUTIONS

Creating your skincare products at home is not just good for your skin. Also an enjoyable activity. You likely have most of the ingredients you need right in your kitchen, for addressing skin concerns. Integrate these five natural recipes into your skincare routine. They're quick and straightforward to make.

1. A face scrub for dull skin

Your skin will feel incredibly smooth. Appear glowing after using this exfoliating scrub; when the water is warm, mix in two teaspoons of sugar. Depending on your skin type, you might need to incorporate ingredients. A splash of lemon juice can help balance skin, while honey and coconut milk work wonders for nourishing and softening skin; for a boost, consider adding oils like hazelnut or sweet almond oil to the mix. Gently massage your face in motion with this DIY scrub. After rinsing off, gently pat your face dry. This scrub works by sloughing off skin cells, revealing your radiance within.

2. A face rinse for brightening up your face

Mix 250 milliliters of mineral water with the juice from one squeezed lemon. Add a few drops of lemon oil, too. The antibacterial and exfoliating properties of lemon can help smooth out flaws on the skin. It's rich in Vitamin C, an antioxidant that can give your skin a glow.

3. A face mask for sensitive skin

When oatmeal is applied to the skin it helps to soothe irritation. It provides relief for inflamed skin in need of calming. To make a paste, mix 1/3 cup of muesli with water. Add a spoonful of each honey and yogurt. This amazing mask is great for treating eczema. You can use it on your body.

4. A face pack for oxidized skin

When it comes to combating skin oxidation, chocolate can be quite beneficial. You can create a mixture by combining a teaspoon of oil with a tablespoon of cream and melting two or three pieces of dark chocolate. Apply this paste onto your face, let it rest for 20 minutes and then rinse off with water. Not only does this treatment help protect your skin. It also leaves behind a lovely chocolate scent that is simply irresistible!

5. A face mask to get soft skin

A large bowl is a spot to mix an egg white, a spoonful of honey, half a spoon of lemon juice and a dollop of yogurt. Honey helps moisturize the skin, leaving it feeling soft and fresh. It's packed with vitamins, minerals and amino acids. The calcium in milk speeds up cell regeneration, while the protein in egg whites helps tighten your skin. It's like having an all-in-one skincare product that does wonders!

Having fun trying out items from around the house for skincare and beauty can be quite enjoyable. These simple skincare recipes using ingredients are beneficial, for all skin types. Not only are these remedies cost-effective and easy to make at home, but they also deliver amazing results. So go ahead. Raid your kitchen if you want healthy skin!

TIPS FOR NATURAL ANTI-AGING AND SKIN HEALTH

Maintaining skin and enhancing aging efforts are influenced by lifestyle choices, skincare regimens and dietary preferences. To achieve skin and support anti-aging without relying on chemical products, consider incorporating the following tips;

1. Protect Your Skin from Sun Damage

Spending time in the sun is a factor in causing skin damage and speeding up the aging process. To shield your skin from the sun's effects, it's important to use sunscreen with SPF 30 daily, even when it's cloudy. Additionally, wearing a hat and sunglasses and avoiding sunlight between 10 AM and 4 PM can help protect you from the sun's rays.

2. Stay Hydrated

Keeping your skin healthy and supple is closely tied to how well-hydrated you are. Make sure to drink water throughout the day to nourish your skin from within. Apart from consuming eight glasses of water each day, it's important to include hydrating foods, like fruits and vegetables, in your diet.

3. Eat a Balanced Diet

Maintaining skin and vitality is aided from within by eating a diet of nutrients. Skin receives advantages from the vitamins, minerals, antioxidants, plant compounds and lean proteins abundant in a diet consisting of fruits, vegetables, good fats and whole grains. To keep the skin soft and hydrated, incorporating omega-3 acids found in walnuts, fish and flaxseeds into your diet can be beneficial.

4. Load Up on Antioxidants

Damage caused by radicals can contribute to skin aging, and antioxidants play a role in shielding the skin from this harm. Including a variety of berries, citrus fruits, leafy greens, nuts, seeds and green tea in your diet can boost your antioxidant intake. These foods are rich in antioxidants. It may help enhance the tone and texture of your skin by combating radicals and supporting collagen production.

5. Practice Good Skincare Habits

To ensure your skin stays healthy and radiant, incorporate cleansing, exfoliating, moisturizing and protecting into your skincare routine. Opt for skincare items containing harmful ingredients to preserve skin health without causing irritation or harm. For hydrated skin, opt for a cleanser, avoid vigorous scrubbing and remember to moisturize regularly.

6. Get Adequate Sleep

To kickstart your skin's rejuvenation process, prioritize a night's rest. For optimal skin appearance, aim for seven to eight hours of sleep each night. Enhance your skin well well-being by cultivating a calming bedtime, steering clear of screens before bedtime and setting up a sleep space.

7. Manage Stress

Chronic stress can speed up the aging process. Damage your skin due, to increased inflammation and oxidative stress. To unwind and reduce stress, consider engaging in activities such as yoga, deep breathing exercises, meditation, or simply immersing yourself in nature. Incorporating stress management practices into your routine can benefit both your skin health and overall well-being.

8. Exercise Regularly

Regular physical activity enhances the health of your skin by boosting blood circulation, oxygen levels and the elimination of toxins. To promote blood flow, collagen production and a radiant complexion, consider engaging in activities like exercises, weightlifting, yoga or any other form of exercise that gets your heart rate up. Aim to incorporate 30 minutes of moderate-intensity exercise into your routine on most days of the week.

9. Limit Alcohol and Tobacco

Using tobacco and alcohol can accelerate skin aging, leading to the development of wrinkles and other visible signs of harm. To safeguard your skin from pollutants and oxidative stress, consider reducing your alcohol intake and quitting smoking. If you find it challenging to quit smoking, explore alternatives such as nicotine replacement therapy or opt for choices like herbal teas or non-alcoholic mocktails.

10. Use Natural Remedies

For keeping your skin hydrated, nourished and shielded, incorporate remedies into your skincare routine. Essential oils, aloe vera, rosehip, coconut, jojoba and shea butter are among the ingredients that can moisturize & soothe irritation and promote skin renewal. To steer clear of aging effects from substances, consider crafting skincare solutions or opting for products with pure botanical elements.

11. Practice Facial Massage

Achieving youthful-looking skin could be the result of incorporating facial massage into your skincare routine. By enhancing drainage, promoting circulation and improving muscle tone, you can reduce puffiness, boost blood flow and achieve a radiant complexion. Whether using your fingertips or a facial roller, gentle massage techniques can work wonders for your skin.

Embracing these recommendations as part of your skincare regimen can lead to anti-aging effects and a luminous complexion at any age. Consistency is key to maintaining these skincare benefits and keeping your skin looking youthful in the run. Commit to an approach that includes lifestyle habits for lasting results.

BOOK 8

Recipes For Health and Wellness

INTRODUCTION

For a variety of health concerns and overall wellness, consider experimenting with tincture, infusion or remedy recipes. Feel free to tweak the amounts of herbs and other components to match your preferences and dietary needs. It's advisable to consult with a herbalist or healthcare before incorporating herbal remedies into your health routine and ensure that you opt for organic top-notch herbs. This is especially crucial if you are expecting a baby or nursing or if you have any existing health issues.

DETAILED HERBAL REMEDY, TINCTURE, AND INFUSION RECIPES

Here are ten detailed and thorough recipes for creating infusions, tinctures and herbal remedies.

1. Lavender Relaxation Tea Infusion

INGREDIENTS

- 1 tablespoon dried lavender flowers
- 1 cup water

INSTRUCTIONS

1. Boil some water in a pot.
2. Arrange the dried lavender blossoms in a teapot or another container that can handle the heat.
3. Drop the flowers into the boiling water, making sure they are fully submerged.
4. Let it sit for 5 to 10 minutes with the lid on to let the lavender steep.
5. Using a fine mesh strainer or tea infuser, pour the infused liquid into a cup.
6. If you prefer, you can add a teaspoon of honey.
7. Enjoy a cup of lavender tea before bedtime when you need to relax.

2. Echinacea Immune-Boosting Tincture

INGREDIENTS

- 1 part dried echinacea root
- 2 parts high-proof alcohol (e.g., vodka, brandy)

INSTRUCTIONS

1. Use a coffee grinder or mortar and pestle to grind the dried echinacea root.
2. Place the echinacea root in a clean glass container. Seal it securely.
3. Add the echinacea root to the alcohol, ensuring it is fully submerged.
4. Seal the container. Shake well to mix the herb with the alcohol.
5. Allow the mixture to sit for four to six weeks in a place, shaking it daily to macerate.
6. The tincture may be transferred to a glass jar after maceration by straining it through cheesecloth using a fine mesh strainer.
7. Label the bottle with the plant name, alcohol ratio and preparation date.
8. To boost your system at signs of cold or flu, consider taking a dropperful of echinacea tincture diluted in water or juice.

3. Rosemary Scalp Stimulating Hair Rinse Infusion

INGREDIENTS

- 2 tablespoons dried rosemary leaves
- 2 cups water

INSTRUCTIONS

1. Heat a pot of water until it starts to bubble
2. Right before the water reaches a boil, add in the dried leaves.
3. Let it gently simmer over heat for ten to fifteen minutes.
4. Once you remove the mixture from the heat, allow it to cool down naturally to room temperature.
5. Before transferring the liquid to another container, strain it using a sieve or cheesecloth.
6. Apply the concoction as a rinse after shampooing your hair and scalp.
7. For promoting blood circulation and encouraging hair growth massage the mixture onto your scalp for a few minutes.
8. Finish off by rinsing with water and styling your hair as usual.

4. Lemon Balm Stress-Relief Tincture

INGREDIENTS

- 1 part dried lemon balm leaves
- 2 parts high-proof alcohol (e.g., vodka, brandy)

INSTRUCTIONS

1. Use a coffee grinder or mortar and pestle to grind or chop the dried lemon balm leaves.
2. Place the lemon balm leaves in a clean glass container. Seal it tightly.
3. Ensure that the lemon balm leaves are fully immersed in alcohol before pouring it over them.
4. To blend the herb with alcohol, seal the container. Shake it thoroughly.
5. Allow the mixture to steep for four to six weeks by shaking the jar in a dark place.
6. Once the steeping time is over, transfer the tincture to a glass container by straining it through cheesecloth using a fine mesh strainer.
7. Label the bottle with the plant's name, alcohol ratio and preparation date.
8. For relaxation, during times of anxiety or stress, consider consuming a dropperful of lemon balm tincture diluted in water or tea.

5. Peppermint Digestive Tonic Infusion

INGREDIENTS

- 1 tablespoon dried peppermint leaves
- 1 cup water

INSTRUCTIONS

1. Fill a pot with water. Heat it until it boils.
2. Place the dried peppermint leaves in a teapot or another container that can withstand heat.
3. Immerse the peppermint leaves completely in the boiling water.
4. Let the peppermint steep for 5 to 10 minutes while keeping the container covered.
5. Use a fine mesh strainer or tea infuser to strain the mixture into a cup.
6. Optionally add some lemon juice to taste.
7. For digestion and reduced gas, consider enjoying this peppermint tonic before or after meals.

6. Calendula Healing Salve

INGREDIENTS

- 1/2 cup dried calendula flowers
- 1 cup carrier oil (e.g., olive oil, coconut oil)
- 2 tablespoons grated beeswax beeswax pellets
- 10 to 20 drops of lavender essential oil

INSTRUCTIONS

1. Move the dried calendula flowers into an airtight glass jar.
2. Add the calendula flowers to the carrier oil, ensuring they are fully immersed.
3. Seal the jar tightly. Place it in a lit spot for four to six weeks to infuse.
4. Transfer the oil into a glass jar after straining it through cheesecloth or a fine sieve at the end of the infusion period.
5. Warm the beeswax beads in the infused oil, stirring slowly using a boiler or heatproof dish over simmering water.
6. Remove from heat. Blend in the essential oil if desired.
7. Fill sanitized jars or tins with the liquid balm.
8. Cover the containers once the balm has cooled down and solidified at room temperature.
9. Label each jar with the salve name, ingredients and production date.
10. Store the salve away from sunlight. Heat in a cool, dark place.
11. Use this healing calendula salve to help heal wounds, cuts, burns or dry skin when needed.

7. Chamomile Relaxing Bath Infusion

INGREDIENTS

- 1/2 cup dried chamomile flowers
- 2 cups hot water
- **Optional:** 1/2 cup Epsom salt or sea salt

INSTRUCTIONS

1. Once the chamomile flowers are dried, place them in a muslin bag or another container that can withstand heat.
2. Submerge the chamomile flowers in boiling water until they are fully covered.
3. Let the water soak up the chamomile essence for 10 to 15 minutes.
4. For added relaxation and relief from muscle tension, consider adding Epsom salt or sea salt to your bathwater.
5. Pour the chamomile infusion into a bathtub filled with water.
6. To relax both physically and mentally, enjoy a 20 to 30-minute soak in the chamomile bath.
7. After showering, gently pat your skin dry with a towel. Apply a layer of lotion or oil.

8. Ginger Digestive Tincture

INGREDIENTS

- 1 part dried ginger root
- 2 parts high-proof alcohol (e.g., vodka, brandy)

INSTRUCTIONS

1. Use a coffee grinder or mortar and pestle to chop or grind the dried ginger root.
2. Take a clean glass jar. Securely cover it with the ginger root.
3. Add the ginger root to the alcohol, ensuring it is completely submerged.
4. To blend the herb with alcohol, seal the container. Give it a shake.
5. Allow the mixture to steep for four to six weeks by shaking the jar in a dark place.
6. Before transferring the tincture to a glass container, strain it through cheesecloth once the steeping time is up.
7. Label the bottle with the plant name, alcohol ratio and preparation date.
8. For aiding digestion and easing nausea, dilute a dropperful of ginger tincture in water or tea and consume before or, after meals.

9. Elderberry Syrup Immune-Boosting Infusion

INGREDIENTS

- 1/2 cup dried elderberries
- 2 cups water
- 1 cup honey

INSTRUCTIONS

1. In a saucepan, mix the water with the dried elderberries.
2. Once the ingredients have boiled, reduce the heat and let it simmer for 30 to 40 minutes.
3. Allow the mixture to cool down before removing it from the heat.
4. After steeping the elderberries, strain the infusion into a container using cheesecloth or a fine mesh strainer.
5. Gently mix the honey into the infusion until it dissolves completely.
6. Transfer the syrup to glass containers before storing it.
7. Remember to label the jars with the syrup name, ingredients and production date.
8. You can store the elderberry syrup in your fridge for around two to three months.
9. For boosting your system and protecting against winter colds and flu consider taking one or two tablespoons of elderberry syrup daily.

10. Turmeric Anti-Inflammatory Tincture

INGREDIENTS

- 1 part dried turmeric root or powder
- 2 parts high-proof alcohol (e.g., vodka, brandy)

INSTRUCTIONS

1. Use a coffee grinder or mortar and pestle to chop or grind the dried turmeric root.
2. Take a clean glass jar. Seal it tightly with either the powder or root inside.
3. Add the turmeric to the alcohol ensuring coverage.
4. To blend the herb with alcohol, close the container. Shake it thoroughly.
5. Shake the jar daily in an area for four to six weeks for maceration.
6. After maceration is finished, transfer the tincture to a glass container by straining it through a fine mesh strainer.
7. Label the bottle with the plant name, alcohol ratio and preparation date.
8. For health benefits and inflammation reduction, dilute one drop of turmeric tincture in one tablespoon of water or juice. Consume orally once daily.

How to properly store and administer these remedies

The effectiveness and safety of remedies rely on how they're properly used and stored. Herbal teas, tinctures and ointments should be. Applied in accordance with these guidelines;

1. Storage of Herbal Teas:

To preserve the potency of dried herbs store them in airtight containers in a place shielded from sunlight and moisture. Preparing teas in advance lets them infuse for a maximum of two days in the refrigerator with a lid on. Remember to write down the herb's name, when it was prepared and any additional details on the label of the container.

2. Administration of Herbal Teas:

Make sure to seek advice from a certified herbalist or healthcare professional for dosage suggestions.

For flavor, prepare your teas freshly whenever you want to enjoy them.

For the taste brew your tea with filtered water or water sourced from a spring.

To prevent consuming any particles it's crucial to strain teas properly to remove any plant residue.

3. Storage of Herbal Tinctures:

To keep tinctures for periods, it's best to store them in dark glass bottles with screw caps. To ensure the tincture's quality lasts, store the bottles in a dark and dry place. Remember to label the bottle with the herb name, alcohol percentage, date of preparation and dosage instructions.

4. Administration of Herbal Tinctures:

For the measurement of tinctures, using a dropper or measuring spoon works well.

If you're concerned about the taste of the tincture, consider mixing it with water, juice or tea before consumption.

Adhere to the recommended dosage provided by an herbalist or healthcare professional. Start with a small amount, adjusting as needed.

To ensure the distribution of the extract remember to give the tincture bottles a good shake before every use.

5. Storage of Herbal Salves:

To maintain the quality and texture of salves, it's best to store them in sealed jars or containers. Prevent. Maintain their integrity by keeping the salve containers in a dry place away from direct sunlight and heat sources. Make sure to label the container with the name of the salve, its ingredients, preparation date and instructions for use.

6. Administration of Herbal Salves:

To maintain the quality and texture of ointments, store them in sealed jars or containers. Prevent them from melting or spoiling by keeping the containers in a place away from direct sunlight and heat. Label the container with the ointment name, ingredients, date of preparation and usage instructions.

7. General Guidelines

To prevent children or pets from consuming medications, be sure to store them in a place out of their reach.

If your herbal remedy develops a smell, molds or separates into parts, it's advisable to discard it.

For guidance on storing, using and dosing remedies, it is recommended to consult with an experienced herbalist or healthcare professional.

CASE STUDIES AND SUCCESS STORIES

Here are some individuals who have experienced benefits from embracing a lifestyle focused on remedies. Their stories showcase the effectiveness of remedies, holistic healthcare and the utilization of herbs and plants to combat illnesses and enhance well-being.

Real-life success stories of natural remedy adopters

1. **Jane's Journey to Wellness with Herbal Remedies:** For years, Jane, who is 45 years old, dealt with headaches. The conventional treatments she tried often came with side effects. Only provided temporary relief. Frustrated by the lack of progress, Jane explored therapies. She started incorporating feverfew, butterbur and ginger into her routine after consulting with an herbalist. Over time, Jane noticed that her headaches became less frequent and less intense. Additionally, she experienced improvements in her health, such as reduced stress levels and better sleep quality. By turning to remedies, Jane regained control of her well-being. I was able to enjoy a more fulfilling life.
2. **John's Journey to Recovery with Plant-Based Medicine:** John, a man in his mid-fifties, was diagnosed with arthritis, a condition characterized by inflammation and persistent discomfort. Dissatisfied with the treatments due to their lack of effectiveness and potential side effects, John explored remedies. He embraced an approach to health incorporating inflammatory herbs such as Boswellia, ginger and turmeric into his daily routine. Alongside exercise stress management techniques and dietary changes,

John experienced improvements over time. His pain reduced mobility. The overall quality of life is enhanced. Through a combination of plant-based remedies and lifestyle adjustments, John did not manage his condition. Also regained control over his well-being.

3. **Sarah's Success with Herbal Remedies for Digestive Health:** For years, Sarah, who is 30 years old, struggled with bloating, gas issues and inconsistent bowel movements. Despite trying over-the-counter remedies and adjusting her diet without success, Sarah felt frustrated and decided to explore a more holistic approach. Seeking advice from an herbalist, she incorporated peppermint, ginger and fennel into her routine. Alongside changes involving fiber-rich meals and eliminating foods that exacerbated her symptoms, Sarah noticed significant improvements in her digestive health within a week. Her overall digestion and bowel regularity saw changes as the frequency and intensity of her issues decreased. Thanks to treatments and lifestyle modifications, Sarah experienced a quality of life with relief from her gastrointestinal concerns.

4. **Mark's Journey to Heart Health with Natural Remedies:** A man named Mark, who is 50 years old, faces a risk of issues due to his elevated cholesterol levels and hypertension. Concerned about the side effects of medications, Mark sought out natural remedies to enhance his heart health. He began incorporating heart herbs like garlic and olive leaf extract into his diet. Additionally, Mark made lifestyle changes by eliminating meat and dairy from his meals, engaging in exercise routines and integrating stress-relieving activities such as yoga and meditation into his daily regimen. Over time, Mark witnessed improvements in both his cholesterol levels and blood pressure readings. His overall cardiovascular well-being showed enhancement, accompanied by a boost in energy and vitality. Through the use of remedies and lifestyle adjustments, Mark successfully enhanced his health status. Reduced the likelihood of developing heart disease.

Lessons learned and tips from their experiences

1. Take a Holistic Approach to Health:

In treating the symptoms, it's important to address the root causes of your health issues. To truly achieve health, you need to understand how the mind, body and spirit are interconnected. For wellness support, explore treatments like nutrition, herbal remedies, stress relief techniques and lifestyle adjustments.

2. Empower Yourself with Knowledge:

Discover all you can about the benefits and applications of plants, herbs and natural remedies. When devising personalized health plans, seek advice from professionals such as nutritionists, holistic doctors or herbal experts. Staying informed about the developments in medicine is crucial for making informed decisions about your well-being.

3. Listen to Your Body:

Pay attention to how your body responds to treatments and actions. Maintaining a health journal can assist you in monitoring your symptoms, development and general well-being over time. Trust your instincts. Adjust your approach as needed to fit your needs and life situations.

4. Practice Patience and Persistence:

Remember to stay patient and persistent when it comes to natural healing methods. Even if you don't notice results, staying dedicated to your remedies, making healthy lifestyle changes and prioritizing self-care can make a difference. Have faith that progress will come through dedication and effort, and take time to acknowledge victories and milestones along your journey to recovery.

5. Prioritize Prevention and Self-Care:

Make sure to focus on healthcare and self-care practices to maintain your health and well-being.

To enhance your immunity, digestion, stress management and overall vitality as a measure, incorporate herbs and natural remedies into your routine.

Engage in activities such as exercise, meditation, relaxation techniques and creative pursuits as forms of self-care that can improve your physical, mental and spiritual well-being.

6. Cultivate a Mindful Lifestyle:

Living in the moment and being aware of your emotions, thoughts, and behavior is a way to incorporate mindfulness into your daily life. Taking time to truly appreciate each mouthful of food and relishing its texture can enhance your eating practice. To improve your well-being, reduce stress levels, and promote relaxation, consider incorporating mindfulness practices such as yoga, deep breathing exercises or meditation into your routine.

7. Embrace the Power of Nature:

Connect with the rejuvenating essence of nature by immersing yourself in its beauty, soaking in the sights and sounds, and simply embracing the world.

Utilize the healing properties of plant-based foods, herbs and botanicals by integrating them into your meals and routines. This can boost your energy levels. Contribute to a life.

Engaging in activities like gardening, foraging herbs or participating in nature-oriented pursuits can foster a sense of kinship with the environment.

BOOK 9

Advanced Herbal Medicine

COMPLEX HERBAL FORMULATIONS AND THEIR THERAPEUTIC USES

Creating blends of herbs that work together harmoniously is the objective of herbal combinations. These formulations are designed to enhance well-being and address health concerns. This article delves deeper into the complexities of mixtures and their therapeutic uses.

1. Synergy and Complementarity:

To enhance the healing properties of herbs, intricate herbal blends leverage their combined strengths and supportive qualities. Due to variations in absorption rates availability in the body or specific target areas, certain herbs can enhance the efficacy of others. Herbal practitioners select herbs for their interactions and complementary roles.

2. Targeted Therapeutic Actions:

For instance, a sophisticated blend could target enhancing the system supporting digestion, relieving stress or regulating equilibrium among various specific health concerns or bodily functions. To address a health issue comprehensively, it is typical to combine herbs with benefits.

3. Adaptogenic and Balancing Effects:

Adaptogenic herbs are frequently included in blends as they assist the body in adapting to stressful circumstances by promoting balance and strength. Adaptogens such as basil, ashwagandha and rhodiola can support the body in managing emotional and environmental pressures.

4. Individualized Formulations:

Tailoring blends to cater to individual needs and health goals is made possible by considering factors such as constitution, symptoms, lifestyle and preferences. Healthcare professionals and herbalists can create concoctions to address the needs of patients, crafting custom blends for optimal efficacy.

5. Traditional Wisdom and Modern Science:

Ancient wisdom and expertise are employed in medicine systems, like Ayurveda, TCM and Western herbalism, to develop intricate formulas. Modern scientific research has validated the uses of herbs by exploring their properties, how they work and their safety profiles. This research does not confirm their effectiveness. Also aids in creating more sophisticated formulations.

6. Quality and Standardization:

To ensure that complex formulations are both efficient and safe, it is essential to use notch ingredients. When you source high-quality herbs from vendors, you can have confidence in the effectiveness, purity and reliability of the components. Standardizing extracts not only ensures consistent therapeutic benefits across different batches but also allows for precise dosing.

7. Holistic Approach to Wellness:

A holistic approach to health that takes into account the interconnectedness of the spirit, mind and body is evident in blends. These remedies not only address symptoms but also aim to enhance well-being, energy levels and ability to bounce back by fostering inner equilibrium and stability.

Integration with Conventional Medicine

People dealing with term or health conditions might find relief from advanced herbal remedies alongside standard medical care and therapies. The primary objectives of healthcare approaches are to improve results and support overall well-being by combining the most effective elements of conventional and natural medicine practices.

1. Immune Support Blend:

INGREDIENTS

- Echinacea purpurea (Echinacea)
- Astragalus membranaceus (Astragalus)
- Sambucus nigra (Elderberry)
- Glycyrrhiza glabra (Licorice)

THERAPEUTIC USES

1. Boosts the body's defenses. Enhances immunity.
2. Supports the system in combating ailments such as the cold and influenza.
3. Reduces inflammation and facilitates recovery post-illness.
4. Enhances being and vitality.

2. Stress Relief Formula:

INGREDIENTS

- Withania somnifera (Ashwagandha)
- Ocimum sanctum (Holy Basil)
- Rhodiola rosea (Rhodiola)
- Melissa officinalis (Lemon Balm)

THERAPEUTIC USES

1. Assists the body in adapting to circumstances and encourages resilience.
2. Regulates cortisol levels down. Supports adrenal performance.
3. Diminishes feelings of anxiety and aids in promoting relaxation.
4. Enhances cognitive abilities, focus and mental sharpness.

3. Digestive Harmony Blend:

INGREDIENTS

- Mentha piperita (Peppermint)
- Zingiber officinale (Ginger)
- Foeniculum vulgare (Fennel)
- Matricaria chamomilla (Chamomile)

THERAPEUTIC USES

1. Supports good. Relieves stomach discomfort.

2. Decreases gas, stomach upset and feeling bloated.
3. Soothes inflammation and muscle spasms, in the system.
4. Promotes digestion and regular bowel movements.

4. Hormonal Balance Formula:

INGREDIENTS

- Vitex agnus-castus (Chaste Tree)
- Angelica sinensis (Dong Quai)
- Actaea racemosa (Black Cohosh)
- Rubus idaeus (Red Raspberry Leaf)

THERAPEUTIC USES

1. It plays a role in regulating cycles and maintaining hormone balance.
2. Helps alleviate symptoms like irritability and mood swings during the syndrome.
3. Enhances. Promotes the health of the reproductive system.
4. Alleviates symptoms such as flashes and night sweats.

5. Energy and Vitality Tonic:

INGREDIENTS

- Panax ginseng (Ginseng)
- Lepidium meyenii (Maca)
- Schisandra chinensis (Schisandra)
- Centella asiatica (Gotu Kola)

THERAPEUTIC USES

1. It gives you a boost. Helps you stay active for a time.
2. Boosts mental. Focus on enhancing abilities. Supports health and reduces fatigue.
3. Prevents burnout. Enhances energy levels, stamina and resilience.

6. Sleep Support Blend:

INGREDIENTS

- Valeriana officinalis (Valerian Root)
- Passiflora incarnata (Passionflower)
- Humulus lupulus (Hops)
- Scutellaria lateriflora (Skullcap)

THERAPEUTIC USES

1. Assists in relaxing and achieving a good night's sleep.
2. It Soothes nerves and reduces stress. Eases thoughts.
3. Especially beneficial for individuals struggling with initiating or maintaining sleep.
4. Supports sleep patterns and the bodys innate cycles.

7. Joint and Muscle Comfort Formula:

INGREDIENTS

- Curcuma longa (Turmeric)
- Boswellia serrata (Boswellia)
- Harpagophytum procumbens (Devil's Claw)
- Salix alba (White Willow Bark)

THERAPEUTIC USES

1. Joint pain and stiffness are eased while inflammation is decreased.
2. Enhances flexibility. Supports the well-being of the system.
3. Eases pain from inflammation and osteoarthritis.
4. Assists in the recovery of muscles and sports-related injuries.

8. Cognitive Function Enhancer:

INGREDIENTS

- Ginkgo biloba (Ginkgo)
- Bacopa monnieri (Bacopa)
- Rosmarinus officinalis (Rosemary)
- Centella asiatica (Gotu Kola)

THERAPEUTIC USES

1. Enhancements in concentration, recollection and general mental sharpness.

2. Boosts brain oxygenation through heightened blood circulation.
3. Averts age-related cognitive. Neurodegenerative conditions.
4. Foster's peak brain. Enriches lucidity.

9. Detoxification and Cleansing Blend:

INGREDIENTS

- Taraxacum officinale (Dandelion Root)
- Silybum marianum (Milk Thistle)
- Arctium lappa (Burdock Root)
- Urtica dioica (Nettle Leaf)

THERAPEUTIC USES

1. Helps in detoxifying the body and supports optimal liver function.
2. Aids, in eliminating toxins and waste products from the body.
3. Protects liver cells, from damage caused by stress.
4. Supports digestion and promotes skin. Boosts overall energy levels.

10. Heart Health Support Formula:

INGREDIENTS

- Crataegus spp. (Hawthorn Berry)
- Allium sativum (Garlic)
- Hibiscus sabdariffa (Hibiscus)
- Leonurus cardiaca (Motherwort)

THERAPEUTIC USES

1. Assists in keeping the heart healthy and decreasing the risk of heart disease.
2. Improves blood circulation. Lowers blood pressure.
3. Manages heartbeat regularity. Fortifies the heart muscle.
4. Maintains the health of blood vessels while reducing cholesterol levels.

Combining herbs for enhanced effects

In medicine, a key aspect is the blending of different plants to enhance their healing properties and promote overall well-being. To achieve outcomes, you might want to try combining the herbs listed below;

1. Synergistic Effects:

When you blend herbs with properties they can create effects that enhance the overall medicinal potency of the herbs. Some herbs may exhibit effectiveness when their synergistic effects are activated, surpassing their benefits. To boost the inflammatory and pain-relieving properties of herbs such as ginger and turmeric, consider combining them.

2. Multi-Faceted Support:

You can offer support for health concerns or bodily functions by blending herbs with different activities. Herbal blends offer aid. Promote overall healing by addressing all aspects of a health issue simultaneously. For instance, a blend of herbs, like holy basil, ashwagandha and Rhodiola, could potentially aid in function, mental focus and stress management.

3. Balancing Formulations:

You can create rounded blends with combinations that support internal balance and help prevent any negative impacts. Some herbs might counteract the effects of others, allowing for treatment methods with reactions. For an effect and to promote relaxation, consider combining nervines (herbs that calm the system) with stimulants, like ginseng.

4. Targeted Support:

One can create blends to target particular health concerns or bodily functions by blending different herbs.

Herbal practitioners can delve into a patient's issues. Enhance their healing process by combining herbs with properties and actions.

For instance, to improve digestion, relieve gas and enhance uptake, consider blending peppermint, fennel and ginger.

5. Individualized Approaches:

Crafting blends to suit the needs, preferences and health goals of individuals is entirely feasible.

By considering factors such as body type, symptoms, and daily habits, experts can adjust the quantity and proportion of herbs in a blend.

Tailoring concoctions to align with each patient's needs can lead to superior treatment outcomes and personalized wellness.

6. Traditional Wisdom and Modern Science:

Decisions on blends stem from a blend of wisdom and modern scientific research considering the combination of plants. Research has validated the healing properties and mechanisms of action of herbs, while traditional herbal practices shed light on how plants interact. By merging knowledge with studies, one can create herbal concoctions that are both safe and productive.

CONCLUSION

Together, as a community, you have embarked on a journey of self-discovery and empowerment. Throughout this exploration of medicine and holistic well-being, you have delved into the profound healing properties of natural remedies, the interconnectedness of mind, body and spirit and practical strategies for reclaiming our health and vitality.

The essence of healing lies in attuning ourselves to the rhythms of nature and heeding the wisdom within our bodies, as outlined in the core tenets of this encyclopedia. Dr Barbara's holistic approach underscores the importance of nurturing our mental and spiritual aspects to achieve optimal health and vitality. Rather than addressing symptoms, true wellness involves addressing root causes to facilitate the body's natural healing processes.

I trust that the knowledge gleaned from this book will accompany you on your journey toward well-being and recovery. Remember that the power to heal yourself and positively impact your life resides within you. Take solace in knowing that many others are also traversing the path towards improved health—be it for ailments, preventive care or overall enhancement.

Throughout your journey to recovery, you might find comfort in Dr. Barbaras's Encyclopaedia of Natural Healing as a companion, a source of inspiration and a practical guide.

I hope that you develop a connection with nature, tune into your body's wisdom, and embrace a lifestyle that nurtures your mind, body and spirit as you integrate natural healing practices into your daily routine. Striving for health and well-being, may you experience joy, vitality and fulfillment. May your journey inspire those around you to embark on their paths of self-discovery and personal growth.

I want to express my gratitude to Dr. Barbara for her dedication, expertise and commitment to remedies. I hope her legacy continues to inspire generations. Let us all approach our quest for health and happiness with courage, compassion and determination as we navigate the terrain of healing.

BOOK 10

Plant-Based Nutrition Basics

INTRODUCTION

Are you ready to embark on a unique culinary journey that nourishes your body, mind, and spirit? Are you seeking recipes that align with the renowned Barbara O'Neill's health principles? Do you yearn to explore the benefits of a plant-based diet? You're in for a treat! This cookbook is a treasure trove of plant-based and wholesome recipes meticulously designed to elevate your health and vitality.

Step into a world of health where the richness of nature meets mindful living. This cookbook, influenced by Barbara O'Neill's holistic approach and her passion for well-being, serves as a roadmap to unlocking the healing power of food.

Barbara O'Neill's philosophy revolves around principles that view the body, mind and spirit as interconnected entities. Unlike medicine that often targets symptoms, O'Neill advocates for addressing root causes to support overall well-being.

Central to O'Neill's teachings is a belief in the healing properties of plants. She encourages us to reconnect with nature's bounty, considering unprocessed, whole foods as valuable allies in fostering health and balance. By aligning our eating choices with the rhythms of the world around us, we nurture not only our bodies but also our emotional and spiritual wellness.

Beyond cooking, O'Neill's vision encompasses an approach to leading a healthy life that emphasizes balance in all aspects. Her teachings underscore the connection between our well-being and the world around us, from prioritizing rest to managing stress and finding joy in everyday activities.

This recipe book goes beyond being a collection of dishes; it encourages you to embark on a comprehensive wellness journey. Each meal celebrates the abundance of nature. Offers an opportunity to tap into the healing properties of food while promoting mindfulness and gratitude in the kitchen.

While some of O'Neill's health assertions have sparked discussions, it is important to approach her teachings with an open mind and consult healthcare professionals before making dietary changes or incorporating herbal remedies. However, the core tenets of her philosophy - embracing a lifestyle, harnessing elements, and aligning our routines with nature's wisdom can serve as valuable guiding principles on the path to well-being.

Now, let's dive into the practicality of the recipes within these pages. From invigorating breakfasts to deeply satisfying meals, each recipe embodies the essence of healthy living. Explore the art of crafting delicious and nutritious dishes that align with your wellness goals. Whether it's a refreshing salad, a hearty breakfast, a satisfying snack, or a guilt-free dessert, every recipe in this cookbook showcases the benefits of plant-based cuisine.

Whether you're a newcomer to plant-based cuisine or a seasoned enthusiast, 'The Dr. Barbara Cookbook' offers a wealth of options for all. Let this cookbook be your trusted companion in nurturing your body, enhancing your well-being, and embracing a lifestyle brimming with energy and vitality. It's not just a cookbook; it's your guide to holistic wellness.

UNDERSTANDING PLANT-BASED NUTRITION

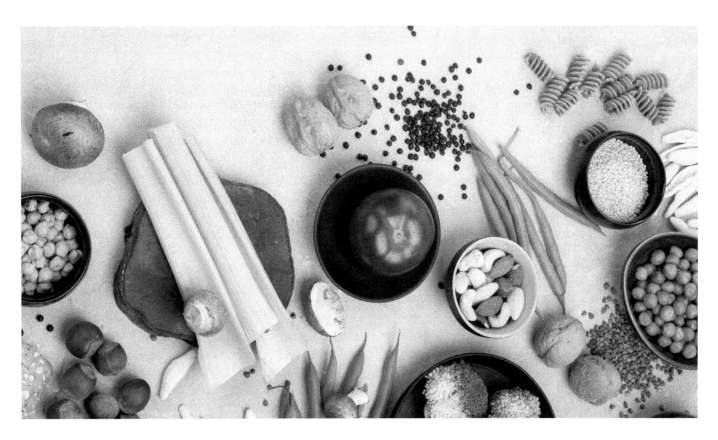

It seems pretty straightforward, or maybe not so much. Switching to a plant-based diet can feel daunting for many people. We are used to our current eating habits and might feel unsure about how to navigate the world of plants. Which ones should we include in our meals, and when? Can we really feel satisfied eating plants? All sorts of questions and worries pop up.

In this chapter, we'll explore together what it's like to follow a plant-based diet. I'll detail what you should and shouldn't eat, and I'll also discuss how adopting this way of eating can positively impact your health and environment. Ultimately, it's all about feeling healthier, looking better, and simply being better, and this dietary choice can help achieve that.

WHAT IS A PLANT-BASED DIET?

"Plant-based" refers to meals made solely from plants or plant-derived sources. Essentially, a plant-based diet excludes honey, eggs, meat, or milk. The fundamental principle of this diet is to consume meals made from natural ingredients and avoid processed, refined, or packaged foods. This means steering clear of takeout and pre-packaged items, like microwave meals.

Eating patterns that are plant-based or plant-forward emphasize foods derived from plants. This includes not only fruits and vegetables but nuts, seeds, legumes, oils, whole grains, and beans. And it does not necessarily mean being vegetarian or vegan and completely giving up meat or dairy products. Instead, it involves opting for food options sourced from plants in proportion to animal-based products.

Here are the various categories to consider:
- Whole grains
- Legumes (such as lentils and beans)
- Vegetables and fruits
- Nuts and seeds (including nut butter)
- Herbs and spices

All these categories together form a whole-foods plant-based diet. The excitement lies in how you prepare them, season them, cook them, and mix and match them to create flavors and variety in your meals. This book includes chapters with plant-based recipes that can inspire you to whip up meals in your kitchen or prepare dishes for your family. By consuming foods like these, you can focus less on tracking carbs, protein and fats forever.

Some individuals may express preferences like "I can't have soy", or "I dislike tofu", etc. The beauty of a food plant-based diet is that if there is a food you don't enjoy, such as soy, you can simply exclude it from your diet. Soy is not an important element of a whole food plant-based diet. You could opt for brown rice over oats. Try quinoa instead of wheat. I'm sure you understand the gist now. It's not a big deal. Just choose something that works for you.

Is Plant-Based Diet Beneficial for the Body?

Indeed, it is. With a variety of food options in this diet, it ensures a rounded and healthy eating pattern that offers numerous health advantages. Legumes, seeds, nuts, vegetables, fruits, and whole grains provide nutrients that are beneficial for the Body's well-being. These natural foods contain healthy nutrients while excluding refined or processed foods high in cholesterol and refined sugars that can be harmful to various body functions. Additionally, carbohydrates that convert into sugar, commonly found in dairy products and bread, are not part of this plan. Consequently, individuals following a plant-based diet can reduce their risk of heart disease, type 2 diabetes, and high cholesterol levels and even lower the likelihood of heart attacks associated with chronic conditions.

The health benefits of any diet depend on the nutritional value of the foods consumed within that diet. In the case of a plant-based diet, whole grains offer carbohydrates for energy production; seeds and nuts provide fats and proteins, while vegetables and fruits supply vital vitamins, minerals and fiber content.

Why it's Important to Reduce Consumption of Processed and Animal-Based Foods

You've likely been told repeatedly that processed food isn't good for you. "Stay away from preservatives; stay away from processed foods." However, the reasons behind why you should steer clear of them and the risks they pose are rarely explained. Let's delve into this further to help you grasp why avoiding these offenders is crucial.

They Have Highly Addictive Properties

As humans, we often find ourselves drawn to foods with addictive qualities, but it is not entirely our fault. Many of the unhealthy snacks we enjoy trigger the release of dopamine in our brains, giving us a feeling of pleasure for a short period of time. This can lead to addictive tendencies, causing individuals to crave even when they don't truly require it. Eliminating triggers can help avoid falling into this cycle.

They are Full of Sugar and High Fructose Corn Syrup

Processed and animal-derived foods contain high amounts of sugars and high fructose corn syrup, which offer little to no benefits. Recent studies confirm held suspicions that modified foods can lead to gut inflammation, hindering the Body's ability to absorb necessary nutrients. The repercussions of absorption, ranging from muscle loss and cognitive cloudiness to weight gain, are significant and cannot be overlooked.

They are Full of Refined Carbs

Processed foods and animal-based products contain a higher amount of carbohydrates. It is true that the Body requires carbohydrates to fuel its functions. However, when carbs are refined, they lose essential nutrients and refining whole grains removes their nutritious components. The result of this refining process is what we call "empty carbs, which can negatively affect metabolism by causing spikes in blood sugar and insulin levels.

They are Full of Artificial Components

When your body ingests artificial substances, it perceives them as foreign entities—essentially, invaders. Your body is not accustomed to identifying substances such as sucralose or artificial sweeteners. Consequently, your body reacts by initiating a response that decreases your immunity and leaves you susceptible to illnesses. The effort and vitality utilized by your body to safeguard your immune system could be diverted elsewhere.

They are Full of Elements that Create a Hyper-Reward Sense in the Body

These ingredients, like MSG, high fructose corn syrup and certain dyes, have properties that can make you crave more. For example, MSG is found in pre-packaged snacks and tricks your taste buds into enjoying the flavor. It's all about how your brain signals pleasure to your taste buds, creating a connection.

This cycle of reward drives you to consume more calories than needed, putting you at risk of overeating.

When it comes to animal protein sources, plant proteins are sometimes labeled as "low quality" because they may lack some amino acids found in animal proteins. However, having an excess of amino acids can actually be harmful to your health. Let's delve into why that's the case.

Animal Protein is Low in Fiber

People often opt for animal protein, and in doing so, they often replace the plant protein they already have. This can be problematic because animal protein tends to lack fiber, antioxidants, and phytonutrients compared to plant-based sources. Fiber deficiency is an issue with many communities not meeting their recommended daily intake. For example, in the United States, the average adult only consumes around 15 grams of fiber per day, falling short of the recommended 38 grams. Inadequate fiber intake has been linked to an increased risk of health conditions such as colon and breast cancers, as well as Crohn's disease, constipation, and heart disease.

Animal Protein Leads to a Rise in IGF-1

Consuming animal-based protein leads to an increase in IGF-1 levels. IGF 1, known as insulin growth factor 1, promotes cell growth and division. While this may seem beneficial, it also triggers the growth of cancer cells. Elevated IGF 1 levels in the bloodstream are linked to risks of cancer development, malignancy, and cell proliferation.

Animal Protein Causes a Spike in Phosphorus

Animal protein is rich in phosphorus. Our bodies regulate phosphorus levels by releasing a hormone known as fibroblast growth factor 23 (FGF23). A 2013 study, "Circulating Fibroblast Growth Factor 23 Is Related with

Angiographic Severity and Extent of Coronary Artery Disease," revealed that this hormone can be detrimental to our blood vessels. Additionally, FGF23 has been linked to irregular enlargement of heart muscles, which poses a risk for heart failure and, in extreme cases, even death.

Considering all the challenges the label of "high quality", for animal protein could be accurately labeled as "high risk." Unlike caffeine, where you might face withdrawal symptoms when you quit entirely, processed foods can be eliminated instantly. The only thing you might long for is the convenience of not having to cook every meal from scratch.

FOODS TO EAT AND AVOID

A variety of foods forms the foundation of a plant-based eating plan. It's crucial to have a grasp of these foods to establish an understanding that you can expand on over time. There are plenty of food options to discover and sample. For now, I'll introduce you to the essentials and tell you what foods to steer clear of.

Foods to Eat

Here's a brief rundown of the food groups you'll savor while following a plant-based eating plan, accompanied by some examples.

Here are some delicious options to include in your diet;

- **Fruits:** There's a variety to choose from, from apples and bananas to grapes, strawberries and citrus fruits.
- **Vegetables:** Load up on peppers, corn, lettuce, spinach, kale, peas, collards and avocados for a mix.
- **Tubers:** Enjoy starchy root vegetables like potatoes, sweet potatoes, yams, cassava (also known as yuca), parsnips, beets, and carrots.
- **Whole grains:** quinoa, brown rice, whole wheat, millet, oats, barley, popcorn and more for added fiber.
- **Legumes:** Include beans of all kinds, along with lentils and pulses, for a protein boost.

Other things you can enjoy include:

- Plant-based proteins such as tempeh or tofu
- Seeds
- Nuts and seed butters
- Spices and herbs
- Unsweetened drinks like tea, sparkling water, coffee, etc.
- Plant-based oils

You can also diversify your meals with nuts, seeds, tofu, tempeh, whole grain flours, breads, and plant-based milks. Just remember moderation is key as these foods are dense in calories and can contribute to weight gain.

Foods to Avoid

Here are some foods to steer clear of when following a plant-based diet;

- **Fast food:** It's best to avoid all types of fast food as they are generally unhealthy, high in fats, and can contribute to obesity.
- **Sweetened drinks:** Sugars in sweetened beverages contain carbohydrates, which can increase the risk of diseases, including diabetes. It's wise to stay away from products with high sugar content, like cakes, cookies, and pastries.
- **Fried foods:** Deep-fried foods are often cooked in oil that's rich in fats, which may not be beneficial for your health.

- **Refined foods:** Refined foods lack essential nutrients and are heavily processed. Opting for whole grains and unprocessed foods is crucial for a diet.
- **Processed foods:** Avoid including processed foods in your plant-based diet. Prepared meals using natural ingredients are preferred over processed options that may lack freshness and nutritional value.

The ideal plan would be to head to the market, pick up some vegetables and fruits, and then return home to experiment with preparing them yourself.

HEALTH BENEFITS OF FOLLOWING A PLANT-BASED DIET

Eating a plant-based diet is actually considered one of the healthiest choices globally. A nutritious vegan diet consists of a variety of fruits and vegetables, whole grains, legumes, and healthy fats like seeds and nuts. These diets are rich in antioxidants, essential minerals, vitamins, and dietary fiber. Now let's explore some of the advantages of following a Plant-Based eating plan.

Reduces Cholesterol

Making eco-friendly choices can greatly reduce the level of LDL cholesterol in your bloodstream, the type that can lead to heart disease and strokes. Skip the butter, opt for plant-based foods instead of fatty meats, and steer clear of dairy and processed products, as they are high in fat and lack fiber. Plant-based diets are completely free of cholesterol, making vegetarian food a healthier option for your heart and overall well-being.

Reduces Blood Pressure

Consuming fatty meats and dairy products thickens your blood, straining your veins. Opting for a plant-based diet that includes plenty of vegetables and fruits and is high in potassium can help regulate blood thickness. That's why individuals following a plant-based lifestyle tend to have lower rates of blood pressure, often referred to as "the silent killer," as per studies published in the Nutrition Review.

Prevents Likelihood of Developing Cancer

Eating a diet high in fats has been linked to an increased risk of cancer. On the other hand, a plant-based diet emphasizes the importance of fiber in maintaining a healthy digestive system and removing harmful substances that could cause harm. Plant-based diets are known for being high in fiber, and low in saturated and trans fats. Often include plenty of fruits, vegetables and other beneficial phytochemicals that can help prevent cancer.

Prevents Cardiovascular Disease

Studies have found that eating a low-fat, plant-based diet reduces cholesterol, aids in weight loss, and decreases blood pressure, ultimately reducing the risk of heart disease.

Maintain Fitness and Aids in Weight Loss

People who follow a plant-based diet generally consume fewer calories. Maintain lower body weights compared to those who don't. While adopting a plant-based diet doesn't guarantee weight loss, it's important to limit your intake of fatty foods, opt for whole grains, include a variety of fruits and vegetables in your meals and choose low-fat or fat-free dairy products. Additionally, it's worth noting that how you cook your food matters – steaming, boiling, grilling, or roasting are better options than frying.

ENVIRONMENTAL BENEFITS OF PLANT-BASED DIET

A plant-based way of living offers various environmental advantages.

Minimizes Greenhouse Gas Emissions

Around the globe, food production contributes to 30% of human greenhouse gas emissions. Among all food sources, meat stands out as the largest contributor. Research indicates that cutting back on meat consumption could help reduce greenhouse gas emissions, promote health, and reduce chronic diseases.

Moreover, studies also suggest that positive environmental effects can be achieved without eliminating meat and dairy products. Embracing plant-based lifestyles that incorporate meat and dairy in moderation can still play a role in reducing greenhouse gas emissions.

Minimizes Usage of Land

Food production plays a role in deforestation, accounting for 80% of it and being the greatest factor in the loss of biodiversity. The intensive use of agricultural land for meat and dairy production poses a threat to the diversity of species. Biodiversity is crucial for ensuring the resilience of our food systems.

Shifting towards plant-based habits would result in less land being allocated for meat and dairy farming, allowing more land to be used for cultivating crops. Research indicates that adopting a plant-based diet can reduce diet-related land use by 76% and also lead to improved health outcomes.

Minimizes Pollution

According to experts, around 35% of plant-warming pollutants are attributed to food production. Moreover, the meat industry is two times more accountable for pollution than the cultivation of fruits, vegetables, and grains. Studies indicate that switching to a plant-based diet could reduce pollution by 49%.

Making changes to one's diet doesn't have to be drastic to impact the environment. Embracing a diet that prioritizes plant-based foods while occasionally incorporating fish, meat, and dairy can still reduce pollution levels.

Water Savage

Adopting plant-based diets could contribute to saving water. Around 24% of the world's freshwater resources are utilized in livestock farming. Interestingly, it requires 23% less water to make 1 kilogram of grain than it does for 1 kilogram of beef. Research indicates that cutting down on animal consumption could lead to a 14% decrease in global water usage. Moreover, plant-based eating habits have the potential to enhance water quality by reducing eutrophication triggered by runoff from animal feed and manure.

Stops Animal Cruelty

It is widely acknowledged that animals raised for food often face mistreatment and lack of legal protection. Opting for ethically sourced meat, seafood, eggs, and poultry while reducing animal product consumption can help reduce the demand for these mistreated animals.

With a growing focus on animal welfare and the negative environmental impact of meat production, there is a rising interest in cultured meat technology. This method of producing meat in a lab setting is seen as an eco-human alternative to traditional meat sourcing. Moreover, plant-based meat substitutes are gaining acceptance in society.

WHY YOU SHOULD ADOPT PLANT-BASED EATING?

Embracing plant-based lifestyles not only benefits our health but also plays a significant role in improving the environment's health. Plant-based diets provide all the nutrients required for health, reduce the risk of various chronic illnesses and use fewer natural resources during production. The interest in plant-based living is on the rise not only for physical well-being but also for environmental sustainability, especially with the worsening impacts of climate change.

On a global scale, climate change poses a threat to food security by affecting the quality and quantity of food produced and distributed. As food demand continues to increase, there are limitations in terms of land, water, and fisheries to meet these growing needs.

Moreover, higher temperatures lead to heat stress among livestock animals, causing a decline in productivity levels in egg and meat quality. This ultimately translates into higher prices at grocery stores for consumers. Transitioning to a plant-based diet could help alleviate some of the pressures that climate change is exerting on our food systems.

TIPS FOR FOLLOWING A PLANT-BASED DIET

If you are thinking about transitioning to a plant-focused diet, there are some easy ways to start. Keep in mind that going plant-based doesn't have to mean being strictly vegetarian or vegan – you can still enjoy dairy, meat, fish, and eggs.

Switch to it gradually by choosing one plant-based meal per week or per day. Consider incorporating a "Meatless Monday" into your meal plan. If having an animal-food-free meal seems daunting, initially, you can include animal products as side dishes. For instance, pair vegetarian chili with a tiny portion of beef, serve pasta with grilled salmon on the side or make a chicken and tofu stir fry. Explore and turn to a plant-based cookbook for ideas and inspiration.

When following a plant-based diet, there are a few nutritional aspects to keep in mind. Plant-based eating may be lacking in nutrients like vitamin B12, zinc, calcium, vitamin D, iron, and omega-3 fatty acids. It's important to ensure you are getting enough of these nutrients by including some animal products in your diet or considering supplementation. Consult with a registered dietitian for advice on planning a plant-based diet that meets your needs effectively.

Switching to a plant-based diet comes with a lot of advantages for your well-being and the planet. As you begin this transition, it's important to take it step by step, try out new ingredients, and consult with a nutrition expert if necessary. In the next chapter, we'll explore the aspects of whole foods to enhance our knowledge of their nutritional benefits. Let's get started!

BOOK 11

The Science of Whole Foods

INTRODUCTION

Each day, we face a variety of food options, which can sometimes make it challenging to decide what to eat. With the abundance of processed foods, the convenience of meals and our busy schedules, many individuals tend to opt for less nutritious choices. Emphasizing the significance of whole foods in our diet is crucial.

This chapter explores the world of whole foods, underscoring its benefits and offering tips for shifting towards a more wholesome eating habit.

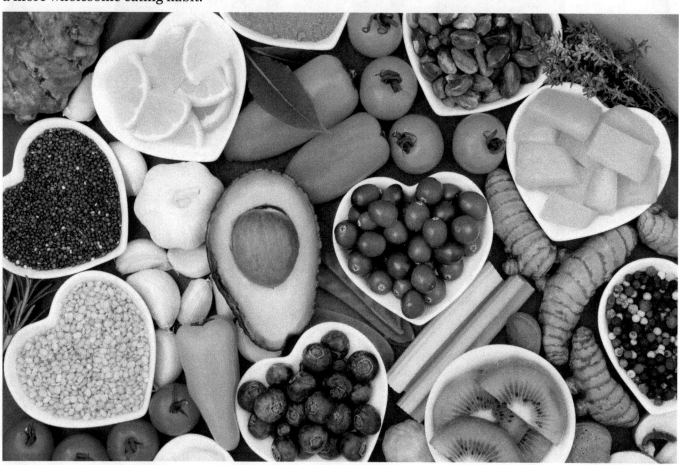

WHAT EXACTLY IS MEANT BY A WHOLE FOODS DIET?

Whole foods refer to those that have been altered or processed little. They remain as close to their natural state as possible. This category includes plant-based foods like fruits and vegetables, legumes, whole grains, nuts and seeds, along with some animal products like lean meats, poultry, fish, and dairy items.

When it comes to nutrition, the choices between processed foods and whole foods can lead to different results. Opting for whole foods over processed ones can significantly affect your health and wellness. Your decisions in the grocery store and kitchen play a role in determining your health. Knowledge about nutrition helps us make informed choices for a longer and healthier life.

EXAMPLE OF WHOLE FOODS

There isn't a proper definition or a set list of whole foods, so opinions may vary on what falls under this category. However, it is generally agreed upon that whole foods include items such as fruits, nuts, vegetables, whole grains, seeds, legumes, unprocessed meats, and fish. On the other hand, processed meals and products with added sugars, fats, salts, or artificial additives are typically not considered whole foods.

A common guideline is that a true whole food will not have an ingredient list. In cases where there is one, like in hummus, whole grain bread, cheese, or natural peanut butter, the list usually consists of minimal additions and primarily other whole food components.

Whole foods can be categorized into food groups:

- Vegetables and fruits of all kinds
- Legumes like chickpeas, lentils, lima beans, split peas, and kidney beans
- Grains such as quinoa, rolled oats, bulgur wheat, wheat, brown rice, barley
- Nuts and seeds like cashews, almonds, peanuts, sunflower seeds, pumpkin seeds
- Animal products, including unprocessed meats, eggs, and some dairy items

WHY SHOULD YOU INCORPORATE WHOLE FOODS INTO YOUR DIET?

Nutritional studies consistently demonstrate that maintaining a rounded diet comprising fruits, grains, vegetables, and legumes yields ample health advantages.

Research conducted at Yale University revealed that the health claims associated with diets like Paleo, low glycemic, and vegan diets were often exaggerated. The one consistent finding was that a diet rich in unprocessed foods mainly sourced from plants is strongly linked to promoting health and preventing diseases.

Numerous research studies have validated that adhering to a whole-food or unprocessed diet can reduce the risks of heart disease, type 2 diabetes, and certain types of cancers. A study from Tufts University in Massachusetts discovered that individuals in their 50s who followed a whole-food diet experienced smaller increases in waist size, blood pressure, and blood sugar levels as they aged.

Another benefit of consuming whole foods is the synergistic effect of the wide range of nutrients present in them.

"Whole foods such as fruits and vegetables are sources of phytochemicals which play a role in reducing the likelihood of diseases and other ailments," explained the researchers.

Fruits and vegetables provide nutrients and fiber in addition to phytochemicals. Consuming these beneficial elements in their natural state ensures their absorption for maximum health benefits.

NUTRITIONAL BENEFITS OF WHOLE FOODS

Whole foods are known for their health advantages. Let's explore the evidence supporting the consumption of whole foods over their processed counterparts.

Nutrient Richness

Whole foods contain nutrients that are crucial for good health. Fruits and vegetables, for instance, are filled with vitamins, fiber, minerals, and antioxidants that help boost the immune system, aid digestion, and lower the likelihood of conditions such as heart disease and cancer. On the other hand, processed foods often lose their nutrients in processing and are full of empty calories, leading to deficiencies in essential nutrients and negative health effects.

Healthy Digestive System

Recent studies indicate that the collection of bacteria in our digestive tract, known as the gut microbiome, impacts our overall well-being. Natural, unprocessed whole foods, those full of fiber, serve as prebiotics that support beneficial gut bacteria and encourage a varied microbiome associated with better digestion, immune system function, and mental health. On the other hand, processed foods containing refined sugars and artificial ingredients disrupt the intricate balance of our gut bacteria, leading to digestive problems, inflammation, and metabolic issues.

Blood Sugar Management

The processed sugars and carbohydrates found in processed foods can disrupt blood sugar levels, causing spikes and subsequent drops that result in feelings of tiredness and irritability. On the other hand, whole foods consist of complex carbs, fiber, and natural sugars that are absorbed gradually, offering lasting energy and averting fluctuations in blood sugar levels. This consistent source of energy contributes to mood balance, cognitive performance, and overall well-being.

Weight Management

Opting for whole foods can significantly impact weight control and body structure. Whole foods are known to be more filling because of their fiber and protein content, keeping you full and hunger-free for long periods and decreasing your overall calorie consumption. Moreover, the nutritional richness of whole foods aids in maintaining metabolic well-being, enhancing energy generation, and fat breakdown. On the other hand, processed foods encourage excessive eating and weight gain as they entice with their addictive flavors, high-calorie content, and lack of satiation.

Disease Prevention and Longevity

Eating whole foods has been shown in studies to help prevent chronic diseases and promote a longer life. These foods are packed with phytonutrients and bioactive compounds that have antioxidants and anti-inflammatory properties, shielding the body from damage caused by stress. On the other hand, consuming many ultra-processed foods has been linked to higher chances of obesity, heart disease, type 2 diabetes, and early death.

HOW WHOLE FOODS CAN HELP NUMBER OF HEALTH ISSUES

Eating a diet rich in whole foods and plant-based ingredients can not only help you maintain a healthy weight but also reduce the chances of developing certain chronic illnesses and alleviate their symptoms, such as:

Heart Disease

An established benefit of Whole-Food, Plant-Based (WFPB) diets is their heart-centered nature, which is influenced by the variety and composition of foods included in the plan.

A detailed study involving over 200,000 individuals found that those who adopted a plant-based diet rich in vegetables, fruits, whole grains, legumes and nuts had a lower chance of developing heart disease compared to those on non-plant-based diets.

On the other hand, plant-based diets, including items like sugary fruit juices, beverages, and refined grains, were associated with a slightly higher risk of heart disease.

Various research studies also suggest that individuals following a plant-based diet may be at a lower risk of getting heart disease when compared to meat eaters.

Making the right food choices is crucial in preventing heart disease, while following a plant-based diet emphasizes the importance of opting for a WFPB diet.

Cancer

Studies indicate that adopting a diet centered around plants could potentially decrease the likelihood of developing specific types of cancer.

Research involving more than 76,000 individuals revealed that adhering to a plant-based diet might be connected to a reduced risk of breast cancer.

Likewise, another investigation demonstrated that consuming higher amounts of plant-based foods was associated with a decreased risk of aggressive types of prostate cancer.

Moreover, an analysis conducted in 2022 suggested that diets emphasizing plant-based foods might be linked to a decreased risk of cancers affecting the digestive system, such as rectal, colon, and colorectal cancers.

Cognitive Decline

Some research indicates that including plenty of vegetables and fruits in your diet could potentially help slow down or prevent cognitive decline and Alzheimer's disease in older individuals.

Diets centered around plants contain a variety of plant compounds and antioxidants, which might contribute to delaying the advancement of Alzheimer's disease and improving cognitive abilities as suggested by laboratory and animal studies.

Numerous studies have shown a link between consuming higher amounts of fruits and vegetables and a decrease in cognitive decline.

An analysis of nine studies involving more than 31,000 participants revealed that a higher intake of fruits and vegetables was connected with a 20% drop in the likelihood of experiencing impairment or dementia.

Additional studies conducted on older individuals have indicated that adopting plant-based patterns could be linked to a lower risk of cognitive impairment as well as a decelerated decline in brain function.

Diabetes

Switching to a whole food plant-based diet could help in managing and lowering the chances of getting diabetes.

Research involving over 200,000 individuals revealed that those who adhered to a plant-based diet had a 34% decreased risk of developing diabetes compared to those who consumed diets devoid of plants.

Moreover, evidence suggests that plant-based diets, when rich in foods like fruits, veggies, nuts, whole grains, and legumes, can help prevent type 2 diabetes.

Furthermore, plant-based eating plans have been proven to enhance blood sugar regulation, weight management, and cholesterol levels in individuals with diabetes.

Ultimately, deciding between whole foods and processed foods goes beyond just personal food choices; it's a crucial decision that can significantly impact your overall well-being and quality of life. Opting for rich whole foods while cutting back on heavily processed junk food enables you to enhance your physical, mental, and emotional vitality.

BOOK 12

Building a Plant-Based Pantry

INTRODUCTION

Keeping your pantry well-stocked can make meal planning easier and help you save time, energy, and money in the long run. Once you have a selection of ingredients and know how to use them, it's simple to prepare a variety of quick, affordable, and nutritious meals. When you go grocery shopping each week, focus on getting fresh ingredients to complement your pantry essentials. If you are unsure about setting up your kitchen for healthy eating that's also sustainable, this chapter offers advice to guide you. So let's get started.

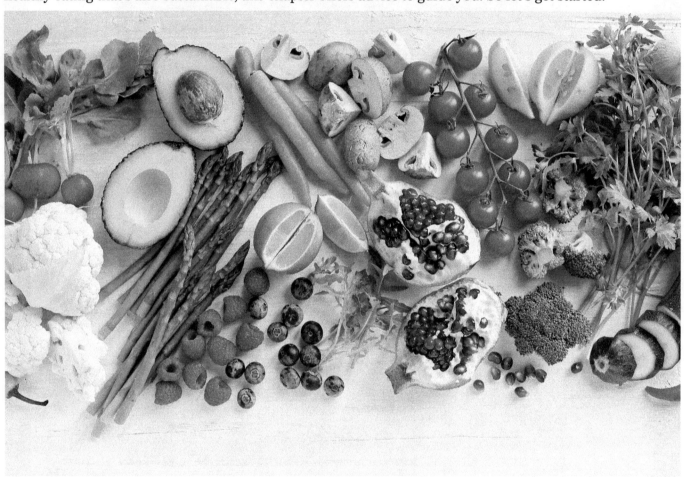

WHY IS IT SO CRUCIAL TO HAVE A WELL-STOCKED PANTRY?

Having a well-stocked supply of plant-based ingredients is crucial for whipping up tasty and nutritious plant-based dishes and snacks. Picture this: you are browsing recipes online or in recipe books, find the one, quickly scan your kitchen for ingredients and feel that rush of excitement when you realize you have got everything you need. A well-stocked kitchen opens up a world of possibilities for cooking.

Here are five solid reasons to keep your pantry well-stocked:

- Lessen the need for frequent grocery store runs, easing the stress of meal prep and saving time.
- Save spending hours in the kitchen.
- **Improve your skills and reduce reliance on takeout, bringing added benefits such as:**
    1. Cost savings (Ever noticed how pricey takeout can be lately?)
    2. Avoidance of earth-crushing plastic containers, and plasticware often found with takeout meals.
    3. Waking up feeling rejuvenated instead of resembling a pufferfish (trust me, restaurant food tends to make my eyes puffy in the morning due to all that salt. And no placing cucumbers on my face doesn't help at all!).
- Cooking plant-based dishes becomes a breeze and more efficient when you always keep essential plant-based ingredients stocked. These versatile ingredients can be used to create a variety of meals.
- It's easier to stick to healthy habits when you have plant-based ingredients on hand. With these ingredients readily available, adopting a plant-based diet becomes nature and can turn into a long-term lifestyle choice.

ESSENTIAL INGREDIENTS TO KEEP IN YOUR PLANT-BASED PANTRY

Whole Grains

Here are some grains that you can enjoy regularly: oats, millet, brown rice, quinoa, and buckwheat. These options are free of gluten and packed with fiber, which can keep you feeling full for a longer period of the day. Don't forget to stock up on whole-wheat pasta or brown rice noodles for quicker meal prep.

Legumes and Beans

Pulses are an important source of protein in a plant-based diet. They are also budget-friendly and versatile. Some of the legumes I enjoy most are red lentils, chickpeas, and mung beans, along with fermented soy options such as tempeh.

Nuts and Seeds

Nuts and seeds are fantastic for adding crunch to meals and as snacks. They can also be used to whip up your nut milks, creamy spreads, and delicious treats. In my pantry, you'll always find a variety of almonds, walnuts, cashews, sunflower seeds, pumpkin seeds, and sesame seeds. They are all best for creating energy balls, too. Additionally, chia seeds and flaxseeds are sources of omega-3 fatty acids that can elevate the nutrition of smoothies and baked goods.

Dried Fruits

Dates and raisins are rich in iron and make great options for snacking, baking, breakfasts or preparing energy balls. Similarly, desiccated or flaked coconut is a wonderful choice for treats or adding to trail mix.

Herbs and Spices

Using a variety of herbs and spices cannot only enhance the flavors of your dishes but also offer potential health benefits. Building a huge herbs and spices collection in your kitchen can help elevate the taste of any meal. While I have my preferences, your choices may vary, such as pepper, cinnamon, cardamom, oregano, cayenne pepper, chili powder or flakes cloves, coriander powder or seeds, cumin powder or seeds, curry powder, fennel seeds, mustard seeds, ginger, smoked paprika, nutmeg, Himalayan salt or sea salt, sweet paprika, thyme, and turmeric. Don't forget to incorporate herbs, like parsley, coriander, or basil whenever you can.

Oils and Vinegars

Use oils in moderation without overheating them where possible. Opt for cold-pressed organic oils when you can. I typically choose coconut oil for cooking because it is more stable and safer when heated. Extra virgin olive oil works well for dressings and recipes that don't involve heat. Toasted sesame oil is perfect for Asian-inspired dishes. Vinegar is also excellent for dressings and giving dishes a flavor. The healthiest option is raw apple cider vinegar (with the mother) since it provides plenty of gut-friendly bacteria.

Baking

Flour plays a main role in baking and whipping up some pancakes. I suggest opting for chickpea flour and buckwheat flour as they are both rich in protein and free from gluten. You can also create oat flour by grinding oats at home. It's always handy to have baking powder, baking soda, and vanilla extract ready for your recipes. Don't forget cacao powder is a must-have ingredient for any chocolate delights!

Sweeteners

I really enjoy using maple syrup as a sweetener. It can be pricey, but I appreciate that a small amount goes a long way. The cost actually makes me savor it mindfully. Brown rice syrup and agave nectar are budget options to consider. Also, blackstrap molasses is rich in iron and gives dishes a treacle taste.

Condiments

In the pantry, it is essential to have items like nut butter, tomato puree, tahini, miso paste, tamari, and harissa. These ingredients really amp up the nutrition and taste of your dressings, dips and sauces. Don't forget to keep some nutritional yeast for that cheesy flavor. When it comes to making soups, stews, or curries, having full-fat coconut milk, chopped tomatoes, and vegetable stock powder on hand is a must.

ADDING FINAL ITEMS TO YOUR GROCERY LIST

There are a couple of things you might need for your kitchen, like plant-based milk and vegetable broth, either homemade or brought from the store. If you feel like trying your hand at making your plant milk with nuts, oats, or seeds, go ahead! If you enjoy making veggie broth from scraps, that's awesome, too! Hey, no pressure if you prefer store-bought options. Just stocking up on plant-based items is already a win.

Whether you decide to make them yourself or buy them from the store, having plenty of broth and plant milk on hand is always handy. Opt for unflavored and unsweetened plant milk, which can be used in all kinds of dishes, savory or sweet.

Let's not forget some soy products that every plant-based kitchen needs, like organic tofu, miso, and tempeh. Remember to refrigerate these items rather than keep them in the pantry. Tofu and tempeh can work wonders as meat substitutes in recipes! Miso, a soy paste, is commonly utilized in creating dressings, sauces and soups, imparting a delightful umami taste. Additionally, there exists a soy alternative crafted from chickpeas for those seeking a soy-free option.

ORGANIZING YOUR PANTRY

Believe me, once you bring those items home from the store, the numbers on the bins won't matter much. You might think you'll remember what's in each one. It is easy to get mixed up. Sure, distinguishing between almonds and cashews is simple. However, when it comes to telling apart wheat berries, einkorn, farro, and kamut, things can get confusing. Why does this all matter? Well, each type of grain has its soaking and cooking requirements along with liquid ratios. When it comes to flours without labels, identifying oats from chickpea or buckwheat flour can be a challenge. Unless you are up for a mystery tour, labeling your grains, flours and legumes is important. Remember to note down when you bought them since they do have expiration dates.

Arrange your ingredients based on an in/ out system so that you use up the older ones first to prevent waste – which isn't good for either the planet or your wallet.

To stay organized, it helps to group ingredients by category. For instance, keep all grains in one place: beans, peas and lentils together, and nuts and seeds in the fridge. Have spices grouped with the most used ones at the front for easy access.

TIPS FOR SOURCING SUSTAINABLE AND ORGANIC PRODUCTS

Here are a few suggestions to assist you in selecting sustainable food options (and boost your mood as well)!

Organic Produce

Organic fruits and vegetables are cultivated without fertilizers, chemicals, food irradiation, or modified ingredients. Choosing organic produce can contribute to minimizing soil erosion and degradation. To ensure that a product is truly organic, check for the "certified organic" symbol, which indicates that it has met the required standards over three years.

Produce in Season

Purchasing fruits and vegetables that are currently in season not only ensures you enjoy the tastiest and freshest produce but also helps you save money. Opting for in-season produce adds diversity to your meals, offering your body an array of essential nutrients that promote good health. Moreover, choosing in-season items contributes to conservation by cutting down on energy usage for storage and transportation.

Locally Grown Food

Consider purchasing your fruits and vegetables from local vendors. Have you thought about visiting the Farmers Market in your area? You can connect with the farmer who is working day and night to grow tasty produce.

By doing you can reduce the travel distance food takes to reach your plate. Less transportation equals fewer harmful pollutants being emitted into the environment.

Animals vs. Plants

Producing animal-based foods consumes more resources than producing plant-based foods. An animal's environmental footprint increases with its size. Larger animals like cattle and sheep are less efficient in converting feed into food, leading to waste and greenhouse gas emissions. Opting for protein sources from smaller animals like poultry and kangaroo is a sustainable choice. On the other hand, grains, fresh vegetables, and legumes have the lowest impact on the environment.

Dietary Variety to Support Biodiversity

Eating different types of food is beneficial not only for getting a range of nutrients but also for promoting crop diversity. This helps protect against harm from pests and weather conditions that might impact crops. For instance, relying heavily on corn cultivation could pose challenges if pests target corn crops exclusively.

Are you all set to stock up your kitchen cabinets?

Get your notepad ready, or just whip out your phone to begin jotting down your list of plant-based groceries. It's important to kick off with the ingredients you are already familiar with and enjoy. As you become at ease with plant-based foods and cooking, think about experimenting with a new ingredient each time you go shopping.

BOOK 13

Dr. Barbara Cookbook

INTRODUCTION

In this chapter, we will explore different plant-based cooking methods that will give you the ability to prepare healthy plant-based dishes with assurance. Whether you are a beginner in plant-based cuisine or aiming to enhance your cooking abilities, learning these basics will guide you towards innovation and mastery. Let's jump in and uncover the wonders of plant-based cooking!

ESSENTIAL COOKING TECHNIQUES EVERY PLANT-BASED CHEF SHOULD MASTER

Enhance your kitchen abilities and self-assurance with these tips for preparing healthy meals as a plant-based home chef.

Steaming

It is known for preserving the most nutrients compared to other cooking methods. To steam your food, simply place it in a steamer basket along with some seasonings over a pot of boiling water. Cover the pot and cook until the veggies are tender. This method is quick, making it ideal for retaining nutrients as the food doesn't lose them to the water and isn't exposed to heat for long. Remember, steamed veggies don't have to be boring! Once they are done steaming, you can add seasonings, sauces, or dressings to enhance their flavor.

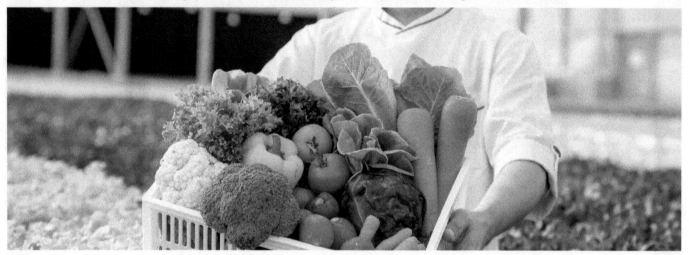

Top picks to experiment with include asparagus, broccoli, green beans, artichokes, sweet potatoes (especially when used in desserts for sweetness or as a binder) and tempeh before incorporating them into any other dishes.

Boiling

Cooking firmer vegetables such as potatoes and dishes like pasta and noodles involves a method where you place the food in boiling water with salt and cook it until it becomes soft. This approach is not commonly utilized in plant-based cuisine, but it is highly effective for softening specific vegetables.

Recommended options to experiment with include potatoes (for mashing on), artichokes, as well as dishes like pasta and noodles.

Simmering

Cooking food in broth, water, or sauce at a lower temperature than boiling is a common method used in vegan cuisine. This technique involves bringing the liquid to a boil and then reducing the heat to maintain a simmer, characterized by slight movement and fewer bubbles compared to boiling. It's particularly popular for creating bean stews and curries, as the cooking process allows the spices, ingredients, and flavors to meld together beautifully.

Some recommended dishes to try with this method include grains like pasta, rice, sauces with tomatoes, green beans, peas, vegetable soups, various legumes such as beans and lentils, tempeh, and tofu in curries, as well as seitan.

Sautéing

When cooking, use a pan to fry the food until it turns a golden color on the outside. You can achieve this by using oil, non-dairy butter, or even dry sautéing without any fats. The food cooks fast due to exposure to the heat of the pan, preserving its crispiness and enhancing the veggie's vibrant colors!

Some top picks to experiment with include mushrooms, onions, snow peas, peppers, snap peas, tofu, fresh corn kernels, tempeh (remember to steam tempeh for 10 minutes before cooking in any way), bok choy, asparagus, spinach, kale, zucchini, sliced leeks, water chestnuts, onions, and artichoke hearts (make sure they are well drained and dried if using canned).

Braising

Great for making one-pot meals and infusing your dish with loads of flavor. To get started, sauté your veggies, add in spices and seasonings, then pour in a liquid for everything to simmer in. The first stage gives your food a color, while the second stage makes it tender and bursting with flavor. You can also try this method in the oven by submerging your food halfway in the flavorful liquid (which will turn into a rich sauce as it reduces), allowing the top part to crisp up nicely.

Some top picks for experimentation include seitan, onions, cabbage, sweet potatoes, kale, artichokes, butternut squash, eggplant, pumpkin, carrots, tempeh, and tofu.

Roasting

Vegetables reach heights of flavor through roasting! Roasting involves cooking your veggies in the oven at 400°F to 425°F, a bit higher temperature than what you'd use for baking a cake. This cooking method brings out the caramelization in the vegetables, enhancing their flavors. It's definitely one of my go-to techniques for preparing veggies;

Recommended options: Potatoes, pumpkin, tofu, garlic, fennel, sweet potatoes, beets, eggplant, carrots, leeks, daikon radish, parsnips, turnips, peppers, pearl onions, cauliflower brussels sprouts, and spaghetti squash. Basically, in everything!

Grilling

Open Grilling is the best way to achieve that char and smoky flavor whether you're cooking plant-based food or not! You can create dishes using a gas or charcoal grill. If you don't have a grill, an indoor cast iron grill pan can work just as well. Have you ever tried grilling corn on the cob indoors? It's a must-try!

Some top picks for grilling include corn on the cob, tomatoes, mini onions, asparagus, eggplant, peppers, zucchini, tempeh, tofu, or seitan, sausages or veggie burgers, pineapple (yes!), mini potatoes, endive, portobello mushrooms, fennel, and bok choy.

Stir-Frying

When cooking in a wok over very high heat with a touch of oil, it's important to keep the food moving constantly. This method results in vibrant colors, a hint of smokiness, and tender yet crispy vegetables.

Some recommendations include onions, peppers, bean sprouts, cabbage, broccoli, water chestnuts, baby corn, green onions, baby bok choy, garlic, carrots, cauliflower, broccolini, edamame, zucchini, tempeh, tofu, pineapple, asparagus, and daikon.

Sweating

It's like sautéing but you do it over low heat to bring out all the flavors from the ingredients.

Some top picks to test out include chopped onions, carrots, garlic, and celery. Great as a base for a variety of cooking methods.

Baking

Vegan sweets have become incredibly popular worldwide! Nowadays, you can organize any dessert. Be sure to bake plant-based treats without eggs. It's a classic, but still great!

FIVE EASY WAYS TO BEGIN ENHANCING YOUR PLANT-BASED COOKING ABILITIES

Tip #1

Explore a new recipe every week, and immerse yourself in the realm of cooking by dedicating a day each week to preparing a new meal. Whether it comes from a recipe book or an online platform, following a recipe can lead to a delightful journey. It not only exposes you to different tastes and methods but also boosts your cooking skills and confidence in the kitchen.

Tip #2

Approach cookbooks and recipes as you would a captivating novel, immersing yourself in the methods, ingredients and taste pairings when you're not actively preparing them. By doing you can enrich your expertise and spark innovation in your cooking endeavors. Embrace different cuisines and culinary approaches to widen your experiences.

Tip #3

Try using unusual ingredients in your cooking. Each week, add a new vegetable, fruit, spice or other unique ingredient to your meals. This not only adds diversity to your diet but also lets you explore different tastes and textures. Experiment with different cooking techniques and combinations to bring out the best in these ingredients.

Tip #4

Get to know how different foods go together by reading recipe books, trying out world dishes, and checking out what's on restaurant menus. Knowing which flavors work well together will help you make harmonious meals with ease. Once you understand food pairings, you'll be able to take your cooking skills up a notch.

Tip #5

Take advantage of cooking demonstrations to improve your cooking skills and learn different techniques. Observing chefs in action can offer knowledge of cooking techniques, ingredient handling, and plating. Whether you watch tutorials, browse YouTube channels or tune into cooking shows, these videos serve as a resource for enhancing your culinary expertise.

By integrating these suggestions into your culinary exploration, you will boost your self-confidence, unleash creativity, and master the art of plant-based cooking, ensuring that each meal brings joy and satisfaction.

Cooking with plant-based ingredients is about embracing flavors, trying out different cooking methods, and ultimately finding joy in the process. So, why not dive in and start experimenting in your kitchen away? Let's get cooking!

BREAKFAST RECIPES

Simple Avocado Toast

PREPARATION TIME: 5 MINUTES
COOK TIMING: 0 MINUTES
SERVES: 2

INGREDIENTS

- 4 slices of cauliflower bread
- 1 sliced avocado
- 3 tbsps of sunflower oil
- Sea salt

INSTRUCTIONS

1. Preheat the oil in a pan. Cook the bread slices for 2 minutes on each side.
2. Season the avocado, with a pinch of salt and place it on top of the bread slices.
3. Pop it in the microwave for 2 minutes then serve immediately.

Nutritional Information: Calories: 140; Fat: 11g; Carbs: 4.6g; Protein: 10.6g

Raspberry and Chia Smoothie Bowl

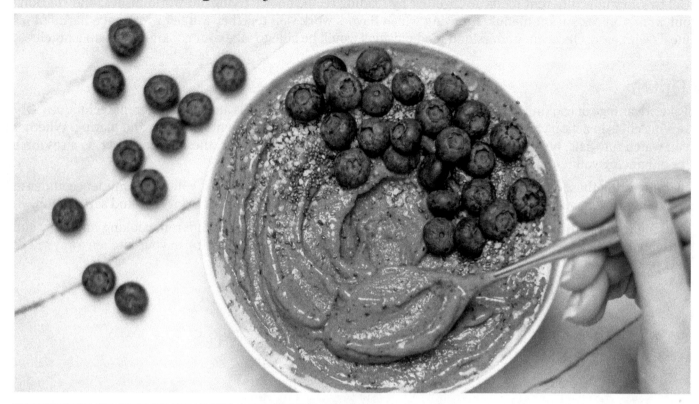

PREPARATION TIME: 5 MINUTES
COOK TIMING: 0 MINUTES
SERVES: 2

INGREDIENTS

- 1 tbsp of pepitas
- 2 small-sized bananas, peeled
- 1 cup of coconut milk
- 2 dates, pitted
- 1 ½ cups of raspberries, fresh or frozen
- 2 tbsps of chia seeds
- 1 tbsp of coconut flakes

INSTRUCTIONS

1. In a blender or food processor, combine the coconut milk with the raspberries, bananas, and dates.
2. Blend until smooth and creamy. Pour the mixture into two bowls.
3. Sprinkle coconut flakes, pepitas, and chia seeds on top of each bowl.
4. Enjoy your meal!

Nutritional Information: Calories: 444; Fat: 11g; Carbs: 41g; Protein: 9.6g

Simple Breakfast Mix

PREPARATION TIME: 5 MINUTES
COOK TIMING: 0 MINUTES
SERVES: 1

INGREDIENTS

- 2 tbsps of unsweetened dark cocoa
- 5 tbsps of flaxseed
- 7 tbsps of hemp seeds
- 2 tbsps of sesame
- 5 tbsps of unsweetened coconut flakes

INSTRUCTIONS

1. Grind the sesame and flaxseed together for 2 minutes then put them in a jar.
2. Mix in the remaining ingredients until they are thoroughly combined.
3. Chill in the refrigerator until it's time to serve.
4. Enjoy your breakfast mix topped with coconut oil.

Nutritional Information: Calories: 150; Fat: 9g; Carbs: 4g; Protein: 8g

Cheeky Cereal

PREPARATION TIME: 5 MINUTES
COOK TIMING: 0 MINUTES
SERVES: 2

INGREDIENTS

- 2 tbsps of flaxseeds
- ¼ cup of slivered almonds
- 1 tbsp of chia seeds
- 10 grams of cocoa nibs
- 1½ cups of unsweetened soymilk

INSTRUCTIONS

1. Place a mixing bowl on a table where you can work comfortably.
2. Combine all the ingredients in the bowl, mix thoroughly and finish by pouring soy milk on top.
3. Serve and enjoy.

Nutritional Information: Calories: 244; Fat: 20g; Carbs: 9.6g; Protein: 6.5g

Oatmeal with Banana and Figs

PREPARATION TIME: 5 MINUTES
COOK TIMING: 15 MINUTES
SERVES: 2

INGREDIENTS

- 1 ½ cups of almond milk
- 1 tbsp of maple syrup
- 1/2 cup of rolled oats
- A pinch of sea salt
- 1/3 teaspoon of cinnamon
- 3 dried figs, chopped
- A pinch of grated nutmeg
- 2 bananas, peeled and sliced

INSTRUCTIONS

1. In a deep pot, heat the milk until it boils quickly.
2. Add the oats, cover the pot, and reduce the heat to medium.
3. Include the nutmeg, salt, and cinnamon. Cook for 12 minutes, stirring occasionally.
4. Transfer the mixture into serving bowls, garnish with figs and bananas, drizzle some maple syrup over each serving, and enjoy while it is warm.
5. Enjoy your meal!

Nutritional Information: Calories: 404; Fat: 5.4g; Carbs: 42g; Protein: 9g

Iced Matcha Latte

PREPARATION TIME: 5 MINUTES
COOK TIMING: 0 MINUTES
SERVES: 2

INGREDIENTS

- 1 tbsp of coconut oil
- 2 ice cubes
- 1 teaspoon of matcha powder
- 1/8 teaspoon of vanilla bean
- 1 cup of unsweetened cashew milk

INSTRUCTIONS

1. Combine all the ingredients in a food processor and blend until you achieve a smooth texture.
2. Pour the mixture into a glass.
3. Serve and enjoy.

Nutritional Information: Calories: 165; Fat: 15g; Carbs: 2.7g; Protein: 2.3g

Oatmeal-Free Breakfast

PREPARATION TIME: 5 MINUTES
COOK TIMING: 15 MINUTES
SERVES: 2

INGREDIENTS

- 3 drops of liquid Stevia
- 1 cup of riced cauliflower
- 3 tbsps of unsweetened shredded coconut
- 1 cup of organic soymilk
- 1/3 cup of fresh organic raspberries

INSTRUCTIONS

1. Combine soy milk and cauliflower rice in a mixing bowl then transfer the blend to a medium pot.
2. Let it cook for 10 minutes before incorporating the raspberries.
3. Crush the raspberries and stir in the liquid stevia and shredded coconut.
4. Cook for another 10 minutes.
5. Serve warm in bowls. Savor your meal.

Nutritional Information: Calories: 325; Fat: 21g; Carbs: 12.8g; Protein: 4.2g

Plant-Powered Pancakes

PREPARATION TIME: 5 MINUTES
COOK TIMING: 15 MINUTES
SERVES: 2 TO 3

INGREDIENTS

- 1 cup of whole-wheat flour
- ½ cup of unsweetened applesauce
- 1 teaspoon of baking powder
- ¼ cup of maple syrup
- 1 teaspoon of vanilla extract
- ½ teaspoon of ground cinnamon
- 1 cup of plant-based milk

INSTRUCTIONS

1. In a mixing bowl, mix together the flour, cinnamon, and baking powder.
2. Add the milk, maple syrup, applesauce, and vanilla and mix until the batter is smooth and no dry lumps of flour are left.
3. Heat a nonstick skillet or griddle on medium heat. Pour ¼ cup of batter for each pancake onto the skillet. Flip the pancake when bubbles form on top and the edges turn brown then cook for another 1 to 2 minutes.
4. Continue this process until you've used up all the batter then serve.

Nutritional Information: Calories: 210; Fat: 2g; Carbs: 34g; Protein: 5g

Banana Nut Smoothie

PREPARATION TIME: 5 MINUTES
COOK TIMING: 0 MINUTES
SERVES: 2 TO 3

INGREDIENTS

- 1 tbsp of almond butter, or sunflower seed butter
- 1 to 2 tbsps of dates, or maple syrup
- 1 banana
- ¼ teaspoon of ground cinnamon
- 1 tbsp of ground flaxseed, or chia, or hemp hearts
- Pinch ground nutmeg
- 1 cup of water
- ½ cup of coconut milk (optional)

INSTRUCTIONS

1. Blend all the ingredients until they form a creamy and smooth mixture, adding water (or non-dairy milk) as required.
2. Serve and enjoy.

Nutritional Information: Calories: 343; Fat: 14g; Carbs: 32g; Protein: 6g

Breakfast Scramble

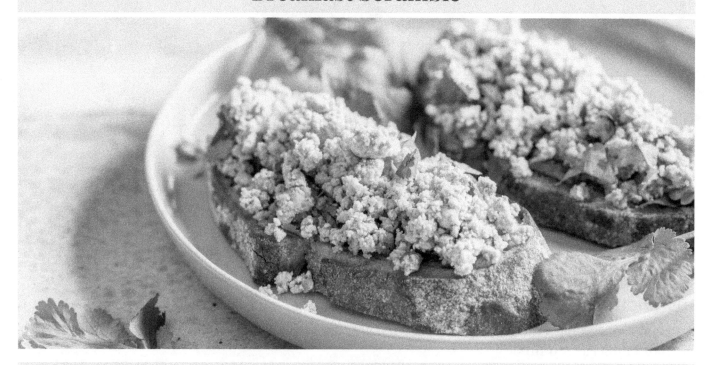

PREPARATION TIME: 5 MINUTES
COOK TIMING: 0 MINUTES
SERVES: 2

INGREDIENTS

- ½ teaspoon of garlic powder
- 1 (14-ounce) package of firm or extra-firm tofu
- ½ bell pepper, diced
- 2 tbsps of nutritional yeast
- ½ teaspoon of onion powder
- 1 cup of fresh spinach
- 4 ounces mushrooms, sliced
- ⅛ teaspoon of freshly ground black pepper
- 1 tbsp of vegetable broth or water

INSTRUCTIONS

1. Start by heating a skillet on low to medium heat.
2. After draining the tofu, put it in the skillet. Use a fork or spoon to mash it. Add in the mushrooms, onion powder, bell pepper, broth, nutritional yeast, garlic powder, and pepper. Let it cook with a lid on for 10 minutes, stirring halfway through.
3. Remove the cover and mix in the spinach. Let it cook for another 5 minutes before serving.

Nutritional Information: Calories: 230; Fat: 10g; Carbs: 12g; Protein: 27g

Cinnamon Apple Toast

PREPARATION TIME: 10 MINUTES
COOK TIMING: 20 MINUTES
SERVES: 1

INGREDIENTS

- 1 tbsp of maple syrup, or coconut sugar
- 1 to 2 teaspoons of coconut oil
- ½ teaspoon of ground cinnamon
- 2 slices of whole-grain bread
- 1 apple, cored and thinly sliced

INSTRUCTIONS

1. In a bowl, combine the cinnamon, coconut oil, and maple syrup. Mix in the apple slices gently with your hands to ensure they are coated.
2. Pan-fry the toast by placing the apple slices in a skillet over medium to high heat and cook for approximately 5 minutes until slightly softened. Then transfer them to a plate.
3. Cook the bread in the skillet for 2 to 3 minutes on each side. Finally, top the toast with the apples. Alternatively, you can opt to bake the toast by rubbing each slice of bread with some of the coconut oil mixture on both sides using your hands.
4. Arrange them on a baking sheet, add the apples on top and place them in an oven or toaster oven preheated to 350°F for 15 to 20 minutes or until the apples have softened.
5. Serve and enjoy.

Nutritional Information: Calories: 187; Fat: 8g; Carbs: 21g; Protein: 4g

Chocolate Chia Pudding

PREPARATION TIME: 5 MINUTES
COOK TIMING: 10 MINUTES
SERVES: 4

INGREDIENTS

- 1 2/3 cups of coconut milk
- 4 tbsps of unsweetened cocoa powder
- A pinch of grated nutmeg
- 1/2 cup of chia seeds
- 4 tbsps of maple syrup
- A pinch of ground cloves
- 1/2 teaspoon of ground cinnamon

INSTRUCTIONS

1. In a bowl, mix together the cocoa powder, milk, maple syrup, and spices until they are thoroughly combined.
2. Next, add the chia seeds and stir well to incorporate. Divide the mixture into four jars, cover them, and refrigerate overnight.
3. When ready to enjoy give it a stir with a spoon before serving. Enjoy your meal!

Nutritional Information: Calories: 346; Fat: 24g; Carbs: 21g; Protein: 6g

Oat and Peanut Butter Breakfast Bar

PREPARATION TIME: 10 MINUTES
COOK TIMING: 0 MINUTES
SERVES: 4

INGREDIENTS

- ½ cup of peanut butter
- 1½ cups date, pit removed
- ½ cup of old-fashioned rolled oats

INSTRUCTIONS

1. Prepare an 8" x 8" baking tin by greasing and lining it with parchment paper then put it aside.
2. Using a food processor, chop the dates until finely chopped.
3. Next, add the peanut butter and oats to the food processor and pulse until well combined.
4. Transfer the mixture to the prepared baking tin and refrigerate or freeze until firm.
5. Once set, serve and enjoy.

Nutritional Information: Calories: 459; Fat: 8.9g; Carbs: 46g; Protein: 7.7g

Berry Blast Smoothie

PREPARATION TIME: 5 MINUTES
COOK TIMING: 0 MINUTES
SERVES: 2

INGREDIENTS

- 1 cup of frozen blackberries
- 1 cup of frozen blueberries
- ¼ cup of Soy Yogurt
- 1 cup of almond milk
- 1 cup of raspberries

INSTRUCTIONS

1. Toss all the ingredients into a blender and blend them together.
2. Then pour the mixture into glasses.
3. Serve and enjoy.

Nutritional Information: Calories: 402; Fat: 27g; Carbs: 31g; Protein: 6.3g

Classic Tofu Scramble

PREPARATION TIME: 5 MINUTES
COOK TIMING: 15 MINUTES
SERVES: 2

INGREDIENTS

- 1 tbsp of olive oil
- 1/2 teaspoon of garlic powder
- 1 cup of baby spinach
- Sea salt and ground black pepper to taste
- 1/2 teaspoon of turmeric powder
- 1 handful of fresh chives, chopped
- 6 ounces of extra-firm tofu, pressed and crumbled
- 1/4 teaspoon of cumin powder

INSTRUCTIONS

1. Start by heating the olive oil in a frying pan on medium heat. Once it is heated, put in the tofu and cook for 8 minutes, stirring occasionally to ensure it cooks evenly.
2. Next, toss in the baby spinach and seasonings. Cook for 1 to 2 minutes.
3. Finish off by topping it with some chives and serve warm.
4. Enjoy your meal!

Nutritional Information: Calories: 202; Fat: 14.3g; Carbs: 7.5g; Protein: 14.6g

Goji Breakfast Bowl

PREPARATION TIME: 10 MINUTES
COOK TIMING: 0 MINUTES
SERVES: 1

INGREDIENTS

- 1 tbsp of chia seeds
- 1 cup of vanilla soy milk
- 1 tbsp of buckwheat
- 2 tbsps of Goji berries
- 1 tbsp of hemp seeds

INSTRUCTIONS

1. Mix buckwheat, chia seeds, hemp seeds, and Goji berries in a bowl.
2. Warm up soy milk in a saucepan until it begins to simmer.
3. Pour the milk over the mixture of seeds and berries.
4. Let it sit for 5 minutes.
5. Serve and enjoy.

Nutritional Information: Calories: 339; Fat: 14.3g; Carbs: 39.8g; Protein: 13.1g

Fig Protein Smoothie

PREPARATION TIME: 5 MINUTES
COOK TIMING: 0 MINUTES
SERVES: 1

INGREDIENTS

- 1 cup of almond milk
- 2 fresh figs
- 1 pitted and dried date
- 2 tbsps of sesame seeds
- ¼ teaspoon of vanilla extract

INSTRUCTIONS

1. Put all the ingredients into the blender.
2. Blend until you get a creamy mixture.

Nutritional Information: Calories: 435; Fat: 18g; Carbs: 46g; Protein: 16.1g

Mixed Berry and Almond Butter Swirl Bowl

PREPARATION TIME: 5 MINUTES
COOK TIMING: 0 MINUTES
SERVES: 2

INGREDIENTS

- 3 scoops of hemp protein powder
- 1 ½ cups of almond milk
- 2 cups of mixed berries, fresh or frozen
- 2 small bananas
- 3 tbsps of smooth almond butter
- 2 tbsps of pepitas
- 3 dates, pitted

INSTRUCTIONS

1. Blend together the almond milk, berries, bananas, and dates in your blender until mixed and smooth. Divide the mixture into three bowls to create servings of the smoothie.
2. Add a dollop of almond butter on top of each bowl. Gently swirl it into the smoothie using a butter knife for a touch.
3. Finish by sprinkling pepitas over each bowl, and chill them before serving.
4. Serve and enjoy.

Nutritional Information: Calories: 397; Fat: 16.3g; Carbs: 42.5g; Protein: 19.6g

Everyday Oats with Coconut and Strawberries

PREPARATION TIME: 5 MINUTES
COOK TIMING: 0 MINUTES
SERVES: 2

INGREDIENTS

- 1 cup of rolled oats
- 1/2 tbsp of coconut oil
- A pinch of flaky sea salt
- 1 cup of water
- 1/4 teaspoon of cardamom
- 1 tbsp of coconut sugar
- 1/8 teaspoon of grated nutmeg
- 2 tbsps of coconut flakes
- 1 cup of coconut milk, sweetened
- 4 tbsps of fresh strawberries

INSTRUCTIONS

1. In a saucepan, heat the coconut oil on medium heat. Next, toast the oats for 3 minutes while stirring constantly.
2. Mix in the salt, nutmeg, cardamom, milk, coconut sugar, and water; cook for 12 minutes or until fully cooked.
3. Serve the mixture in bowls; garnish with coconut flakes and fresh strawberries. Enjoy your meal!

Nutritional Information: Calories: 457; Fat: 14.4g; Carbs: 46.3g; Protein: 17.3g

Peaches and Cream Oats

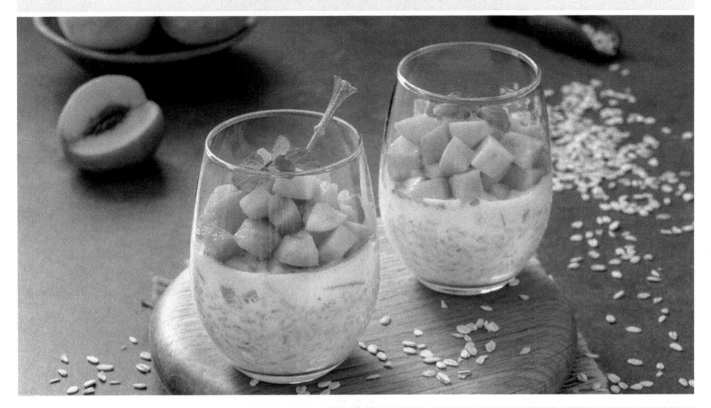

PREPARATION TIME: 5 MINUTES
COOK TIMING: 15 MINUTES
SERVES: 2

INGREDIENTS

- ½ vanilla bean
- 1 cup of coconut milk
- 2 peaches, chopped
- 1 cup of steel-cut oats
- 2 cups of water

INSTRUCTIONS

1. Place the peaches in a saucepan.
2. Combine coconut milk, vanilla bean, oats, and water. Cook for 5 to 10 minutes.
3. Serve and enjoy.

Nutritional Information: Calories: 130; Fat: 2g; Carbs: 5g; Protein: 3g

Frosty Hemp and Blackberry Smoothie Bowl

PREPARATION TIME: 5 MINUTES
COOK TIMING: 0 MINUTES
SERVES: 2

INGREDIENTS

- 2 small-sized bananas, frozen
- 1/2 cup of coconut milk
- 1 cup of coconut yogurt
- 2 tbsps of hemp seeds
- 1 cup of blackberries, frozen
- 4 tbsps of granola

INSTRUCTIONS

1. Blend all the ingredients in your blender making sure to keep the liquids at the bottom to assist in breaking down the fruits.
2. Transfer your smoothie into serving bowls.
3. Top each bowl with granola and extra frozen berries if you'd like.
4. Serve and enjoy.

Nutritional Information: Calories: 362; Fat: 9.1g; Carbs: 44g; Protein: 22.1g

Buckwheat Porridge with Apples and Almonds

PREPARATION TIME: 5 MINUTES
COOK TIMING: 20 MINUTES
SERVES: 3

INGREDIENTS

- 1/4 teaspoon of sea salt
- 1 cup of rice milk
- 3 tbsps of agave syrup
- 1 cup of apples, cored and diced
- 3 tbsps of almonds, slivered
- 1 cup of buckwheat groats, toasted
- 2 tbsps of coconut flakes
- 3/4 cup of water
- 2 tbsps of hemp seeds

INSTRUCTIONS

1. Let's start by heating the buckwheat groats, milk, water, and salt in a saucepan until they boils. Then, reduce the heat to a simmer. Cook for around 13 minutes until they are nice and soft.
2. Next, add in the syrup and portion out the porridge into three bowls.
3. Finally, top each serving with some apples, coconut, almonds, and hemp seeds.
4. Serve and enjoy!

Nutritional Information: Calories: 377; Fat: 8.8g; Carbs: 40g; Protein: 10.1g

Tropical Paradise Smoothie

PREPARATION TIME: 5 MINUTES
COOK TIMING: 0 MINUTES
SERVES: 2

INGREDIENTS

- ½ cup of diced fresh mango
- 1 thinly sliced frozen peeled banana
- 4 to 5 ice cubes
- ¾ cup of pineapple chunks
- 1 tbsp of chia seeds
- 1/8 teaspoon of ground ginger
- 2 tbsps of toasted shredded coconut, for topping
- 1 cup of full-fat coconut milk

INSTRUCTIONS

1. Combine all the listed ingredients in the blender, excluding the toasted coconuts.
2. Blend until smooth.
3. Finish by sprinkling the toasted coconuts on top of the glasses before serving.

Nutritional Information: Calories: 359; Fat: 26g; Carbs: 33.3g; Protein: 8g

Chocolate Oat Smoothie

PREPARATION TIME: 5 MINUTES
COOK TIMING: 0 MINUTES
SERVES: 1

INGREDIENTS

- 1 ½ tbsps of cocoa powder, unsweetened
- 1/8 teaspoon of sea salt
- 1 teaspoon of flax seeds
- ¼ cup of rolled oats
- 1 large frozen banana
- 1/8 teaspoon of cinnamon
- 2 tbsps of almond butter
- ¼ teaspoon of vanilla extract, unsweetened
- 1 cup of coconut milk, unsweetened

INSTRUCTIONS

1. Put all the ingredients into a food processor or blender then blend on high speed for 2 to 3 minutes until you achieve a smooth consistency.
2. Transfer the blended mixture into a glass. Serve it.

Nutritional Information: Calories: 262; Fat: 7.3g; Carbs: 45g; Protein: 8.1g

Raw Morning Pudding

PREPARATION TIME: 5 MINUTES
COOK TIMING: 0 MINUTES
SERVES: 3

INGREDIENTS

- 3 tbsps of agave syrup
- 1/2 cup of instant oats
- A pinch of flaky salt
- 2 ½ cups of almond milk
- 1/4 teaspoon of ground cardamom
- 1/2 teaspoon of vanilla essence
- 1/4 teaspoon of crystalized ginger
- A pinch of grated nutmeg
- 1/2 cup of chia seeds

INSTRUCTIONS

1. Mix the agave syrup, milk, and spices in a bowl until they are thoroughly combined.
2. Gently add the oats and chia seeds, stirring to ensure everything is mixed well. Divide the mixture into three jars, cover them and refrigerate overnight.
3. When ready to enjoy give it a stir with a spoon before serving. Enjoy your meal!

Nutritional Information: Calories: 364; Fat: 10.5g; Carbs: 41g; Protein: 9g

Peach Crumble Shake

PREPARATION TIME: 5 MINUTES
COOK TIMING: 0 MINUTES
SERVES: 1

INGREDIENTS

- ¼ cup of rolled oats
- 1 tbsp of chia seeds
- ½ cup of water
- 2 peaches, pitted, sliced
- 1 Medjool date, pitted
- ½ teaspoon of vanilla extract, unsweetened
- 2 tbsps of lemon juice
- 1 tbsp of coconut butter
- ¾ teaspoon of ground cinnamon
- 1 cup of coconut milk, unsweetened

INSTRUCTIONS

1. Combine all the ingredients in a blender. Blend on for 2 to 3 minutes until you achieve a smooth consistency.
2. Transfer the blended mixture into a glass. Serve.

Nutritional Information: Calories: 270; Fat: 4g; Carbs: 28g; Protein: 25g

Banana Cream Pie Chia Pudding

PREPARATION TIME: 5 MINUTES
COOK TIMING: 0 MINUTES
SERVES: 2

INGREDIENTS

- 1 tbsp of agave or maple syrup
- 1/2 cup of almond milk
- Coconut flakes, for garnishing
- 1 teaspoon of cinnamon
- 1/2 cup of full-fat coconut milk
- 1 banana, mashed
- 1/4 cup of chia seeds
- 1 banana, chopped for garnishing

INSTRUCTIONS

1. Combine the coconut milk, chia seeds, cinnamon, almond milk, agave, and mashed banana in a bowl. Stir until everything is well-combined.
2. Cover the bowl securely. Refrigerate, for 1 hour to set.
3. Divide the chia pudding into two cups and garnish with sliced bananas and coconut flakes.

Nutritional Information: Calories: 321; Fat: 17g; Carbs: 34g; Protein: 5g

Oatmeal-Banana Pancakes

PREPARATION TIME: 5 MINUTES
COOK TIMING: 0 MINUTES
SERVES: 2

INGREDIENTS

- 3/4 cup of almond milk
- 1 banana
- 1/2 cup of almond flour
- 2 tbsps of maple syrup
- 1/2 cup of old-fashioned oatmeal
- 1 teaspoon of vanilla concentrate
- 1/4 teaspoon of salt
- 1/2 teaspoon of ground cinnamon
- Non-stick cooking spray
- 1/2 teaspoon of baking powder

INSTRUCTIONS

1. Start by putting oats in a blender and blending them into a powder. Add almond milk, almond flour, maple syrup, banana, vanilla extract, baking powder, cinnamon, and salt; mix until everything is well combined. Allow the mixture to rest until it thickens which usually takes 10 minutes.
2. Next, heat a skillet over medium to high heat and lightly grease it with cooking spray. Pour 1/4 cup of the mixture onto the skillet. Cook until bubbles form on the surface and the edges become dry typically for about 3 to 4 minutes.
3. Flip the pancake. Continue cooking until it caramelizes on the other side, usually for about 2 to 3 minutes. Repeat this process with the remaining batter.

Nutritional Information: Calories: 340; Fat: 17.9g; Carbs: 25g; Protein: 9.7g

Pumpkin Spice Protein Oatmeal

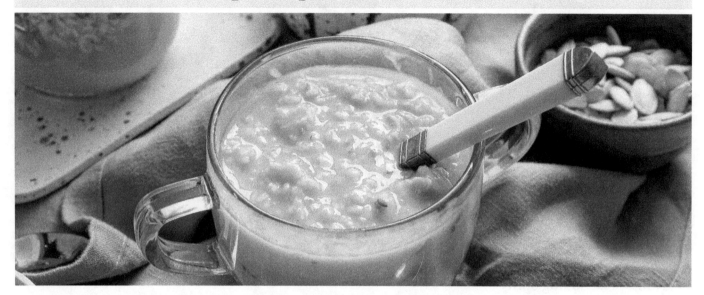

PREPARATION TIME: 5 MINUTES
COOK TIMING: 5 MINUTES
SERVES: 1

INGREDIENTS

- 2 tbsps of steel-cut oats
- ½ tbsp of maple syrup
- 1 scoop of vegan protein
- 3 tbsps of pumpkin puree
- 1 tbsp of chia seeds
- ½ teaspoon of ginger, ground
- 1 cup of water, hot
- ¼ teaspoon of nutmeg, ground
- 1 tbsp of pecans, chopped

INSTRUCTIONS

1. Start by mixing the pumpkin puree, oats, water, nutmeg, chia seeds, ginger, and cinnamon in a mixing bowl until they're well combined.
2. Place the mixture in the microwave. Heat it on high for 2 minutes.
3. After heating, stir in the protein powder into the oatmeal, mix thoroughly.
4. If needed, add more water to achieve your desired consistency.
5. Continue stirring until the protein powder is fully dissolved.
6. Finally, transfer the oatmeal to a serving bowl. Garnish with chopped pecans and a drizzle of maple syrup.

Nutritional Information: Calories: 332; Fat: 13g; Carbs: 32g; Protein: 23g

Chocolate Quinoa Breakfast Bowl

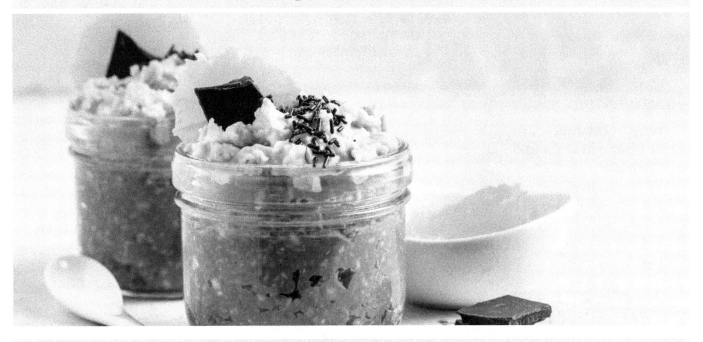

PREPARATION TIME: 5 MINUTES
COOK TIMING: 30 MINUTES
SERVES: 2

INGREDIENTS

- 2 tbsps of walnuts
- 1 teaspoon of ground cinnamon
- ¼ cup of raspberries
- 1 cup of non-dairy milk
- 1 large banana
- 2 to 3 tbsps of unsweetened cocoa powder or carob
- 1 cup of quinoa
- 1 to 2 tbsps of almond butter, or other seed or nut butter
- 1 cup of water
- 1 tbsp of ground flaxseed, or hemp or chia seeds

INSTRUCTIONS

1. Combine the quinoa, cinnamon, milk and water in a large saucepan. Bring to a boil, then reduce the heat and let it simmer covered for about 25 to 30 minutes.
2. While the quinoa is simmering, mash and blend the banana in a bowl. Add cocoa powder, almond butter and flaxseed to the mashed banana.
3. When ready to serve, place 1 cup of quinoa in a bowl. Top it with half of the pudding mixture, along with half of the walnuts and raspberries.

Nutritional Information: Calories: 392; Fat: 19g; Carbs: 49g; Protein: 12g

Baked Banana French Toast with Raspberry Syrup

PREPARATION TIME: 10 MINUTES
COOK TIMING: 30 MINUTES
SERVES: 4

INGREDIENTS

- 1 cup of coconut milk
- ¼ teaspoon of ground nutmeg
- 1 banana
- ½ teaspoon of ground cinnamon
- 1½ teaspoons of arrowroot powder, or flour
- 1 teaspoon of pure vanilla extract
- 8 slices of whole-grain bread
- Pinch sea salt

For the Raspberry Syrup:
- 1 cup of fresh or frozen raspberries, or other berries
- 2 tbsps of water, or pure fruit juice
- 1 to 2 tbsps of maple syrup, or coconut sugar (optional)

INSTRUCTIONS

1. Preheat your oven to 350°F.
2. Take a bowl and thoroughly mash the banana until smooth. Add the coconut milk, arrowroot, vanilla, cinnamon, nutmeg, and salt to make a mixture.
3. Dunk the bread slices in the banana mixture. Arrange them in a 13 by 9-inch baking dish. Ensure they cover the bottom of the dish without stacking on top of each other. Pour any remaining banana mixture over the bread before placing it in the oven.
4. Bake, for 30 minutes until the tops are lightly browned.
5. When ready, serve with raspberry syrup drizzled on top.

Nutritional Information: Calories: 166; Fat: 7g; Carbs: 23g; Protein: 5g

Chocolate Peanut Butter Smoothie

PREPARATION TIME: 5 MINUTES
COOK TIMING: 0 MINUTES
SERVES: 3 TO 4

INGREDIENTS

- ½ cup of non-dairy milk (optional)
- 1 tbsp of maple syrup (optional)
- 1 banana
- 1 tbsp of flaxseed, or chia seeds
- ¼ cup of rolled oats, or 1 scoop of plant protein powder
- 1 tbsp of peanut butter, or almond butter
- 1 cup of alfalfa sprouts, or spinach, chopped (optional)
- 1 tbsp of unsweetened cocoa powder
- 1 cup of water
- Bonus Boosters (Optional)
- 1 teaspoon of cocoa nibs
- 1 teaspoon of maca powder

INSTRUCTIONS

1. Blend all ingredients in a blender until you achieve a smooth consistency. If necessary, you can gradually add water or non-dairy milk to reach the desired texture.
2. Feel free to incorporate any enhancements you prefer. Blend again until everything is well mixed.
3. Serve and enjoy.

Nutritional Information: Calories: 474; Fat: 16g; Carbs: 69g; Protein: 13g

Chickpea Scramble

PREPARATION TIME: 5 MINUTES
COOK TIMING: 15 MINUTES
SERVES: 1

INGREDIENTS

- ½ cup of chopped zucchini
- 1 teaspoon of olive oil, or 1 tbsp of vegetable broth or water
- ½ cup of mushrooms, sliced
- 1 teaspoon of turmeric
- Pinch sea salt
- ½ cup of chickpeas (cooked or canned)
- 1 teaspoon of smoked paprika, or regular paprika
- ½ cup of cherry tomatoes, chopped
- 1 tbsp of nutritional yeast (optional)
- ¼ cup of fresh parsley, chopped
- Freshly ground black pepper

INSTRUCTIONS

1. Begin by heating a skillet over medium to high heat. Once the skillet is hot, pour in the olive oil and add mushrooms along with a pinch of sea salt to assist in softening them. Sauté the mixture, stirring occasionally, for approximately 7 to 8 minutes.
2. Then, introduce the zucchini into the skillet.
3. If you are using canned chickpeas, ensure to rinse and drain them. Proceed to mash the chickpeas using a potato masher, fork, or your hands, and add them to the skillet. Cook until they are heated through.
4. Sprinkle turmeric, paprika, and nutritional yeast over the chickpeas. Thoroughly mix.
5. Lastly, add pepper, cherry tomatoes, and fresh parsley towards the end, just enough to warm through. Remember to reserve some parsley for garnishing purposes.
6. Serve and relish.

Nutritional Information: Calories: 265; Fat: 8g; Carbs: 37g; Protein: 16g

Fruity Granola

PREPARATION TIME: 15 MINUTES
COOK TIMING: 45 MINUTES
SERVES: 2

INGREDIENTS

- ½ cup of goji berries (optional)
- 1¼ cups of pure fruit juice (apple, cranberry, or something similar)
- 2 cups of rolled oats
- ½ cup of almonds, chopped
- 1 tbsp of ground cinnamon
- ½ cup of unsweetened shredded coconut
- 1 teaspoon of ground ginger (optional)
- ¾ cup of whole-grain flour
- ½ cup of pumpkin seeds
- ½ cup of sunflower seeds, or walnuts, chopped
- ½ cup of raisins, or dried cranberries

INSTRUCTIONS

1. Preheat your oven to 350°F.
2. Combine together oats, flour, cinnamon, ginger, almonds, sunflower seeds, pumpkin seeds and coconut in a bowl.
3. Sprinkle the juice over the mixture. Stir until it is just moistened. Adjust the liquid amount based on how the oats and flour soak.
4. Spread the granola evenly on a baking sheet for crunchiness. Bake in the oven for 15 minutes before flipping it with a spatula to ensure drying. Continue baking until it reaches your desired level of crunchiness around 30 minutes more.
5. Remove the granola from the oven. Mix in raisins and goji berries if desired.
6. Store any leftovers in a container for up to two weeks.

Nutritional Information: Calories: 398; Fat: 25g; Carbs: 39g; Protein: 11g

Avocado Walnut Sandwich

PREPARATION TIME: 10 MINUTES
COOK TIMING: 10 MINUTES
SERVES: 4

INGREDIENTS

For the spread:
- 1 garlic clove, minced
- ½ teaspoon of dill, dried
- 2 tbsps of lemon juice, fresh
- ¼ cup of water
- 2 tbsps of carrot, minced
- 1 cup of walnuts
- 2 tbsps of red bell pepper, minced
- ¼ teaspoon of sea salt
- 2 tbsps of nutritional yeast
- 1/8 teaspoon of black pepper
- 2 tbsps of sundried tomatoes, chopped

For the sandwich:
- 8 sprouted grain bread slices
- 1 cup of carrot, shredded
- 1 large tomato, sliced
- 2 cups of mixed greens
- 1 large avocado, sliced

INSTRUCTIONS

1. Start by combining yeast, water, walnuts, salt, lemon juice, and pepper in a food processor until you achieve a smooth consistency.
2. Move the mixture to a bowl. Mix in the remaining ingredients.
3. Mix thoroughly ad hen apply the walnut paste onto the bread slices. Add all sandwich fillings.
4. Finally, assemble the sandwich.
5. Serve and enjoy.

Nutritional Information: Calories: 541; Fat: 29.8g; Carbs: 50g; Protein: 22.6g

Strawberry, Banana, and Coconut Shake

PREPARATION TIME: 5 MINUTES
COOK TIMING: 0 MINUTES
SERVES: 1

INGREDIENTS

- 1/2 cup of coconut milk, unsweetened
- 1 tbsp of coconut flakes
- 1 1/2 cups of frozen banana slices
- 1/4 cup of strawberries for topping
- 8 strawberries, sliced

INSTRUCTIONS

1. Put all the ingredients into a food processor or blender.
2. Blend at high speed for 2 to 3 minutes until smooth.
3. Transfer the blended mixture into a glass. Serve.

Nutritional Information: Calories: 335; Fat: 5g; Carbs: 55g; Protein: 4g

Spiced Orange Breakfast Couscous

PREPARATION TIME: 5 MINUTES
COOK TIMING: 10 MINUTES
SERVES: 4

INGREDIENTS

- 1½ cups of couscous
- ½ cup of chopped almonds or other nuts or seeds
- 1 teaspoon of ground cinnamon
- ¼ teaspoon of ground cloves
- 3 cups of orange juice
- ½ cup of dried fruit, such as raisins or apricots

INSTRUCTIONS

1. In a saucepan, heat the orange juice until it boils. Then mix in the couscous along with some cinnamon and cloves before taking it off the heat. Cover the pan with a lid. Let it sit for 5 minutes until the couscous becomes soft.
2. Use a fork to fluff up the couscous and then add in dried fruit and nuts.
3. Serve and enjoy.

Nutritional Information: Calories: 150; Fat: 2g; Carbs: 6g; Protein: 5g

Banana Bread

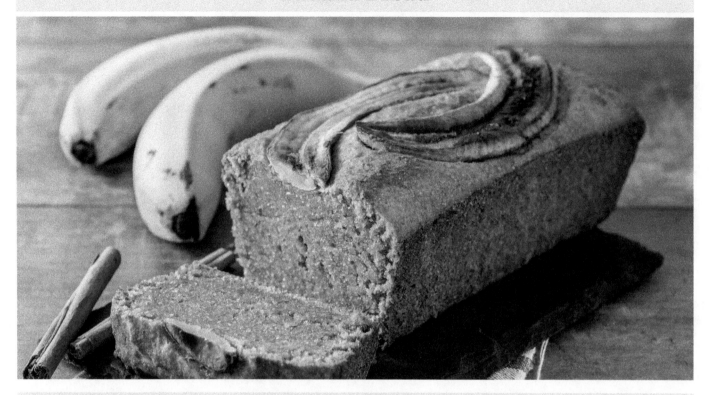

PREPARATION TIME: 15 MINUTES
COOK TIMING: 1 HOUR
SERVES: 6

INGREDIENTS

- ⅓ cup of olive oil
- 4 bananas
- 2 ½ cups of almond flour
- 4 flax eggs
- ½ tbsp of baking soda

INSTRUCTIONS

1. Preheat your oven to 350°F.
2. Lightly grease a loaf pan.
3. Cut the bananas into slices, about a quarter inch thick.
4. Put the sliced bananas in a bowl.
5. Combine almond flour, flax eggs, olive oil and baking soda in the bowl.
6. Stir with a spoon until mixed.
7. Pour the mixture into the loaf pan.
8. Bake for 1 hour.
9. Take it out of the oven. Allow it to cool at room temperature.
10. Serve and enjoy.

Nutritional Information: Calories: 106; Fat: 17.9g; Carbs: 12.1g; Protein: 5.3g

Pumpkin Pie Smoothie

PREPARATION TIME: 5 MINUTES
COOK TIMING: 0 MINUTES
SERVES: 4

INGREDIENTS

- 1 clove
- 175g of raw pumpkin
- 4 dates
- 1/8 teaspoon of nutmeg
- 1 banana
- 1/8 teaspoon of ground ginger
- 500 ml of cashew milk
- 1 teaspoon of ground cinnamon
- Ice, as needed

INSTRUCTIONS

1. Put all the ingredients into the blender.
2. Blend them on high speed until they become smooth.
3. Serve and enjoy.

Nutritional Information: Calories: 148; Fat: 2g; Carbs: 24.9g; Protein: 3.6g

Breakfast Parfaits

PREPARATION TIME: 15 MINUTES
COOK TIMING: 0 MINUTES
SERVES: 2

INGREDIENTS

- 1 cup of sliced strawberries or other seasonal berries
- 1 14-ounce can of coconut milk, refrigerated overnight
- ½ cup of walnuts
- 1 cup of granola

INSTRUCTIONS

1. Pour out the liquid from the canned coconut milk and keep the solid part.
2. In two parfait glasses, alternate layers of coconut cream, granola, walnuts, and strawberries.
3. Serve and enjoy.

Nutritional Information: Calories: 150; Fat: 4g; Carbs: 60g; Protein: 6g

SOUPS AND SALADS

Loaded Kale Salad

PREPARATION TIME: 10 MINUTES
COOK TIMING: 0 MINUTES
SERVES: 4

INGREDIENTS

- **Quinoa:**
- ¾ cups of quinoa, cooked and drained
- **Vegetables:**
- 2 tbsps of water
- 1 whole beet, sliced
- ½ teaspoon of curry powder
- 1 ripe avocado, cubed
- 8 cups of kale, chopped
- ½ cup of cherry tomatoes, chopped
- ¼ cup of hemp seeds
- 4 large carrots, halved and chopped
- ½ cup of sprouts
- 1 pinch of salt
- **Dressing:**
- ⅓ cup of tahini
- 3 tbsps of lemon juice
- 1 pinch of salt
- ¼ cup of water
- 1 to 2 tbsps of maple syrup

INSTRUCTIONS

1. Mix together all the ingredients for the dressing in a bowl.
2. Next, in a bowl, gently mix the quinoa, vegetables, and dressing.
3. Ensure everything is well combined, before chilling in the refrigerator.
4. Serve and enjoy.

Nutritional Information: Calories: 72; Fat: 15.4g; Carbs: 28.5g; Protein: 7.9g

Classic Lentil Soup with Swiss Chard

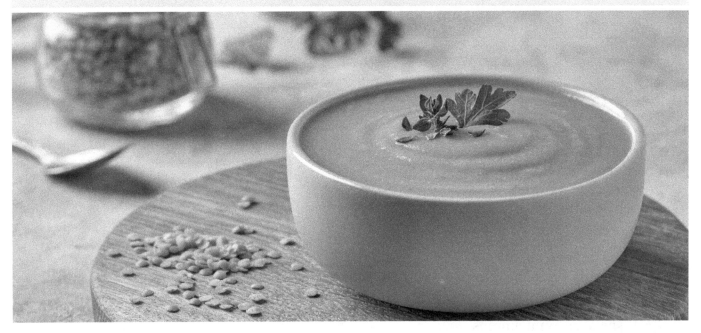

PREPARATION TIME: 5 MINUTES
COOK TIMING: 25 MINUTES
SERVES: 5

INGREDIENTS

- 1 white onion, chopped
- 1 ¼ cups of brown lentils, soaked overnight and rinsed
- 1 teaspoon of garlic, minced
- 2 large carrots, chopped
- 1 parsnip, chopped
- 2 stalks of celery, chopped
- 5 cups of roasted vegetable broth
- 2 bay leaves
- 1/2 teaspoon of dried thyme
- 2 tbsps of olive oil
- 1/4 teaspoon of ground cumin
- 2 cups of Swiss chard, torn into pieces

INSTRUCTIONS

1. In a pot, warm up the oil over medium heat.
2. Next, sauté the veggies and spices for around 3 minutes until they soften right.
3. Pour in the veggie broth and lentils and bring it to a boil. Then, reduce the heat to simmer and toss in the bay leaves. Let it simmer for 15 minutes or until the lentils are nice and tender.
4. Add the Swiss chard, cover, and simmer for an additional 5 minutes or until the chard wilts.
5. Serve in bowls and enjoy.

Nutritional Information: Calories: 148; Fat: 7.2g; Carbs: 14.6g; Protein: 7.7g

Roasted Fennel Salad

PREPARATION TIME: 10 MINUTES
COOK TIMING: 20 MINUTES
SERVES: 4

INGREDIENTS

Fennel:
- 1 tbsp of avocado oil
- 1 bulb fennel fronds, sliced
- 1 tbsp of curry powder
- 1 pinch of salt

Salad:
- 1 red bell pepper, sliced
- 5 cups of salad greens

Dressing:
- 1½ tbsps of coconut aminos
- ¼ cup of tahini
- 1 tbsp of freshly minced rosemary
- 1½ teaspoons of apple cider vinegar
- 1 pinch salt
- 3 cloves of garlic, minced
- 1½ tbsps of lemon juice
- 5 tbsps of water to thin

INSTRUCTIONS

1. Start by preheating your oven to 375°F.
2. Take a baking sheet and coat it with a layer of oil. Place the fennel on the baking sheet. Sprinkle some salt, curry powder, and oil over it.
3. Let the curried fennel bake in the oven for 20 minutes.
4. Next, mix all the ingredients for the dressing in a bowl.
5. In a salad bowl, combine all the vegetables, roasted fennel, and dressing. Mix everything thoroughly before refrigerating to cool.
6. Once chilled, serve and enjoy!

Nutritional Information: Calories: 205; Fat: 22.7g; Carbs: 26.1g; Protein: 5.2g

Cannellini Bean Soup with Kale

PREPARATION TIME: 5 MINUTES
COOK TIMING: 25 MINUTES
SERVES: 5

INGREDIENTS

- 1/2 teaspoon of ginger, minced
- 1 red onion, chopped
- 1/2 teaspoon of cumin seeds
- 1 carrot, trimmed and chopped
- 1 tbsp of olive oil
- 2 garlic cloves, minced 5 cups vegetable broth
- 1 parsnip, trimmed and chopped
- 12 ounces of Cannellini beans, drained
- Sea salt and ground black pepper, to taste
- 2 cups of kale, torn into pieces

INSTRUCTIONS

1. In a pot, heat the olive oil over medium to high heat.
2. Next, sauté the ginger and cumin for a minute.
3. Then, add the carrot, onion, and parsnip; cook for 3 minutes or until the vegetables are just tender.
4. Add the garlic. Cook for another minute until fragrant.
5. After that, pour in the vegetable broth and bring it to a boil. Reduce the heat to a simmer and let it simmer for 10 minutes.
6. Mix in the Cannellini beans and kale; let it simmer until the kale wilts and everything is heated through. Season with salt and pepper to your liking.
7. Serve hot in bowls.
8. Enjoy your meal!

Nutritional Information: Calories: 188; Fat: 4.7g; Carbs: 24.5g; Protein: 11.1g

Quinoa and Black Bean Salad

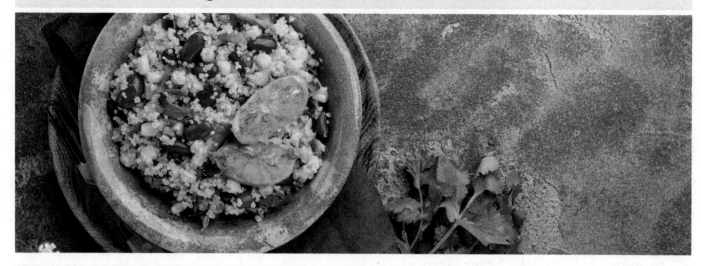

PREPARATION TIME: 15 MINUTES
COOK TIMING: 0 MINUTES
SERVES: 4

INGREDIENTS

- 1 tbsp of apple cider vinegar
- 2 cups of water
- 16 ounces of canned black beans, drained
- 2 Roma tomatoes, sliced
- 1 red onion, thinly sliced
- 2 tbsps of fresh cilantro, chopped
- 1 cucumber, seeded and chopped
- 2 cloves of garlic, pressed or minced
- 1 cup of quinoa, rinsed
- 2 Italian peppers, seeded and sliced
- 1/4 cup of olive oil
- Sea salt and ground black pepper, to taste
- 1 lemon, freshly squeezed
- 1/2 teaspoon of dried dill weed
- 2 tbsps of fresh parsley, chopped
- 1/2 teaspoon of dried oregano

INSTRUCTIONS

1. Put the water and quinoa in a pot. Bring it to a boil, then reduce the heat to a simmer.
2. Allow it to simmer for 13 minutes until the quinoa has soaked up all the water; use a fork to fluff the quinoa and let it cool down completely.
3. Next, move the quinoa into a bowl.
4. Mix the rest of the ingredients into the bowl. Toss everything together thoroughly.
5. Enjoy your meal!

Nutritional Information: Calories: 433; Fat: 17.3g; Carbs: 57g; Protein: 15.1g

Creamy Pumpkin and Toasted Walnut Soup

PREPARATION TIME: 15 MINUTES
COOK TIMING: 30 MINUTES
SERVES: 4

INGREDIENTS

- 1 small pie pumpkin, peeled, seeded, and chopped (around 6 cups)
- ¼ cup of toasted walnuts
- 1 teaspoon of olive oil
- 4 cups of water, or vegetable stock
- 1 onion, diced
- 2 to 3 teaspoons of ground sage
- ¼ teaspoon of sea salt
- 2 to 3 tbsps of nutritional yeast
- Freshly ground black pepper
- 1 cup of non-dairy milk, or 1 tbsp of nut or seed butter plus 1 cup of water or stock

INSTRUCTIONS

1. Start by placing a saucepan over medium heat and sauté the pumpkin in the oil with some salt until it softens slightly, which should take about 10 minutes.
2. Next, add the onion and cook until it also softens a bit around 5 minutes.
3. Pour in the water and bring it to a boil. Reduce the heat to a simmer, cover the pot and let it cook for 15 to 20 minutes until the pumpkin is tender when tested with a fork.
4. Mix in the nutritional yeast, sage, and non-dairy milk. Blend the soup using an immersion blender or a regular blender until smooth.
5. Serve with some toasted walnuts on top, along with a sprinkle of pepper for flavor.
6. Serve and enjoy.

Nutritional Information: Calories: 236; Fat: 12g; Carbs: 29g; Protein: 10.6g

Classic Roasted Pepper Salad

PREPARATION TIME: 5 MINUTES
COOK TIMING: 15 MINUTES
SERVES: 3

INGREDIENTS

- 2 tbsps of fresh parsley, chopped
- 6 bell peppers
- Sea salt and freshly cracked black pepper, to taste
- 3 garlic cloves, finely chopped
- 1/2 teaspoon of red pepper flakes
- 3 tbsps of extra-virgin olive oil
- 6 tbsps of pine nuts, roughly chopped
- 3 teaspoons of red wine vinegar

INSTRUCTIONS

1. Broil the peppers on a baking sheet lined with parchment paper for 10 minutes, making sure to turn the pan halfway through cooking time to ensure even charring on all sides.
2. Next, wrap the peppers in plastic wrap to allow them to steam.
3. Remove the skin, seeds and cores before slicing the peppers into strips and mixing them with the other ingredients. Refrigerate until you're ready to enjoy.
4. Enjoy your meal!

Nutritional Information: Calories: 178; Fat: 14.4g; Carbs: 11.8g; Protein: 2.4g

Roasted Beet and Avocado Salad

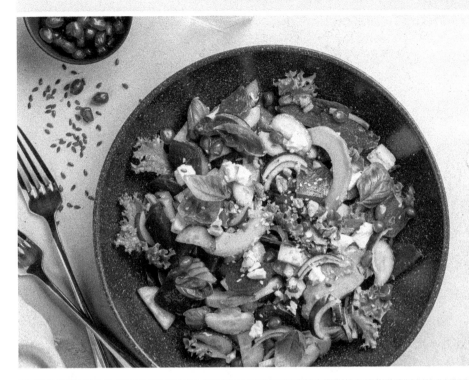

PREPARATION TIME: 10 MINUTES
COOK TIMING: 30 MINUTES
SERVES: 2

INGREDIENTS

- 2 cups of mixed greens
- 1 teaspoon of olive oil
- 2 tbsps of chopped almonds, sunflower seeds, or pumpkin seeds (toasted or raw)
- A pinch of sea salt
- 2 beets, peeled and thinly sliced
- 1 avocado
- 3 to 4 tbsps of Creamy Balsamic Dressing

INSTRUCTIONS

1. Preheat your oven to 400°F.
2. Combine the beets, oil, and salt in a bowl and gently toss the beets to coat them. Place them in a layer in a baking dish and bake for 20 to 30 minutes until they are tender and have a lightly browned edge.
3. While the beets are cooking, halve the avocado. Remove the pit and scoop out the flesh carefully. Cut it into crescent shapes.
4. Once the beets are ready, arrange slices on two plates. Place a smaller size of avocado slice on each beet slice. Add a portion of mixed greens on top.
5. Drizzle dressing over the dish and sprinkle some chopped almonds for flavor.

Nutritional Information: Calories: 167; Fat: 13g; Carbs: 15g; Protein: 4g

Moroccan Aubergine Salad

PREPARATION TIME: 30 MINUTES
COOK TIMING: 15 MINUTES
SERVES: 2

INGREDIENTS

- 1 teaspoon of olive oil
- ½ teaspoon of ground cumin
- 1 eggplant, diced
- 2 cups of spinach, chopped
- ¼ teaspoon of turmeric
- 1 tbsp of chopped green olives
- ¼ teaspoon of ground nutmeg
- Pinch sea salt
- 2 tbsps of capers
- ½ teaspoon of ground ginger
- 1 garlic clove, pressed
- Handful of fresh mint, finely chopped
- 1 lemon, half zested and juiced, half cut into wedges

INSTRUCTIONS

1. Heat the oil in a skillet over medium heat, then sauté the eggplant until it softens slightly, approximately 5 minutes. Mix in the cumin, nutmeg, ginger, turmeric, and salt and continue cooking until the eggplant becomes very soft, around 10 minutes.
2. Next, add the lemon zest and juice, capers, garlic, olives, and mint. Sauté for another minute or two to blend all the flavors.
3. Place a handful of spinach on each plate. Spoon the eggplant mixture on top. Serve with a lemon wedge for squeezing juice over the greens.

Nutritional Information: Calories: 97; Fat: 4g; Carbs: 16g; Protein: 4g

Green Lentil Salad

PREPARATION TIME: 5 MINUTES
COOK TIMING: 20 MINUTES
SERVES: 5

INGREDIENTS

- 2 cups of arugula
- 1 cup of baby spinach
- 1 ½ cups of green lentils, rinsed
- 1/4 cup of fresh basil, chopped
- 2 cups of Romaine lettuce, torn into pieces
- 1/2 cup of shallots, chopped
- Sea salt and ground black pepper, to taste
- 1/4 cup of oil-packed sun-dried tomatoes, rinsed and chopped
- 5 tbsps of extra-virgin olive oil
- 2 garlic of cloves, finely chopped
- 3 tbsps of fresh lemon juice

INSTRUCTIONS

1. In a saucepan, heat 4 ½ cups of water and red lentils until boiling.
2. Reduce the heat to low and simmer the lentils for about 15 to 17 minutes until they are tender but not overly soft. Drain and allow them to cool completely.
3. Put the lentils in a bowl; mix them with the rest of the ingredients until everything is well mixed.
4. Enjoy your dish either chilled or at room temperature.

Nutritional Information: Calories: 349; Fat: 15.1g; Carbs: 40.9g; Protein: 15.4g

Hearty Winter Quinoa Soup

PREPARATION TIME: 5 MINUTES
COOK TIMING: 25 MINUTES
SERVES: 4

INGREDIENTS

- 2 carrots, peeled and chopped
- Sea salt and ground black pepper, to taste
- 2 tbsps of olive oil
- 1 onion, chopped
- 2 tbsps of Italian parsley, chopped
- 1 celery stalk, chopped
- 4 garlic cloves, pressed or minced
- 1 parsnip, chopped
- 1 bay laurel
- 2 cups of Swiss chard, tough ribs removed and torn into pieces
- 1 cup of yellow squash, chopped
- 4 cups of roasted vegetable broth
- 1 cup of quinoa
- 2 medium tomatoes, crushed

INSTRUCTIONS

1. In a saucepan, heat the olive oil over medium to high heat.
2. Next, sauté the onion, celery, carrot, parsnip, and yellow squash for around 3 minutes until they are just soft.
3. Add the garlic and cook for another minute until it smells fragrant.
4. Then, add the vegetable broth, pepper, tomatoes, quinoa, salt, and bay leaf; bring it to a boil. Lower the heat immediately to simmer and let it cook for 13 minutes.
5. Mix in the Swiss chard; continue simmering until the chard wilts.
6. Serve in individual bowls topped with parsley.
7. Enjoy your meal!

Nutritional Information: Calories: 328; Fat: 11.1g; Carbs: 44.1g; Protein: 13.3g

Tomato Pumpkin Soup

PREPARATION TIME: 10 MINUTES
COOK TIMING: 20 MINUTES
SERVES: 4

INGREDIENTS

- 1/2 cup of tomato, chopped
- 2 cups of pumpkin, diced
- 1/2 cup of onion, chopped
- 2 cups of vegetable stock
- 1/2 teaspoon of garlic, minced
- 1 teaspoon of olive oil
- 1 1/2 teaspoons of curry powder
- 1/2 teaspoon of paprika

INSTRUCTIONS

1. In a saucepan, heat some oil, garlic and onion together for 3 minutes on medium heat.
2. Next, put all the ingredients in the saucepan. Let it come to a boil.
3. Lower the heat, cover the pan and let it simmer for 10 minutes.
4. Puree the soup until it is nice and smooth.
5. Stir it. Serve while it is warm.

Nutritional Information: Calories: 70; Fat: 2.7g; Carbs: 13.8g; Protein: 2g

Chilled Avocado Mint Soup

PREPARATION TIME: 10 MINUTES
COOK TIMING: 0 MINUTES
SERVES: 2

INGREDIENTS

- 1 cup of coconut milk
- 2 romaine lettuce leaves
- 1 medium avocado, peeled, pitted, and cut into pieces
- 20 fresh mint leaves
- 1/8 teaspoon of salt
- 1 tbsp of fresh lime juice

INSTRUCTIONS

1. Combine all the ingredients in the blender and mix until you achieve a smooth consistency. The soup should have a thick texture, not like a puree.
2. Pour the mixture into serving bowls. Let it chill in the refrigerator for 10 minutes.
3. Stir it before serving it.

Nutritional Information: Calories: 268; Fat: 25.6g; Carbs: 11.2g; Protein: 2.7g

Cream of Green Bean Soup

PREPARATION TIME: 5 MINUTES
COOK TIMING: 35 MINUTES
SERVES: 4

INGREDIENTS

- 1 onion, chopped
- 2 russet potatoes, peeled and diced
- 1 tbsp of sesame oil
- 2 garlic cloves, chopped 4 cups vegetable broth
- 1 pound of green beans, trimmed
- 1 cup of full-fat coconut milk
- Sea salt and ground black pepper, to season
- 1 green pepper, seeded and chopped

INSTRUCTIONS

1. In a heavy-bottomed pot, warm the oil over medium to high heat.
2. Next, sauté the onions, peppers, and potatoes for around 5 minutes, stirring occasionally.
3. Add the garlic. Cook for another minute until it releases its aroma.
4. Then, add the vegetable broth, salt, green beans, and black pepper; bring it to a boil. Reduce the heat to a simmer immediately, and let it cook for 20 minutes.
5. Use an immersion blender to blend the green bean mixture until smooth and consistent.
6. Pour back the blended mixture into the pot. Mix in the coconut milk and let it simmer until heated through for about 5 minutes.
7. Serve hot in serving bowls, and enjoy your meal!

Nutritional Information: Calories: 410; Fat: 19.6g; Carbs: 45.6g; Protein: 13.3g

Cauliflower Spinach Soup

PREPARATION TIME: 20 MINUTES
COOK TIMING: 30 MINUTES
SERVES: 5

INGREDIENTS

- 5 oz. of fresh spinach, chopped
- 1/2 cup of unsweetened coconut milk
- 5 watercress, chopped
- 1 lb. of cauliflower, chopped
- 8 cups of vegetable stock
- Salt

INSTRUCTIONS

1. Place both the stock and cauliflower into a saucepan, then bring them to a boil over medium heat for about 15 minutes.
2. Next, toss in the spinach and watercress. Let it all cook for an additional 10 minutes.
3. Once done, take it off the heat. Blend the soup using an immersion blender until it is nice and smooth.
4. Pour in the coconut milk. Give it a good stir.
5. Season with some salt to taste.
6. Finally, mix everything together. Serve while hot.

Nutritional Information: Calories: 153; Fat: 8.3g; Carbs: 14.7g; Protein: 11.9g

Cherry Tomato Salad with Soy Chorizo

PREPARATION TIME: 5 MINUTES
COOK TIMING: 10 MINUTES
SERVES: 4

INGREDIENTS

- 2 ½ cups of cherry tomatoes, halved
- 4 soy chorizo, chopped
- 2 teaspoons of red wine vinegar
- 3 tbsps of sliced black olives to garnish
- 2 tbsps of chopped cilantro
- 1 small red onion, finely chopped
- 2 ½ tbsps of olive oil
- Salt and freshly ground black pepper to taste

INSTRUCTIONS

1. Start by heating half a tbsp of olive oil in a skillet over medium heat. Fry the soy chorizo until it turns brown, then turn off the heat.
2. In a salad bowl, mix together the remaining olive oil and vinegar. Add in the onion, tomatoes, cilantro, and the fried soy chorizo. Toss everything with the dressing and season using salt and pepper.
3. Finish off by garnishing with olives before serving.

Nutritional Information: Calories: 138; Fat: 8.9g; Carbs: 9g; Protein: 7.10g

Creamy Squash Soup

PREPARATION TIME: 15 MINUTES
COOK TIMING: 25 MINUTES
SERVES: 5

INGREDIENTS

- 1 tbsp of coconut oil
- 3 cups of butternut squash, chopped
- 1 teaspoon of dried onion flakes
- 1 ½ cups of unsweetened coconut milk
- 1 tbsp of curry powder
- 1 garlic clove
- 4 cups of water
- 1 teaspoon of kosher salt

INSTRUCTIONS

1. In a saucepan, add the squash, coconut oil, garlic, onion flakes, curry powder, water, and salt. Heat on high heat until it boils.
2. Reduce the heat to medium. Let it simmer for 20 minutes.
3. Use a blender to puree the soup until smooth. Return the soup to the saucepan, mix in coconut milk, and cook for 2 minutes.
4. Stir it and serve hot.

Nutritional Information: Calories: 146; Fat: 12.6g; Carbs: 24.6g; Protein: 2g

Roasted Carrot Soup

PREPARATION TIME: 10 MINUTES
COOK TIMING: 45 MINUTES
SERVES: 4

INGREDIENTS

- 2 tbsps of fresh cilantro, roughly chopped
- 1 ½ pounds of carrots
- 2 cloves of garlic, minced
- 1 yellow onion, chopped
- 1/3 teaspoon of ground cumin
- 4 tbsps of olive oil
- 1/2 teaspoon of turmeric powder
- 4 cups of vegetable stock
- Sea salt and white pepper, to taste
- 2 teaspoons of lemon juice

INSTRUCTIONS

1. Preheat your oven to 400°F.
2. Next, place the carrots on a baking sheet lined with parchment paper and toss them with 2 tbsps of olive oil.
3. Roast the carrots until they become soft, which usually takes 35 minutes.
4. In a heavy-bottomed pot, heat the remaining 2 tbsps of olive oil. Then sauté the onion and garlic until they release their aroma, about 3 minutes.
5. Add cumin, salt, vegetable stock, pepper, turmeric, and roasted carrots to the pot. Let it simmer for another 12 minutes.
6. Use an immersion blender to puree the soup. Before serving drizzle some lemon juice over it. Garnish with cilantro leaves.
7. Enjoy your meal!

Nutritional Information: Calories: 264; Fat: 18.4g; Carbs: 20.1g; Protein: 7.4g

Rocket Chickpeas Salad

PREPARATION TIME: 5 MINUTES
COOK TIMING: 0 MINUTES
SERVES: 2

INGREDIENTS

- 2 handfuls of rocket
- 1 avocado, cut into small pieces
- 1 chopped red chili
- 400g can of chickpeas, drained and rinsed
- 1 teaspoon of cumin seeds
- 3 chopped roasted red peppers
- ½ finely chopped red onion
- **1 lime:** plus wedges for serving
- Olive oil

INSTRUCTIONS

1. Combine onions, ripe avocado, bell peppers, chickpeas, and chili in a mixing bowl.
2. In a bowl, whisk together two tbsps of olive oil with lime juice, adding seasoning and cumin seeds for flavor.
3. Carefully fold the dressing into the vegetable mixture until combined.
4. Divide the chickpea salad on a bed of rockets into two serving plates.

Nutritional Information: Calories: 486; Fat: 26.2g; Carbs: 60.4g; Protein: 18.3g

Classic Cream of Broccoli Soup

PREPARATION TIME: 5 MINUTES
COOK TIMING: 35 MINUTES
SERVES: 4

INGREDIENTS

- 3 cups of vegetable broth
- 1 pound of broccoli florets
- 2 tbsps of olive oil
- 1 parsnip, chopped
- 1 celery rib, chopped
- 1/2 teaspoon of dried dill
- 1 onion, chopped
- 1/2 teaspoon of dried oregano
- 1 cup of full-fat coconut milk
- Sea salt and ground black pepper, to taste
- 1 teaspoon of garlic, chopped
- 2 tbsps of flaxseed meal

INSTRUCTIONS

1. In a heavy-bottomed pot, heat up the oil over medium to high heat.
2. Proceed to cook the broccoli, celery, onion, and parsnip for 5 minutes, stirring occasionally.
3. Add the garlic and sauté for 1 minute until its aroma is released.
4. Then incorporate the vegetable broth, salt, dill, oregano, and black pepper. Bring it to a boil. Immediately reduce the heat to a simmer. Allow it to cook for approximately 20 minutes.
5. Using an immersion blender, blend the soup until smooth and uniform in consistency.
6. Return the blended mixture to the pot. Stir in the flaxseed meal and coconut milk; continue to simmer until heated through for 5 minutes.
7. Serve the soup in four bowls. Enjoy each spoonful!

Nutritional Information: Calories: 334; Fat: 24.5g; Carbs: 22.5g; Protein: 10.2g

Tarragon Cauli Salad

PREPARATION TIME: 5 MINUTES
COOK TIMING: 0 MINUTES
SERVES: 2

INGREDIENTS

- 1 tbsp of olive oil
- Salt, as needed
- 1 cup of cauliflower florets
- Pepper, as needed
- **For The Tarragon Dressing:**
- 2 tbsps of olive oil
- ½ bunch of tarragon
- 1 teaspoon of Dijon mustard
- ½ cup of baby spinach
- 1 tbsp of lemon juice
- ½ teaspoon of salt
- 2 teaspoons of capers

INSTRUCTIONS

1. Preheat your oven to 375 degrees Celsius.
2. Spread out the cauliflower florets on a baking sheet.
3. Drizzle some oil and season with salt and pepper.
4. Bake in the oven for 25 to 30 minutes until they are tender.
5. Combine all the ingredients for the tarragon dressing in a bowl with water.
6. Transfer the mixture to a blender and blend until smooth and thick.
7. Toss the cauliflower in the dressing and mix well.
8. Enjoy.

Nutritional Information: Calories: 178; Fat: 14.22g; Carbs: 9.6g; Protein: 4g

Old-Fashioned Green Bean Salad

PREPARATION TIME: 5 MINUTES
COOK TIMING: 0 MINUTES
SERVES: 4

INGREDIENTS

- 1 teaspoon of deli mustard
- 1/2 cup of scallions, chopped
- 1 Persian cucumber, sliced
- 2 cups of grape tomatoes, halved
- 1 teaspoon of garlic, minced
- 1/4 cup of olive oil
- 2 tbsps of tamari sauce
- 1 ½ pounds of green beans, trimmed
- 2 tbsps of lemon juice
- 1/4 teaspoon of cumin powder
- 1 tbsp of apple cider vinegar
- 1/2 teaspoon of dried thyme
- Sea salt and ground black pepper, to taste

INSTRUCTIONS

1. Cook the beans in a pot of salted water until they are slightly tender, around 2 minutes.
2. After draining and allowing the beans to cool down completely, place them in a bowl and mix them with the rest of the ingredients.
3. Enjoy your meal!

Nutritional Information: Calories: 240; Fat: 14.1g; Carbs: 29g; Protein: 4.4g

Italian-Style Cremini Mushroom Soup

PREPARATION TIME: 5 MINUTES
COOK TIMING: 15 MINUTES
SERVES: 3

INGREDIENTS

- 1 white onion, chopped
- 3 tbsps of vegan butter
- 1 red bell pepper, chopped
- 3 cups of cremini mushrooms, chopped
- 1 heaping tbsp of fresh chives, roughly chopped
- 2 tbsps of almond flour
- 1 teaspoon of Italian herb mix
- 3 cups of water
- Sea salt and ground black pepper, to taste
- 1/2 teaspoon of garlic, pressed

INSTRUCTIONS

1. In a pot, melt the plant-based butter over high heat.
2. Once it's hot, cook the onion and bell pepper for around 3 minutes until they become tender.
3. Next, add the garlic and Cremini mushrooms. Keep cooking until the mushrooms are soft. Sprinkle the almond meal over the mushrooms. Continue cooking for a minute.
4. Then, mix in all the ingredients. Allow it to simmer with the lid on and continue cooking for another 5 to 6 minutes until the liquid slightly thickens.
5. Serve in three soup bowls and garnish with chives. Enjoy your meal!

Nutritional Information: Calories: 154; Fat: 12.3g; Carbs: 10g; Protein: 4.4g

Creamy Avocado Salad with Herb Dressing

PREPARATION TIME: 5 MINUTES
COOK TIMING: 0 MINUTES
SERVES: 4

INGREDIENTS

- 1/2 teaspoon dried basil
- 1 garlic clove, chopped
- 1/8 teaspoon freshly ground black pepper
- 1/3 cup olive oil
- 1 tablespoon chopped shallot
- 1/4 teaspoon brown sugar (optional)
- 3 tablespoons white wine vinegar
- 1/2 cup frozen baby peas, thawed
- 1 medium head romaine lettuce, cut into 1/4-inch strips
- 12 ripe grape tomatoes, halved
- 8 kalamata olives, pitted
- 1/2 teaspoon salt
- 1 ripe Hass avocado

INSTRUCTIONS

1. In a blender or food processor, combine salt, garlic, sugar (if using), shallot, basil, pepper, and vinegar until a paste forms. Then add the oil and blend until creamy. Set aside.
2. In a large bowl, mix lettuce, tomatoes, peas, and olives together. Remove the pit from the avocado, peel it, and cut it into 1/2-inch cubes. Add the avocado to the bowl.
3. Pour the dressing over the salad ingredients, tossing gently to coat everything lightly.
4. Serve and enjoy!

Nutritional Information: Calories: 272; Fat: 24g; Carbs: 11 g; Protein: 3g

Quinoa and Avocado Salad

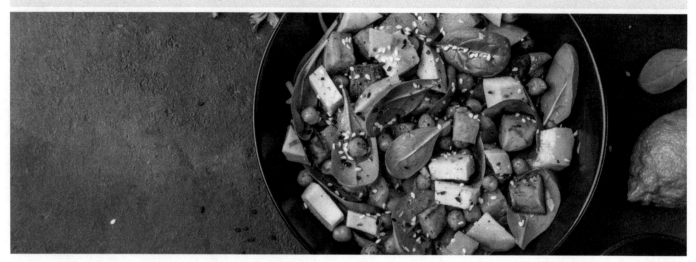

PREPARATION TIME: 5 MINUTES
COOK TIMING: 0 MINUTES
SERVES: 4

INGREDIENTS

- 1 onion, chopped
- 2 roasted peppers, cut into strips
- 1 cup of quinoa, rinsed
- 2 tbsps of parsley, chopped
- 1 tomato, diced
- 2 tbsps of basil, chopped
- 1/4 cup of extra-virgin olive oil
- Sea salt and freshly ground black pepper, to season
- 2 tbsps of lemon juice
- 1/4 teaspoon of cayenne pepper
- 1 avocado, peeled, pitted and sliced
- 2 tbsps of red wine vinegar
- 1 tbsp of sesame seeds, toasted

INSTRUCTIONS

1. Start by putting the water and quinoa in a pot and bring it to a boil. Then, reduce the heat to a simmer.
2. Let it cook for 13 minutes until the quinoa has soaked up all the water. Use a fork to fluff up the quinoa, then allow it to cool down completely.
3. Next, transfer the quinoa into a bowl.
4. Combine the onion, tomato, roasted peppers, parsley and basil in the salad bowl. In another bowl, mix together the olive oil, lemon juice, vinegar, salt, cayenne pepper, and black pepper.
5. Drizzle the dressing over your salad, tossing everything well. Finally, top it off with slices of avocado and sprinkle toasted seeds on top.

Nutritional Information: Calories: 399; Fat: 24.3g; Carbs: 38.5g; Protein: 8.4g

Red Bean and Corn Salad

PREPARATION TIME: 5 MINUTES
COOK TIMING: 0 MINUTES
SERVES: 4

INGREDIENTS

- 8 cups of chopped romaine lettuce
- 2 (14.5-ounce cans of kidney beans, rinsed and drained
- 1 teaspoon of chili powder
- 2 cups of frozen corn, thawed, or 2 cups of canned corn, drained
- ¼ cup of Cashew Cream or other salad dressing
- 1 cup of cooked farro, barley, or rice (optional)

INSTRUCTIONS

1. Let's get the ingredients ready to cook.
2. Get four large glass quart jars lined up.
3. In a bowl, mix the cream with chili powder. Put one tbsp of cream into each jar. Add ¾ cup of kidney beans, ½ cup of corn, ¼ cup of farro (if you have it) and 2 cups of romaine lettuce into each jar, pressing it down to make it all fit. Seal the lids securely, or enjoy right away.

Nutritional Information: Calories: 303; Fat: 9g; Carbs: 45g; Protein: 14g

Spring Vegetable Soup

PREPARATION TIME: 10 MINUTES
COOK TIMING: 20 MINUTES
SERVES: 4

INGREDIENTS

- 3 cups of green beans, chopped
- 1 cup of pearl onions, peeled and halved
- 2 cups of seaweed mix (or spinach
- 1 tbsp of garlic powder
- 2 cups of asparagus, chopped
- 4 cups of vegetable stock
- Salt and freshly ground white pepper to taste

INSTRUCTIONS

1. In a pot, pour addvegetable broth, green beans, asparagus, and pearl onions. Sprinkle with garlic powder, salt, and white pepper.
2. Cover the pot and let it cook over medium heat until the vegetables are tender, about 10 to 15 minutes.
3. Mix in some seaweed blend. Adjust the seasoning with salt and white pepper.
4. Spoon into serving bowls.
5. Enjoy with a side of whole-wheat bread.

Nutritional Information: Calories: 196; Fat: 11.9g; Carbs: 11g; Protein: 7g

Kidney Bean and Potato Soup

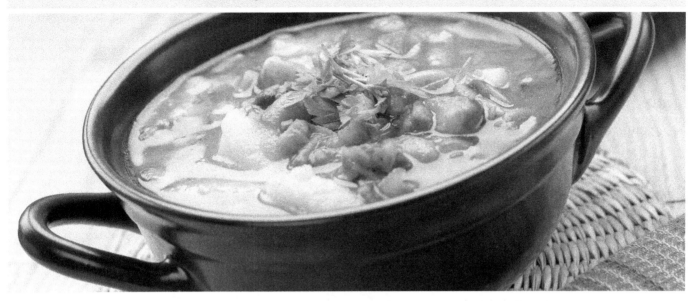

PREPARATION TIME: 5 MINUTES
COOK TIMING: 0 MINUTES
SERVES: 4

INGREDIENTS

- 1 onion, chopped
- 2 tbsps of olive oil
- 1 pound of potatoes, peeled and diced
- 2 garlic cloves, minced 1 teaspoon paprika
- 1 medium celery stalks, chopped
- 4 cups of water
- 16 ounces of canned kidney beans, drained
- 2 tbsps of vegan bouillon powder
- Sea salt and ground black pepper, to taste
- 2 cups of baby spinach

INSTRUCTIONS

1. In a heavy-bottomed pot, warm the olive oil over medium to high heat.
2. Next, cook the onion, potatoes, and celery for around 5 minutes until the onion becomes see-through and soft.
3. Add the garlic. Cook for another minute until it releases an aroma.
4. Then mix in the paprika, water, and vegan bouillon powder, bringing it to a boil. Lower the heat to a simmer and let it simmer for 15 minutes.
5. Stir in the navy beans and spinach, and simmer for 5 minutes until everything is heated through. Season with salt and pepper according to your preference.
6. Scoop into serving bowls individually. Serve while hot.
7. Enjoy your meal!

Nutritional Information: Calories: 266; Fat: 7.7g; Carbs: 41.3g; Protein: 9.3g

Creamy Golden Veggie Soup

PREPARATION TIME: 5 MINUTES
COOK TIMING: 45 MINUTES
SERVES: 4

INGREDIENTS

- 3 cups of vegetable stock
- 1 yellow onion, chopped
- 2 pounds of butternut squash, peeled, seeded and diced
- 1 parsnip, trimmed and sliced
- 2 tbsps of avocado oil
- 1 teaspoon of ginger and garlic paste
- 2 Yukon Gold potatoes, peeled and diced
- 1 teaspoon of turmeric powder
- 1 teaspoon of fennel seeds
- 1/2 teaspoon of pumpkin pie spice
- 2 tbsps of pepitas
- 1/2 teaspoon of chili powder
- Kosher salt and ground black pepper, to taste
- 1 cup of full-fat coconut milk

INSTRUCTIONS

1. In a heavy-bottomed pot, heat the oil over medium to high heat. Next, cook the onion, butternut squash, potatoes, and parsnip for around 10 minutes, stirring occasionally to ensure they cook evenly.
2. Add the ginger and garlic paste. Continue cooking for 1 minute until it becomes fragrant.
3. Then mix in the turmeric powder, fennel seeds, chili powder, pumpkin pie spice, salt, black pepper, and vegetable stock; bring it to a boil. Reduce the heat to low immediately, and let it simmer for 25 minutes.
4. Blend the soup with an immersion blender until smooth and consistent.
5. Return the blended mixture to the pot. Stir in the coconut milk. Let it simmer until heated through for about 5 minutes.
6. Serve in bowls topped with pepitas.
7. Enjoy your meal!

Nutritional Information: Calories: 550; Fat: 27.2g; Carbs: 60g; Protein: 13.6g

Greek Orzo and Bean Salad

PREPARATION TIME: 10 MINUTES
COOK TIMING: 0 MINUTES
SERVES: 4

INGREDIENTS

- 1 cup of canned kidney beans, drained
- 10 ounces of orzo
- 1 cup of canned sweet corn, drained
- 1 green chili pepper, seeded and diced
- 1 small red onion, thinly sliced
- 1 cup of grape tomatoes, halved
- 2 bell peppers, seeded and diced
- 1 tbsp of fresh parsley, chopped
- 1 tbsp of capers, drained
- 1 cup of canned green beans, drained
- 1 tbsp of fresh chervil, chopped
- 1/2 teaspoon of red pepper flakes, crushed
- 1 tbsp of fresh basil, chopped
- 4 tbsps of extra-virgin olive oil
- Sea salt and ground black pepper, to season
- 1 cup of figs, sliced
- 2 tbsps of fresh lemon juice
- 1 teaspoon of garlic powder
- 1 small sweet onion, thinly sliced
- 1 tbsp of fresh oregano, chopped

INSTRUCTIONS

1. Prepare the orzo as instructed on the package. After cooking, rinse thoroughly. Allow it to cool down completely before transferring it to a salad bowl.
2. Next, combine the beans, corn, onions, capers, tomatoes, peppers, and herbs in the salad bowl.
3. Whisk together olive oil, salt, black pepper, lemon juice, red pepper flakes, and garlic powder to make a dressing for your salad. Drizzle the dressing over the salad and garnish with sliced figs. Enjoy your meal!

Nutritional Information: Calories: 565; Fat: 15.4g; Carbs: 56g; Protein: 17.5g

MAIN DISHES

Curried Mango Chickpea Wrap

PREPARATION TIME: 15 MINUTES
COOK TIMING: 0 MINUTES
SERVES: 2

INGREDIENTS

- 1 red bell pepper, seeded and diced small
- 3 to 4 tbsps of water
- Zest and juice of 1 lime
- ¼ teaspoon of sea salt
- 1 (14-ounce) can of chickpeas, rinsed and drained, or 1½ cups cooked
- 1 to 2 cups of shredded green leaf lettuce
- 3 tbsps of tahini
- 1 cup of diced mango
- ½ cup of fresh cilantro, chopped
- 1 tbsp of curry powder
- 3 large whole-grain wraps

INSTRUCTIONS

1. Mix the tahini, lime zest and juice, curry powder and salt in a bowl until it becomes creamy and thick. You can add 3 to 4 tbsps of water to make it thin it, if needed or blend everything together. The flavor should be strong and salty to enhance the salad.
2. Combine the chickpeas, bell pepper, mango, and cilantro with the tahini dressing.
3. Place the salad in the middle of the wraps, sprinkle shredded lettuce on top, roll them up and savor every bite.

Nutritional Information: Calories: 437; Fat: 8g; Carbs: 69g; Protein: 15g

Sushi Bowl

PREPARATION TIME: 15 MINUTES
COOK TIMING: 20 MINUTES
SERVES: 1

INGREDIENTS

- ¼ cup of sliced avocado
- ¾ cup of cooked brown rice, or quinoa, millet, or other whole-grain
- 1 tbsp of sesame seeds (toasted)
- ¼ cup of sliced bell pepper
- ½ cup of shelled edamame beans (fresh or frozen)
- 1 to 2 tbsps of tamari
- ¼ cup of fresh cilantro, chopped
- 1 scallion, chopped
- ¼ nori sheet
- ½ cup of chopped spinach

INSTRUCTIONS

1. Steam or thaw edamame beans, then combine them with rice, spinach, avocado, cilantro, bell pepper, and scallions in a bowl.
2. Use scissors to cut the nori into ribbons and scatter them over the bowl.
3. Finish off by drizzling some tamari on top and sprinkling sesame seeds over it.

Nutritional Information: Calories: 467; Fat: 20g; Carbs: 56g; Protein: 22g

Sweet Potato Patties

PREPARATION TIME: 15 MINUTES
COOK TIMING: 20 MINUTES
SERVES: 3

INGREDIENTS

- ½ cup of diced onion
- 1 cup of grated sweet potato
- 1 to 2 tbsps of nutritional yeast (optional)
- A pinch of sea salt
- 1 teaspoon of olive oil
- ¼ cup of fresh parsley, finely chopped
- 1 tbsp of dried dill, or 2 tbsps fresh
- ½ cup of whole-grain flour, or gluten-free flour. or bread crumbs
- 1 cup of cooked brown rice, fully cooled

INSTRUCTIONS

1. Mix the rice, sweet potato, onion, and salt in a bowl. Let it rest for a while to allow the salt to extract moisture from the potato and onion.
2. Add the parsley, dill, and nutritional yeast (if desired). Mix in flour to create a sticky batter, adding a tbsp or two of water if needed.
3. Shape the mixture into balls. Gently flatten them into patties.
4. Heat a skillet over medium heat, then add the oil. Cook for 7 to 10 minutes on one side, then flip and cook for another 5 to 7 minutes.
5. Serve and enjoy.

Nutritional Information: Calories: 146; Fat: 2g; Carbs: 29g; Protein: 6g

Vietnamese Summer Rolls

PREPARATION TIME: 30 MINUTES
COOK TIMING: 0 MINUTES
SERVES: 5

INGREDIENTS

- 10 palm-size lettuce leaves (cut into smaller chunks)
- 2 carrots, grated or julienned
- 10-round rice roll wraps
- ½ cucumber, julienned
- 1 mango, sliced after peeling into long and thin pieces
- ½ cup of Peanut Sauce
- 3 scallions, sliced into quarters
- ¼ cup of fresh basil, cilantro, mint, or parsley leaves (or a combo)
- 1 cup of bean sprouts

INSTRUCTIONS

1. Place a plate filled with room-temperature water and immerse a rice roll wrap in it to soften it. Let it soak for a few minutes until it becomes very soft. Remove it from the water, let it drain briefly, and then transfer it to a dry plate.
2. Arrange 2 basil leaves and a lettuce leaf down the middle of the wrap. Top with carrots, mango, cucumber, scallions, and bean sprouts without overfilling to ease rolling.
3. Fold the bottom edges of the rice wrap, then fold one side over the filling and tuck it in underneath. Gently press with your hands before rolling towards the end. Allow the wraps to set and adhere together before serving.
4. Slice each wrap in half. Serve alongside Peanut Sauce for dipping.

Nutritional Information: Calories: 110; Fat: 5g; Carbs: 8g; Protein: 3g

Greek-Style Eggplant Skillet

PREPARATION TIME: 5 MINUTES
COOK TIMING: 15 MINUTES
SERVES: 4

INGREDIENTS

- 2 ounces of Kalamata olives, pitted and sliced
- 1 ½ pounds of eggplant, peeled and sliced
- 4 tbsps of olive oil
- 1 teaspoon of garlic, minced
- 1/4 teaspoon of ground bay leaf
- Sea salt and ground black pepper, to taste
- 1 teaspoon of cayenne pepper
- 1/2 teaspoon of dried oregano
- 1 tomato, crushed

INSTRUCTIONS

1. Start by heating the oil in a sauté pan on medium heat.
2. Cook the eggplant for 9 minutes until it is just tender.
3. Next, mix in all the ingredients, cover the pan, and let it cook for 2 to 3 minutes until everything is fully cooked. Serve it warm.

Nutritional Information: Calories: 195; Fat: 16.1g; Carbs: 13.4g; Protein: 2.4g

Pesto and Sun-dried Tomato Quinoa

PREPARATION TIME: 10 MINUTES
COOK TIMING: 20 MINUTES
SERVES: 1

INGREDIENTS

- 2 cups of cooked quinoa
- 1 teaspoon of olive oil, or 1 tbsp of vegetable broth or water
- 2 tbsps of chopped sun-dried tomatoes
- 1 tomato, chopped
- 1 garlic clove, minced
- 1 cup of chopped zucchini
- 1 cup of chopped spinach
- Pinch sea salt
- 1 cup of chopped onion
- 2 to 3 tbsps of Basil Pesto

INSTRUCTIONS

1. Start by heating the oil in a skillet over medium to high heat. Sauté the onion for 5 minutes until it softens.
2. Next, add the garlic, followed by the zucchini and a pinch of salt.
3. Once the zucchini has slightly softened after around 5 minutes, remove the skillet from heat. Incorporate both sun-dried tomatoes. Mix well before adding the pesto sauce. Ensure all vegetables are evenly coated.
4. Arrange a bed of spinach followed by quinoa, and then top it off with the zucchini mixture on a plate for a meal. Enjoy!

Nutritional Information: Calories: 535; Fat: 23g; Carbs: 59g; Protein: 20g

Olive and White Bean Pasta

PREPARATION TIME: 10 MINUTES
COOK TIMING: 20 MINUTES
SERVES: 1

INGREDIENTS

- ½ cup of spinach
- A pinch of sea salt
- ½ cup of cooked cannellini beans
- 1 teaspoon of olive oil, or 1 tbsp of vegetable broth
- ¼ cup of thinly sliced red bell pepper
- 2 or 3 black olives, pitted and chopped
- ¼ cup of thinly sliced zucchini
- 1 tbsp of balsamic vinegar
- ½ cup of whole-grain pasta
- 1 tbsp of nutritional yeast

INSTRUCTIONS

1. Start by boiling a pot of water, then cook the pasta with some salt until it is just tender, according to the package instructions.
2. While the pasta is cooking, heat some oil in a skillet. Sauté the bell pepper and zucchini lightly for about 7 to 8 minutes.
3. Add the beans and let them warm up for 2 minutes, then add the spinach until it wilts. Finish off by drizzling some vinegar over it.
4. When serving, top or mix the pasta with the bean mixture and sprinkle with olives and nutritional yeast.

Nutritional Information: Calories: 387; Fat: 17g; Carbs: 42g; Protein: 18g

Blackeyed Peas Burritos

PREPARATION TIME: 10 MINUTES
COOK TIMING: 30 TO 40 MINUTES
SERVES: 6

INGREDIENTS

- 1 bell pepper, diced and seeded, any color
- 1 (14-ounce) can of blackeyed peas, rinsed and drained, or 1½ cups of cooked
- 1 teaspoon of olive oil, or water or vegetable broth
- 2 garlic cloves, minced
- 1 chopped zucchini
- 2 teaspoons of chili powder
- 1 red onion, diced
- 6 whole-grain tortillas, or corn tortillas
- Pinch sea salt
- 1 tomato, diced

INSTRUCTIONS

1. Preheat your oven to 325°F.
2. In a pan over medium heat, heat some olive oil and cook the onion until it becomes soft, around 5 minutes. Add the garlic and cook it briefly.
3. Next, add the zucchini to the pan and sauté until it turns tender, around 5 minutes. Then, toss in the bell pepper and tomato. Cook for another minute or two.
4. Once the tomato is heated through, mix in the chili powder, salt, and black-eyed peas. Stir everything well.
5. Spoon some of the pea mixture into each tortilla, fold in the sides, and roll them up into burritos.
6. Arrange the burritos with their seams facing down in a baking dish. Pour any remaining juices from the pan over them. Bake in the oven for 20 to 30 minutes.
7. Serve and enjoy.

Nutritional Information: Calories: 334; Fat: 6g; Carbs: 58g; Protein: 12 g

Falafel Burgers

PREPARATION TIME: 15 MINUTES
COOK TIMING: 30 MINUTES
SERVES: 8

INGREDIENTS

- ¼ cup of vegetable broth
- 2 teaspoons of onion powder
- ¼ cup of chopped fresh parsley
- 2 cups of cooked brown rice
- 1 tbsp of freshly squeezed lemon juice
- 2 teaspoons of garlic powder
- 1½ teaspoons of ground cumin
- 3 cups of cooked chickpeas
- ¼ teaspoon of freshly ground black pepper
- Whole-Wheat Pita Pockets or whole-wheat buns
- 1 teaspoon of ground coriander
- Lettuce, onion, and tomato, for topping (optional)

INSTRUCTIONS

1. Preheat your oven to 425°F. Prepare a baking sheet with parchment paper.
2. Combine chickpeas, rice, broth, parsley, lemon juice, garlic powder, onion powder, cumin, coriander, and pepper in a food processor or blender. Blend on low for around 30 to 45 seconds until the mixture can be shaped into patties easily, without turning into hummus. Remember to pause and scrape down the sides as needed.
3. Take out about half a cup of the chickpea mixture. Shape it into a patty before placing it on the baking sheet. Repeat this process until you have used up all of the chickpea mixture.
4. Bake for 15 minutes initially. Then, flip the patties over and bake for 12 to 15 minutes more until cooked through. Serve them in pita pockets or buns, with your desired toppings.

Nutritional Information: Calories: 230; Fat: 4g; Carbs: 44g; Protein: 10g

Savory Sweet Potato Casserole

PREPARATION TIME: 15 MINUTES
COOK TIMING: 30 MINUTES
SERVES: 6

INGREDIENTS

- 1 tbsp of dried sage
- 8 sweet potatoes, cooked (see here)
- 1 teaspoon of dried thyme
- ½ cup of vegetable broth
- 1 teaspoon of dried rosemary

INSTRUCTIONS

1. Preheat your oven to 375°F.
2. Peel off and discard the skin from the cooked potatoes, then place them in a baking dish. Use a fork or potato masher to mash the potatoes, then mix in the broth, thyme, sage, and rosemary.
3. Cook in the oven for 30 minutes.
4. Serve and enjoy.

Nutritional Information: Calories: 154; Fat: 2g; Carbs: 35g; Protein: 3g

Oil-Free Rice-and-Vegetable Stir-Fry

PREPARATION TIME: 5 MINUTES
COOK TIMING: 20 MINUTES
SERVES: 4

INGREDIENTS

- 4 cups of brown rice, cooked
- 2 cups of green peas (fresh or frozen)
- 1 teaspoon of garlic powder
- 2 cups of green beans (fresh or frozen)
- 1 teaspoon of onion powder
- ¼ cup of vegetable broth or water

INSTRUCTIONS

1. Heat a saucepan over medium heat.
2. Combine the peas, garlic powder, green beans, broth, and onion powder in the saucepan and stir well. Simmer for 8 minutes, stirring occasionally, until the veggies are tender but still crisp. If anything starts to stick, add a bit of broth or water.
3. Uncover the pan and mix in the cooked brown rice. Continue cooking for another 5 minutes, stirring now and then.
4. Serve hot and enjoy.

Nutritional Information: Calories: 233; Fat: 2g; Carbs: 48g; Protein: 8g

Mango-Ginger Chickpea Curry

PREPARATION TIME: 5 MINUTES
COOK TIMING: 30 MINUTES
SERVES: 6

INGREDIENTS

- 2 cups of mango chunks (fresh or frozen)
- 1 teaspoon of garlic powder
- 2 cups of plant-based milk
- 1 tbsp of curry powder
- 3 cups of cooked chickpeas
- 1 tbsp of ground ginger
- 2 tbsps of maple syrup
- 1 teaspoon of ground coriander
- ⅛ teaspoon of ground cinnamon
- 1 teaspoon of onion powder

INSTRUCTIONS

1. Start by heating a stockpot on medium heat.
2. Add the chickpeas, mango, milk, onion powder, maple syrup, curry powder, ginger, coriander, garlic powder, and cinnamon to the pot. Cook for 10 minutes, stirring it through.
3. Continue cooking for another 5 minutes, stirring every couple of minutes. Then, it's ready to be served.

Nutritional Information: Calories: 219; Fat: 4g; Carbs: 38g; Protein: 8g

Rice with Asparagus and Cauliflower

PREPARATION TIME: 10 MINUTES
COOK TIMING: 20 MINUTES
SERVES: 2

INGREDIENTS

- 1 tbsp of olive oil
- 3 ounces of asparagus
- 1/3 teaspoon of salt
- 2 ounces of tomato sauce
- 1/2 cup of brown rice
- 3/4 cup of water
- 1/4 teaspoon of ground black pepper
- 3 ounces of cauliflower, chopped
- 1/4 teaspoon of garlic powder

INSTRUCTIONS

1. Grab a saucepan, place it on the stove over medium heat and add some oil along with the asparagus and cauliflower. Sauté them for about 5 to 7 minutes until they turn brown.
2. Season the veggies with garlic powder, salt, and black pepper. Stir in some tomato sauce and let it cook for a minute.
3. Next, add the rice and pour in some water. Mix everything well, cover the pan with a lid and let it cook for 10 to 12 minutes until the rice absorbs all the liquid and becomes tender.
4. Once ready, take the pan off the heat. Fluff up the rice using a fork before serving.

Nutritional Information: Calories: 257; Fat: 5g; Carbs: 40g; Protein: 4g

Swiss Chard Skillet

PREPARATION TIME: 5 MINUTES
COOK TIMING: 15 MINUTES
SERVES: 4

INGREDIENTS

- 1 cup of vegetable broth
- 1 shallot, thinly sliced
- 2 pounds of Swiss chard, tough stalks removed, torn into pieces
- 1 red bell pepper, seeded and diced
- 4 garlic cloves, chopped
- Sea salt and ground black pepper, to taste
- 3 tbsps of olive oil

INSTRUCTIONS

1. In a saucepan, warm up the oil on medium to high heat.
2. Next, sauté the shallot and pepper for around 3 minutes until they are soft. Then sauté the garlic for a minute until it smells nice.
3. Pour in the broth and Swiss chard. Let it come to a boil, then lower the heat to simmer and keep cooking for another 10 minutes.
4. Season with salt and pepper according to your taste. Serve while it is still warm.
5. Enjoy your meal!

Nutritional Information: Calories: 169; Fat: 11.1g; Carbs: 14.9g; Protein: 6.3g

Avocado Bread with Chickpeas

PREPARATION TIME: 5 MINUTES
COOK TIMING: 5 MINUTES
SERVES: 2

INGREDIENTS

- 1 tbsp of lime juice
- 1/2 of avocado, peeled, pitted
- 1 teaspoon of apple cider vinegar
- 1/4 teaspoon of salt
- 4 tbsps of canned chickpeas, liquid reserved
- 1 teaspoon of olive oil
- 1/4 teaspoon of paprika
- 2 slices of bread, toasted

INSTRUCTIONS

1. Get a skillet, put it on the stove over medium heat and pour in some oil. Once it is hot, toss in the chickpeas. Cook them for 2 minutes.
2. Sprinkle the chickpeas with paprika and salt, mix to coat them evenly, and then take the pan off the heat.
3. In a bowl, smash an avocado with a fork, drizzle lime juice and vinegar over it and mix everything well.
4. Spread the avocado on slices of bread and top it with the chickpeas.
5. Serve and enjoy.

Nutritional Information: Calories: 235; Fat: 5g; Carbs: 31g; Protein: 6g

Chili Sin Carne

PREPARATION TIME: 5 MINUTES
COOK TIMING: 30 MINUTES
SERVES: 6

INGREDIENTS

- 28 ounces of tinned chopped tomatoes
- 1 cup of vegetable stock
- 2 tbsps of olive oil
- 1 pound of frozen soy mince
- 2 garlic cloves, minced
- 1 tin (14 ounces) red kidney beans, drained and rinsed
- ½ ounce of split red lentils
- 1 red onion, thinly sliced
- 2 celery stalks, chopped
- 1 teaspoon of ground cumin
- 2 carrots, peeled and chopped
- 1 teaspoon of chili powder
- 2 red peppers, chopped
- Salt and pepper to taste

INSTRUCTIONS

1. Heat the pan with some oil on a medium heat. Cook the carrots, peppers, celery, garlic, and onion until they become soft after a few minutes.
2. Mix in some pepper, salt, and one teaspoon each of chili powder and cumin.
3. Combine lentils, vegetable broth, red kidney beans, diced tomatoes, and frozen soy crumbles. Let everything simmer for around 25 minutes.
4. If desired, serve with brown rice and fresh coriander leaves torn on top (optional).
5. Finish off with a drizzle of lime juice. Enjoy your meal!

Nutritional Information: Calories: 340; Fat: 18g; Carbs: 42 g; Protein: 25g

Brown Rice with Vegetables and Tofu

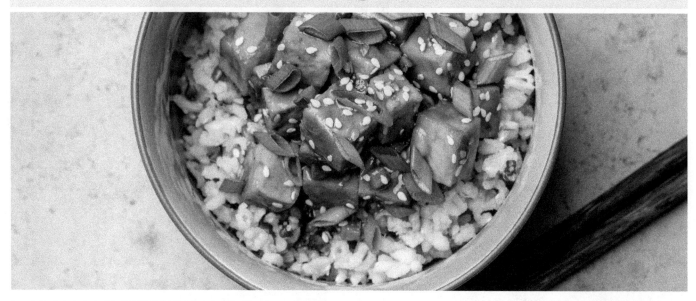

PREPARATION TIME: 10 MINUTES
COOK TIMING: 35 MINUTES
SERVES: 4

INGREDIENTS

- 2 (1/2) cups of water
- 1 cup of spring onions, chopped
- 4 teaspoons of sesame oil
- 1 carrot, trimmed and sliced
- 2 tbsps of soy sauce
- 1 celery rib, sliced
- 1/4 cup of dry white wine
- 2 spring garlic stalks, minced
- 10 ounces of tofu, cubed
- 1 (1/2) cups of long-grain brown rice, rinsed thoroughly
- 2 tbsps of tahini
- 1 tbsp of lemon juice

INSTRUCTIONS

1. In a saucepan or wok, heat 2 teaspoons of oil on medium to high heat. Next, sauté the garlic, carrot, onion, and celery for around 3 minutes, stirring to ensure everything cooks evenly.
2. Deglaze the pan with wine. Move the vegetables to one side of the wok. Then add the remaining oil and stir fry the tofu for 8 minutes, stirring from time to time.
3. Bring 2.5 cups of water to a boil on medium to high heat. Reduce to a simmer. Cook the rice until tender for 30 minutes, fluffing it up and mixing in soy sauce and tahini.
4. Combine the vegetables and tofu with the rice; squeeze some lemon juice over it and serve while warm. Enjoy your meal!

Nutritional Information: Calories: 410; Fat: 13.2g; Carbs: 60g; Protein: 14.3g

Veggie Curry

PREPARATION TIME: 10 MINUTES
COOK TIMING: 40 TO 50 MINUTES
SERVES: 4

INGREDIENTS

- ¾ cup of peas
- 14 ounces of canned coconut milk
- 1 cup of veggie stock
- Cooking spray
- ¼ cup of green curry paste
- 1 tbsp of ginger, grated
- ½ teaspoon of turmeric
- 1 tbsp of coconut sugar
- 16 ounces of firm tofu, pressed and cubed
- 1 yellow onion, chopped
- 1 ½ cups of red bell pepper, chopped
- 1 eggplant, chopped
- A pinch of salt

INSTRUCTIONS

1. Place the coconut milk into your pot.
2. In the pot, combine ginger, broth, curry paste, turmeric, coconut sugar, onion, peas, bell pepper, salt, and eggplant chunks. Mix well, cover, and cook for 40 to 50 minutes.
3. In the meantime, spray a pan with cooking spray. Heat it over high heat.
4. Cook tofu pieces in the pan until they turn brown on both sides.
5. Serve the tofu in bowls topped with the cooked curry mixture.
6. Enjoy.

Nutritional Information: Calories: 200; Fat: 4g; Carbs: 10g; Protein: 9g

Barley Pilaf with Wild Mushrooms

PREPARATION TIME: 5 MINUTES
COOK TIMING: 40 MINUTES
SERVES: 4

INGREDIENTS

- 1 cup of medium pearl barley, rinsed
- 1 small onion, chopped
- 2 tbsps of vegan butter
- 1 teaspoon of garlic, minced
- 1 pound of wild mushrooms, sliced
- 2 ¾ cups of vegetable broth
- 1 jalapeno pepper, seeded and minced

INSTRUCTIONS

1. Heat the vegan butter in a saucepan over medium heat until it melts.
2. Sauté the onion for 3 minutes until it becomes tender. Then add the garlic, jalapeno pepper, and mushrooms. Continue cooking for 2 minutes until they release their aroma.
3. Stir in the barley and broth, cover the pan, and let it simmer for about 30 minutes. Once all the liquid is absorbed, allow the barley to sit for 10 minutes before fluffing it with a fork.
4. Taste the dish. Adjust the seasonings as needed.
5. Enjoy your meal!

Nutritional Information: Calories: 288; Fat: 7.7g; Carbs: 45.3g; Protein: 12.1g

Potage au Quinoa

PREPARATION TIME: 5 MINUTES
COOK TIMING: 25 MINUTES
SERVES: 4

INGREDIENTS

- 1 jalapeno pepper, seeded and chopped
- 4 medium potatoes, peeled and diced
- 1 carrot, trimmed and diced
- 1 cup of quinoa
- 2 tbsps of olive oil
- 1 onion, chopped
- 4 cups of vegetable broth
- 1 parsnip, trimmed and diced
- Sea salt and ground white pepper, to taste

INSTRUCTIONS

1. In a heavy-bottomed pot, heat the oil over medium to high heat. Cook the onion, potatoes, parsnip, carrots, and pepper for about 5 minutes until they become tender.
2. Pour in the vegetable broth and quinoa; let it come to a boil.
3. Reduce the heat to a simmer. Cook for about 15 minutes until the quinoa is soft.
4. Season with salt and pepper as per your liking. Blend your soup using an immersion blender.
5. Warm up the potage again before serving, and savor it!

Nutritional Information: Calories: 466; Fat: 11.1g; Carbs: 57g; Protein: 16.1g

Old-Fashioned Pilaf

PREPARATION TIME: 5 MINUTES
COOK TIMING: 45 MINUTES
SERVES: 4

INGREDIENTS

- 2 bell peppers, seeded and sliced
- 1 shallot, sliced
- 3 cloves of garlic, minced
- 2 tbsps of sesame oil
- 10 ounces of oyster mushrooms, cleaned and sliced
- 2 tomatoes, pureed
- 1 cup of sweet corn kernels
- 2 cups of vegetable broth
- Salt and black pepper, to taste
- 1 cup of green peas
- 2 cups of brown rice

INSTRUCTIONS

1. Start by heating the oil in a saucepan over medium to high heat.
2. Once it is hot, sauté the shallot and peppers for around 3 minutes until they're just soft.
3. Next, add the garlic and oyster mushrooms. Continue to cook for a minute until they release their fragrant aroma.
4. In a casserole dish, lightly coated with oil, layer the rice first, followed by the mushroom mixture, tomatoes, broth, salt, black pepper, corn and green peas.
5. Cover it up. Bake at 375°F for 40 minutes. Remember to stir it.
6. Enjoy your meal!

Nutritional Information: Calories: 532; Fat: 11.4g; Carbs: 56g; Protein: 16.3g

Barley with Portobello Mushrooms and Chard

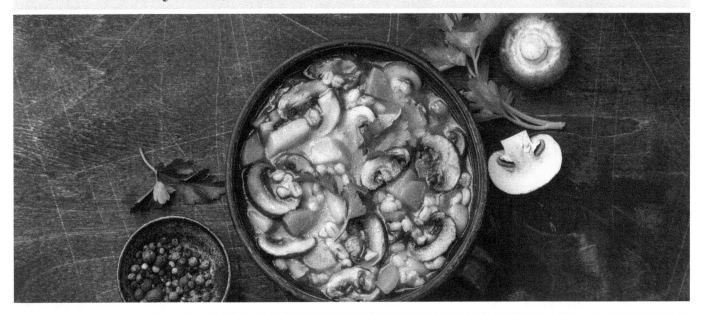

PREPARATION TIME: 5 MINUTES
COOK TIMING: 35 MINUTES
SERVES: 4

INGREDIENTS

- 4 cups of Swiss chard, torn into pieces
- 1 onion, chopped
- 12 ounces of Portobello mushrooms, sliced
- 3 cloves of garlic, minced
- 1 cup of pearl barley
- 4 cups of vegetable broth
- 1/2 cup of dry white wine
- Sea salt and ground black pepper, to taste
- 1 teaspoon of dried oregano
- 4 tbsps of olive oil
- 1 teaspoon of dried thyme

INSTRUCTIONS

1. Heat some olive oil in a saucepan over medium to high heat. Once it is hot, sauté the onion until it's just tender which should take 3 minutes.
2. Next, add the garlic and mushrooms. Continue cooking for another 2 minutes until they release their flavors.
3. Pour in the vegetable broth, barley, black pepper, wine, salt, oregano and thyme. Cover the pan. Let it simmer gently for around 25 minutes.
4. Lastly, stir in the Swiss chard. Cook for 5 to 6 minutes until it wilts.
5. Serve and enjoy!

Nutritional Information: Calories: 389; Fat: 15.9g; Carbs: 49.3g; Protein: 13.3g

Traditional Tuscan Bean Stew

PREPARATION TIME: 10 MINUTES
COOK TIMING: 25 MINUTES
SERVES: 5

INGREDIENTS

- 1 cup of crostini
- 1 medium leek, chopped
- 2 cups of Lacinato kale, torn into pieces
- 1 celery with leaves, chopped
- 3 tbsps of olive oil
- 1 zucchini, diced
- 3 garlic cloves, crushed
- 1 Italian pepper, sliced
- 2 bay leaves
- Kosher salt and ground black pepper, to taste
- 1 teaspoon of cayenne pepper
- 2 cups of vegetable broth
- 1 (28-ounce) can of tomatoes, crushed
- 2 (15-ounce) cans of Great Northern beans, drained

INSTRUCTIONS

1. In a heavy-bottomed pot, warm up the oil on medium heat.
2. Once it's hot, cook the leek, zucchini, celery, and pepper for around 4 minutes.
3. Sauté the garlic and bay leaves for a minute or so.
4. Mix in the spices, broth, tomatoes, and canned beans. Let it simmer, stirring occasionally, for 15 minutes or until fully cooked.
5. Add the Lacinato kale and let it simmer further for 4 minutes while stirring occasionally.
6. Serve with crostini on top.
7. Enjoy your meal!

Nutritional Information: Calories: 388; Fat: 10.3g; Carbs: 57.3g; Protein: 19.5g

Beluga Lentil and Vegetable Mélange

PREPARATION TIME: 5 MINUTES
COOK TIMING: 25 MINUTES
SERVES: 5

INGREDIENTS

- 1 ½ cups of beluga lentils, soaked overnight and drained
- 1 teaspoon of ginger, minced
- 3 tbsps of coconut oil
- 1 onion, minced
- 1 carrot, trimmed and chopped
- 2 cups of Swiss chard
- 1 parsnip, trimmed and chopped
- 1 cup of vegetable broth
- 2 cloves of garlic, minced
- Sea salt and ground black pepper, to taste
- 1 large-sized zucchini, diced
- 2 bell peppers, seeded and chopped
- 1 cup of tomato sauce

INSTRUCTIONS

1. In a saucepan, heat the coconut oil until it starts to sizzle.
2. Next, sauté the onion, bell pepper, carrot, and parsnip until they become tender.
3. Then, stir in the ginger and garlic. Continue cooking for another half a minute.
4. After that season with salt and black pepper, add in the zucchini, tomato sauce, vegetable broth, and lentils.
5. Let it all simmer for 20 minutes until everything is cooked through.
6. Finally, mix in the Swiss chard; cover the pot and let it simmer for around 5 minutes.
7. Enjoy your meal!

Nutritional Information: Calories: 382; Fat: 9.3g; Carbs: 59g; Protein: 17.2g

Green Lentil Stew with Collard Greens

PREPARATION TIME: 5 MINUTES
COOK TIMING: 30 MINUTES
SERVES: 5

INGREDIENTS

- 1 cup of tomato sauce
- 1 cup of frozen corn
- 2 tbsps of coconut oil
- 1 onion, chopped
- 2 carrots, chopped
- 1 bell pepper, chopped
- 2 sweet potatoes, peeled and diced
- 1 celery, chopped
- 2 cloves of garlic
- 1 ½ cups of green lentils
- 1 cup of collard greens, torn into pieces
- 1 tbsp of Italian herb mix
- 5 cups of vegetable broth
- 1 parsnip, chopped

INSTRUCTIONS

1. In a saucepan, heat the oil until it starts to sizzle.
2. Next, sauté the onion, potatoes, parsnip, bell pepper, carrots, and celery until they become tender.
3. Throw in the garlic. Keep cooking for another half a minute.
4. Then mix in the green lentils, tomato sauce, Italian herb mix, and vegetable broth; allow it to simmer for approximately 20 minutes until everything is fully cooked.
5. Toss in the corn and collard greens; cover and let it simmer for 5 minutes.
6. Enjoy your meal!

Nutritional Information: Calories: 415; Fat: 6.6g; Carbs: 51g; Protein: 18.4g

Classic Italian Minestrone

PREPARATION TIME: 5 MINUTES
COOK TIMING: 30 MINUTES
SERVES: 5

INGREDIENTS

- 2 tbsps of olive oil
- 1 cup of whole-wheat pasta
- 2 carrots, sliced
- 1 tbsp of fresh basil leaves, chopped
- 4 cloves garlic, minced
- 1 large onion, diced
- 5 cups of vegetable broth
- 1 (28-ounce) can of tomatoes, crushed
- 1 large zucchini, diced
- 1 tbsp of fresh oregano leaves, chopped
- 1 (15-ounce) can of white beans, drained
- 1 tbsp of fresh Italian parsley, chopped

INSTRUCTIONS

1. Heat the oil in a saucepan until hot. Next, sauté the onions and carrots until tender.
2. Include the uncooked pasta, garlic, and broth; allow it to simmer for approximately 15 minutes.
3. Mix in the beans, tomatoes, zucchini, and spices. Cook with a lid on for about 10 minutes until everything is cooked through.
4. Top it off with some herbs for added flavor.
5. Enjoy your meal!

Nutritional Information: Calories: 305; Fat: 8.6g; Carbs: 45.1g; Protein: 14.2g

Mexican-Style Bean Bowl

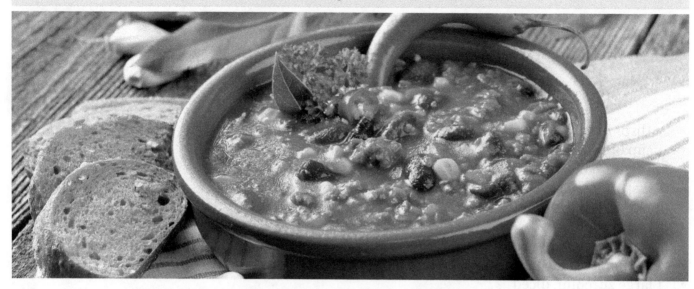

PREPARATION TIME: 5 MINUTES
COOK TIMING: 0 MINUTES
SERVES: 6

INGREDIENTS

- 1 cup of cherry tomatoes, halved
- 1 pound of red beans, soaked overnight and drained
- 2 roasted bell peppers, sliced
- 1 chili pepper, finely chopped
- Sea salt and ground black, to taste
- 1 red onion, chopped
- 1/4 cup of fresh cilantro, chopped
- 1 cup of canned corn kernels, drained
- 2 tbsps of fresh lemon juice
- 1/4 cup of fresh parsley, chopped
- 1 teaspoon of Mexican oregano
- 1/3 cup of extra-virgin olive oil
- 1 avocado, peeled, pitted and sliced
- 1/4 cup of red wine vinegar

INSTRUCTIONS

1. Place the beans and cover in water. Bring it to a boil.
2. Let it simmer for around 10 minutes. Reduce the heat. Cook for 50 to 55 minutes until the beans are soft.
3. Once cooled, move the beans to a bowl.
4. Mix in all the ingredients. Toss well.
5. Serve at room temperature.

Nutritional Information: Calories: 465; Fat: 17.9g; Carbs: 60.4g; Protein: 20.2g

Chickpea Garden Vegetable Medley

PREPARATION TIME: 5 MINUTES
COOK TIMING: 30 MINUTES
SERVES: 4

INGREDIENTS

- 3 cloves of garlic, minced
- 1 onion, finely chopped
- 1 bell pepper, chopped
- 2 tbsps of olive oil
- 1 fennel bulb, chopped
- 2 tbsps of fresh basil, roughly chopped
- 1 teaspoon of paprika
- 2 tbsps of fresh parsley, roughly chopped
- 14 ounces of canned chickpeas, drained
- 2 tbsps of fresh coriander, roughly chopped
- Kosher salt and ground black pepper, to taste
- 2 cups of vegetable broth
- 1/2 teaspoon of cayenne pepper
- 2 ripe tomatoes, pureed
- 1 avocado, peeled and sliced

INSTRUCTIONS

1. In a heavy-bottomed pot, heat the oil on medium heat. Once it's hot, cook the onion, bell pepper, and fennel bulb for about 4 minutes.
2. Sauté the garlic for a minute until it smells aromatic.
3. Add the tomatoes, fresh herbs, cayenne pepper, broth, chickpeas, salt, black pepper, and paprika. Stir and let it simmer for 20 minutes until it is fully cooked.
4. Taste it and adjust the seasonings as needed. Serve with slices of avocado on top.
5. Enjoy your meal!

Nutritional Information: Calories: 369; Fat: 18.1g; Carbs: 43.5g; Protein: 13.2g

Old-Fashioned Lentil and Vegetable Stew

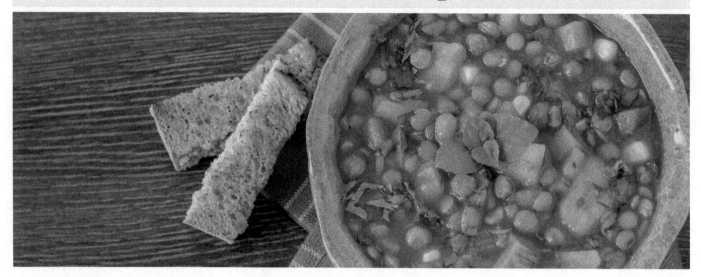

PREPARATION TIME: 5 MINUTES
COOK TIMING: 25 MINUTES
SERVES: 5

INGREDIENTS

- 3 cloves of garlic, minced
- 1 large onion, chopped
- 3 tbsps of olive oil
- 1 carrot, chopped
- 1 avocado, sliced
- 1 habanero pepper, chopped
- Kosher salt and black pepper, to taste
- 1 teaspoon of ground cumin
- 3/4 pound of dry red lentils, soaked overnight and drained
- 1 teaspoon of smoked paprika
- 1 (28-ounce) can of tomatoes, crushed
- 2 tbsps of tomato ketchup
- 1 bell pepper, diced
- 4 cups of vegetable broth

INSTRUCTIONS

1. In a heavy-bottomed pot, heat the oil on medium heat. When it is hot, cook the carrots, onion, and peppers for about 4 minutes.
2. Sauté the garlic for a minute.
3. Mix in the spices, broth, tomatoes, ketchup, and canned lentils. Allow it to simmer while stirring occasionally for 20 minutes or until fully cooked.
4. Serve topped with avocado.
5. Enjoy your meal!

Nutritional Information: Calories: 475; Fat: 17.3g; Carbs: 61.4g; Protein: 23.7g

Brown Lentil Bowl

PREPARATION TIME: 5 MINUTES
COOK TIMING: 25 MINUTES
SERVES: 4

INGREDIENTS

- 2 cups of arugula
- 1 cup of brown lentils, soaked overnight and drained
- 2 cups of brown rice, cooked
- 1 zucchini, diced
- 2 cups of Romaine lettuce, torn into pieces
- 1 cucumber, sliced 1 bell pepper, sliced
- 3 cups of water
- 1 red onion, chopped
- 4 tbsps of olive oil
- 1 tbsp of rice vinegar
- 2 tbsps of lemon juice
- 1 teaspoon of garlic, minced
- 2 tbsps of soy sauce
- 1/2 teaspoon of dried oregano
- Sea salt and ground black pepper, to taste
- 1/2 teaspoon of ground cumin

INSTRUCTIONS

1. Put the brown lentils and water in a saucepan. Bring to a boil on high heat, then lower the heat to simmer for about 20 minutes until they are soft.
2. Transfer the cooked lentils to a salad bowl and allow them to cool down completely.
3. Mix in all the remaining ingredients and toss well to combine. Serve either at room temperature or chilled. Enjoy your meal!

Nutritional Information: Calories: 452; Fat: 16.6g; Carbs: 59.7g; Protein: 16.4g

HEALTHY SIDES AND SNACKS

Roasted Carrots with Herbs

PREPARATION TIME: 5 MINUTES
COOK TIMING: 25 MINUTES
SERVES: 6

INGREDIENTS

- 2 tbsps of fresh parsley, chopped
- 4 tbsps of olive oil
- 2 tbsps of fresh chives, chopped
- 1 teaspoon of granulated garlic
- 2 pounds of carrots, trimmed and halved lengthwise
- 1 teaspoon of paprika
- 2 tbsps of fresh cilantro, chopped
- Sea salt and freshly ground black pepper

INSTRUCTIONS

1. Begin by preheating your oven to 400°F.
2. Mix the carrots with some olive oil, granulated garlic, paprika, salt and black pepper. Place them in a layer on a baking sheet lined with parchment paper.
3. Roast the carrots in the preheated oven for 20 minutes until they are tender when pierced with a fork.
4. After roasting, toss the carrots with some fresh herbs.
5. Serve right away. Enjoy your meal!

Nutritional Information: Calories: 217; Fat: 14.4g; Carbs: 22.4g; Protein: 2.3g

Easy Braised Green Beans

PREPARATION TIME: 5 MINUTES
COOK TIMING: 20 MINUTES
SERVES: 4

INGREDIENTS

- 1 carrot, cut into matchsticks
- 4 tbsps of olive oil
- 1 ½ pounds of green beans, trimmed
- 1 lemon, cut into wedges
- 4 garlic cloves, peeled
- 1 ½ cups of vegetable broth
- 1 bay laurel
- Sea salt and ground black pepper, to taste

INSTRUCTIONS

1. Heat the olive oil in a saucepan on medium heat.
2. Once it is hot, sauté the carrots and green beans for 5 minutes, stirring occasionally to ensure they cook evenly.
3. Next, toss in the garlic and bay leaf. Continue cooking for another minute until you can smell the aromas.
4. Pour in the broth, salt, and black pepper, cover it up and let it simmer for around 9 to 10 minutes or until the green beans are nice and tender.
5. Give it a taste, adjust the seasonings as needed and serve with some lemon wedges.
6. Enjoy your meal!

Nutritional Information: Calories: 207; Fat: 14.5g; Carbs: 16.5g; Protein: 5.3g

Braised Kale with Sesame Seeds

PREPARATION TIME: 5 MINUTES
COOK TIMING: 10 MINUTES
SERVES: 4

INGREDIENTS

- 4 tbsps of sesame seeds, lightly toasted
- 1 cup of vegetable broth
- 4 tbsps of olive oil
- 1 pound of kale, cleaned, tough stems removed, torn into pieces
- 6 garlic cloves, chopped
- Kosher salt and ground black pepper, to taste
- 1 teaspoon of paprika

INSTRUCTIONS

1. In a saucepan, bring the vegetable broth to a boil. Add the kale leaves. Reduce the heat to a simmer. Allow it to cook for 5 minutes until the kale becomes tender; set aside.
2. Next, heat some oil in the pot over medium heat. Once it is hot, sauté the garlic for around 30 seconds until it releases its fragrance.
3. Then, mix in the reserved kale along with salt, paprika, and black pepper. Let it cook for a few minutes until everything is heated through.
4. Finish off by sprinkling some toasted sesame seeds on top as a garnish before serving right away.
5. Enjoy your meal!

Nutritional Information: Calories: 247; Fat: 19.9g; Carbs: 13.9g; Protein: 8.3g

Sautéed Zucchini with Herbs

PREPARATION TIME: 5 MINUTES
COOK TIMING: 10 MINUTES
SERVES: 4

INGREDIENTS

- 2 tbsps of olive oil
- 1/2 teaspoon of dried rosemary
- 1 onion, sliced
- 1 ½ pounds of zucchini, sliced
- 1 teaspoon of cayenne pepper
- Sea salt and fresh ground black pepper, to taste
- 1/2 teaspoon of dried basil
- 2 garlic cloves, minced
- 1/2 teaspoon of dried oregano

INSTRUCTIONS

1. Start by heating the olive oil in a saucepan on medium to high heat. Cook the onion until it softens which should take, about 3 minutes.
2. Next, sauté the garlic until it becomes fragrant, around 1 minute.
3. Introduce the zucchini and spices into the pan. Continue cooking for another 6 minutes until everything's tender.
4. Taste the dish. Adjust the seasonings to your liking. Enjoy your meal!

Nutritional Information: Calories: 99; Fat: 7.4g; Carbs: 6g; Protein: 4.3g

Sautéed Cauliflower with Sesame Seeds

PREPARATION TIME: 5 MINUTES
COOK TIMING: 15 MINUTES
SERVES: 4

INGREDIENTS

- 2 tbsps of sesame seeds, lightly toasted
- 4 tbsps of olive oil
- 1 cup of vegetable broth
- 2 scallion stalks, chopped
- 1 ½ pounds of cauliflower florets
- 4 garlic cloves, minced
- Sea salt and freshly ground black pepper, to taste

INSTRUCTIONS

1. In a saucepan, heat the broth until it boils.
2. Next, toss in the cauliflower and cook for around 6 minutes until it's soft when pierced with a fork. Set it aside.
3. After that, heat the olive oil hot and sauté the scallions and garlic for a minute until they are tender and smell nice.
4. Mix in the cauliflower you saved earlier then add some salt and black pepper. Let it simmer for 5 minutes or until everything is heated through.
5. Sprinkle with toasted seeds and serve right away.

Nutritional Information: Calories: 217; Fat: 17g; Carbs: 13.2g; Protein: 7.1g

Sautéed Turnip Greens

PREPARATION TIME: 5 MINUTES
COOK TIMING: 10 MINUTES
SERVES: 4

INGREDIENTS

- 1/4 cup of vegetable broth
- 2 tbsps of olive oil
- 1 ½ pounds of turnip greens cleaned and chopped
- 1 onion, sliced
- 1/4 cup of dry white wine
- 2 garlic cloves, sliced
- 1/2 teaspoon of dried oregano
- Kosher salt and ground black pepper, to taste
- 1 teaspoon of dried parsley flakes

INSTRUCTIONS

1. In a skillet, warm up the oil over medium heat.
2. Then, cook the onion for about 3 to 4 minutes until it is soft and see-through.
3. Then, add the garlic and cook for another 30 seconds until it smells fragrant.
4. Mix in the turnip greens, oregano, broth, wine, and parsley; continue sautéing for 6 minutes until they are fully wilted.
5. Season with salt and pepper to your liking. Serve while it is still warm.
6. Enjoy your meal!

Nutritional Information: Calories: 140; Fat: 8.8g; Carbs: 13g; Protein: 4.4g

Yukon Gold Mashed Potatoes

PREPARATION TIME: 5 MINUTES
COOK TIMING: 20 MINUTES
SERVES: 5

INGREDIENTS

- 1/2 cup of soy milk
- 2 pounds of Yukon Gold potatoes, peeled and diced
- Sea salt and red pepper flakes, to taste
- 3 tbsps of vegan butter
- 1 clove of garlic, pressed
- 2 tbsps of scallions, sliced

INSTRUCTIONS

1. Please make sure the potatoes are submerged in an inch or two of cold water.
2. Allow the potatoes to simmer in the boiling water for 20 minutes.
3. Next, blend the potatoes, with salt, garlic, red pepper, butter and milk until you achieve your desired texture.
4. Finally, serve with a sprinkle of scallions.
5. Enjoy your meal!

Nutritional Information: Calories: 221; Fat: 7.9g; Carbs: 34.1g; Protein: 4.7g

Aromatic Sautéed Swiss Chard

PREPARATION TIME: 5 MINUTES
COOK TIMING: 15 MINUTES
SERVES: 4

INGREDIENTS

- 1 ½ pounds of Swiss chard, torn into pieces, remove the tough stalks
- 2 cloves of garlic, sliced
- 1 onion, chopped
- 1 thyme sprig
- Sea salt and ground black pepper, to season
- 1 cup of vegetable broth
- 2 tbsps of vegan butter
- 1 bay leaf
- 2 rosemary sprigs
- 1 teaspoon of celery seeds
- 1/2 teaspoon of mustard seeds

INSTRUCTIONS

1. Start by melting the plant-based butter in a saucepan on medium heat.
2. Next, cook the onion for 3 minutes until it becomes soft and see-through; then sauté the garlic for around 1 minute until it releases its aroma.
3. Combine all of the remaining ingredients and reduce the heat to a simmer; cover the mixture and allow it to simmer for 10 minutes until everything is fully cooked.
4. Enjoy your meal!

Nutritional Information: Calories: 124; Fat: 6.7g; Carbs: 11.1g; Protein: 5g

Classic Sautéed Bell Peppers

PREPARATION TIME: 5 MINUTES
COOK TIMING: 15 MINUTES
SERVES: 2

INGREDIENTS

- 2 cloves of garlic, minced
- 4 bell peppers, seeded and sliced into strips
- 2 tbsps of fresh cilantro, roughly chopped
- Salt and freshly ground black pepper, to taste
- 1 teaspoon of cayenne pepper
- 3 tbsps of olive oil
- 4 tbsps of dry white wine

INSTRUCTIONS

1. Heat the oil in a saucepan over medium heat. Sauté the peppers until they are soft and aromatic which should take 4 minutes.
2. Next, cook the garlic until it releases its aroma for around 1 minute.
3. Season with black pepper, salt, and cayenne pepper. Continue cooking while adding wine for another 6 minutes until everything is tender and fully cooked.
4. Adjust the seasonings as needed.
5. Finish by garnishing with cilantro before serving.
6. Enjoy your meal!

Nutritional Information: Calories: 154; Fat: 13.7g; Carbs: 2.9g; Protein: 0.5g

Roasted Garden Vegetables

PREPARATION TIME: 5 MINUTES
COOK TIMING: 40 MINUTES
SERVES: 4

INGREDIENTS

- 4 sweet potatoes, peeled and cut into one-inch pieces
- 1 teaspoon of dried rosemary
- 1/2 cup of carrots, peeled and cut into one-inch pieces
- 1 teaspoon of paprika
- 2 medium onions, cut into wedges
- 1 pound of butternut squash, peeled and cut into one-inch pieces
- 4 tbsps of olive oil
- 1 teaspoon of granulated garlic
- Kosher salt and freshly ground black pepper, to taste
- 1 teaspoon of mustard seeds

INSTRUCTIONS

1. Begin by preheating your oven to 420 degrees Fahrenheit.
2. Mix the vegetables with the olive oil and seasonings. Place them on a baking sheet lined with parchment paper.
3. Roast for around 25 minutes.
4. Stir the vegetables and keep cooking for another 20 minutes.
5. Serve and enjoy.

Nutritional Information: Calories: 311; Fat: 14.1g; Carbs: 45.2g; Protein: 3.9g

Herb Cauliflower Mash

PREPARATION TIME: 5 MINUTES
COOK TIMING: 20 MINUTES
SERVES: 4

INGREDIENTS

- 4 tbsps of vegan butter
- 2 tbsps of fresh parsley, roughly chopped
- 4 cloves of garlic, sliced
- 1/4 cup of plain oat milk, unsweetened
- Sea salt and ground black pepper, to taste
- 1 ½ pounds of cauliflower florets

INSTRUCTIONS

1. Steam the cauliflower pieces for 20 minutes then allow them to cool.
2. In a saucepan, melt the plant-based butter over high heat. Next, sauté the garlic for around 1 minute until fragrant.
3. Transfer the steamed cauliflower to a food processor along with the sautéed garlic, pepper, salt, and oat milk.
4. Blend until smooth and creamy.
5. Finish by topping with parsley leaves before serving.

Nutritional Information: Calories: 167; Fat: 13g; Carbs: 11.3g; Protein: 4.4g

Creamy Rosemary Broccoli Mash

PREPARATION TIME: 5 MINUTES
COOK TIMING: 15 MINUTES
SERVES: 4

INGREDIENTS

- 3 tbsps of vegan butter
- 1 ½ pounds of broccoli florets
- 4 cloves of garlic, chopped
- Sea salt and red pepper, to taste
- 2 sprigs of fresh rosemary, leaves picked and chopped
- 1/4 cup of soy milk, unsweetened

INSTRUCTIONS

1. Steam the broccoli pieces for 10 minutes. Let them cool.
2. In a saucepan, melt vegan butter over high heat; then sauté the garlic and rosemary until fragrant, about 1 minute.
3. Combine the steamed broccoli with the sautéed garlic and rosemary, pepper, salt, and milk in a food processor.
4. Blend until smooth. If desired, top with herbs before serving hot.
5. Enjoy your meal!

Nutritional Information: Calories: 155; Fat: 9.8g; Carbs: 14.1g; Protein: 5.7g

Carrot Energy Balls

PREPARATION TIME: 5 MINUTES
COOK TIMING: 0 MINUTES
SERVES: 8

INGREDIENTS

- 1 ½ cups of old-fashioned oats
- 1 large carrot, grated carrot
- 1/2 teaspoon of ground cinnamon
- 1 cup of raisins 1 cup dates, pitied
- 1/4 teaspoon of ground cloves
- 1 cup of coconut flakes

INSTRUCTIONS

1. In your food processor, pulse all the ingredients until they come together to form a consistent mixture.
2. Form the dough into balls. Keep them in the refrigerator until you are prepared to serve.
3. Enjoy your meal!

Nutritional Information: Calories: 495; Fat: 21.1g; Carbs: 58.4g; Protein: 22.1g

Oven-Baked Kale Chips

PREPARATION TIME: 5 MINUTES
COOK TIMING: 20 MINUTES
SERVES: 8

INGREDIENTS

- 1/2 teaspoon of mustard seeds
- 2 bunches of kale, leaves separated
- 1/2 teaspoon of celery seeds
- 2 tbsps of olive oil
- 1/2 teaspoon of dried oregano
- 1 teaspoon of garlic powder
- 1/4 teaspoon of ground cumin
- Coarse sea salt and ground black pepper, to taste

INSTRUCTIONS

1. Begin by preheating your oven to 340°F.
2. Prepare a baking sheet by lining it with parchment paper.
3. Mix the kale leaves with the remaining ingredients until they are evenly coated.
4. Place the baking sheet in the oven and bake for approximately 13 minutes, remembering to rotate the pan occasionally.
5. Enjoy your meal!

Nutritional Information: Calories: 65; Fat: 3.9g; Carbs: 5.3g; Protein: 2.4g

Peppery Hummus Dip

PREPARATION TIME: 10 MINUTES
COOK TIMING: 0 MINUTES
SERVES: 8

INGREDIENTS

- 2 tbsps of olive oil
- 20 ounces of canned or boiled chickpeas, drained
- 2 garlic cloves, minced
- 1/2 teaspoon of paprika
- 2 tbsps of lemon juice, freshly squeezed
- 1/2 cup of chickpea liquid
- 2 red roasted peppers, seeded and sliced
- 1/4 cup of tahini
- Sea salt and ground black pepper, to taste
- 1 teaspoon of dried basil

INSTRUCTIONS

1. Mix all the ingredients in a blender or food processor, excluding the oil, until you achieve your desired texture.
2. Chill in the refrigerator until you are ready to enjoy it.
3. Pair with toasted pita slices or chips, if you like.
4. Enjoy your meal!

Nutritional Information: Calories: 155; Fat: 7.9g; Carbs: 17.4g; Protein: 5.9g

Roasted Chickpeas

PREPARATION TIME: 5 MINUTES
COOK TIMING: 30 MINUTES
SERVES: 2

INGREDIENTS

- 1 teaspoon of curry powder
- 2 cups of canned chickpeas, drained
- 1/2 teaspoon of paprika
- 2 tbsps of olive oil
- 1/2 teaspoon of garlic powder
- Sea salt and red pepper, to taste
- 1 teaspoon of garam masala

INSTRUCTIONS

1. Pat dry the chickpeas with paper towels.
2. Drizzle some olive oil over the chickpeas.
3. Place the chickpeas in an oven at 400°F.
4. Roast for approximately 25 minutes, giving them a toss once or twice during cooking.
5. Mix your chickpeas with the spices.
6. Savor the flavors!

Nutritional Information: Calories: 223; Fat: 6.4g; Carbs: 32.2g; Protein: 10.4g

Traditional Baba Ganoush

PREPARATION TIME: 5 MINUTES
COOK TIMING: 25 MINUTES
SERVES: 8

INGREDIENTS

- 3 tbsps of olive oil
- 1 pound of eggplant, cut into rounds
- 3 tbsps of tahini
- 1/4 teaspoon of ground cloves
- 1 teaspoon of coarse sea salt
- 2 cloves of garlic, minced
- 1/2 teaspoon of ground cumin
- 3 tbsps of fresh lime juice
- 2 tbsps of fresh parsley, roughly chopped

INSTRUCTIONS

1. Rub the sea salt over the slices of eggplant.
2. Next, place them in a strainer. Allow them to rest for 15 minutes. Drain, rinse and gently dry with kitchen towels.
3. Roast the eggplant until the skin darkens; then peel it. Place it in your food processor bowl.
4. Combine olive oil, lime juice, cloves, tahini, garlic, and cumin. Blend until everything is thoroughly mixed.
5. Finish off with a sprinkle of parsley leaves for added flavor.
6. Enjoy your dish!

Nutritional Information: Calories: 104; Fat: 8.2g; Carbs: 5.3g; Protein: 1.6g

Roasted Cauliflower Dip

PREPARATION TIME: 5 MINUTES
COOK TIMING: 25 MINUTES
SERVES: 7

INGREDIENTS

- 1/4 cup of olive oil
- 1 pound of cauliflower florets
- 1/2 teaspoon of paprika
- 2 cloves of garlic, minced
- Sea salt and ground black pepper, to taste
- 2 tbsps of fresh lime juice
- 4 tbsps of tahini

INSTRUCTIONS

1. Begin by preheating your oven to 420°F.
2. Mix the cauliflower florets with the olive oil. Place them on a baking sheet lined with parchment paper.
3. Bake for 25 minutes. Until the cauliflower is tender.
4. Next, blend the cauliflower with the ingredients, adding cooking liquid as necessary.
5. Add a touch of oil for flavor if you like.
6. Enjoy your meal!

Nutritional Information: Calories: 142; Fat: 12.5g; Carbs: 6.3g; Protein: 2.9g

Easy Zucchini Roll-Ups

PREPARATION TIME: 10 MINUTES
COOK TIMING: 0 MINUTES
SERVES: 5

INGREDIENTS

- 2 tbsps of fresh parsley, chopped
- 1 medium tomato, chopped
- 1/4 teaspoon of oregano
- 1 cup of hummus, preferably homemade
- 1/2 teaspoon of cayenne pepper
- 1 teaspoon of mustard
- Sea salt and ground black pepper, to taste
- 2 tbsps of fresh basil, chopped
- 1 large zucchini, cut into strips

INSTRUCTIONS

1. In a bowl, mix together the hummus, salt, tomato, cayenne, mustard, oregano, pepper, and black pepper until combined.
2. Spread the filling evenly among the zucchini strips.
3. Roll up the zucchini and top it off with basil and parsley.
4. Enjoy your meal!

Nutritional Information: Calories: 99; Fat: 4.4g; Carbs: 12.1g; Protein: 3.1g

Oven-Roasted Button Mushrooms

PREPARATION TIME: 5 MINUTES
COOK TIMING: 20 MINUTES
SERVES: 4

INGREDIENTS

- 3 tbsps of olive oil
- 1 ½ pounds of button mushrooms, cleaned
- 1 teaspoon of dried oregano
- 3 garlic of cloves, minced
- 1 teaspoon of dried basil
- Kosher salt and ground black pepper, to taste
- 1/2 teaspoon of dried rosemary

INSTRUCTIONS

1. Mix the mushrooms with the remaining ingredients.
2. Place the mushrooms on a baking sheet lined with parchment paper.
3. Cook the mushrooms in the oven preheated to 420°F for around 20 minutes until they are soft and aromatic.
4. Transfer the mushrooms to a serving dish.
5. Enjoy them with toothpicks.

Nutritional Information: Calories: 136; Fat: 10.5g; Carbs: 7.6g; Protein: 5.6g

Hummus Avocado Boats

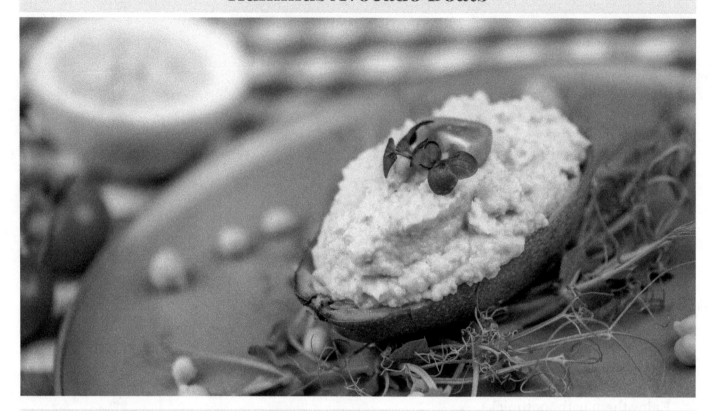

PREPARATION TIME: 10 MINUTES
COOK TIMING: 0 MINUTES
SERVES: 4

INGREDIENTS

- 2 ripe avocados, halved and pitted
- 1 tbsp of fresh lemon juice
- 1 medium tomato, chopped
- Sea salt and ground black pepper, to taste
- 1 tbsp of tahini
- 1/2 teaspoon of turmeric powder
- 8 ounces of hummus
- 1/2 teaspoon of cayenne pepper
- 1 garlic clove, minced

INSTRUCTIONS

1. Drizzle the squeezed lemon juice on the avocado halves, then combine the hummus, garlic, tomato, salt, turmeric powder, black pepper, cayenne pepper, and tahini.
2. Fill your avocados with this mixture. Serve right away.

Nutritional Information: Calories: 297; Fat: 21.2g; Carbs: 23.9g; Protein: 6g

Lettuce Wraps with Hummus and Avocado

PREPARATION TIME: 5 MINUTES
COOK TIMING: 0 MINUTES
SERVES: 2

INGREDIENTS

- 1 medium avocado, pitted and diced
- 1/2 cup of hummus
- 1 teaspoon of garlic, minced
- 1 carrot, shredded
- 1 teaspoon of white vinegar
- 1 head of butter lettuce, separated into leaves
- 1 teaspoon of soy sauce
- 1 tomato, chopped
- 1 teaspoon of agave syrup
- 1 teaspoon of ginger, freshly grated
- Kosher salt and ground black pepper, to taste
- 1 tbsp of Sriracha sauce

INSTRUCTIONS

1. Mix the hummus, tomato, carrot and avocado together thoroughly.
2. Combine vinegar soy sauce, agave syrup, Sriracha sauce, garlic, ginger, salt and black pepper.
3. Distribute the filling among lettuce leaves, roll them up, and serve with sauce on the side.
4. Enjoy your meal!

Nutritional Information: Calories: 115; Fat: 6.9g; Carbs: 11.6g; Protein: 2.6g

Baked Zucchini Chips

PREPARATION TIME: 5 MINUTES
COOK TIMING: 0 MINUTES
SERVES: 7

INGREDIENTS

- 1/2 teaspoon of dried oregano
- 1 pound of zucchini, cut into 1/8-inch thick slices
- Sea salt and ground black pepper, to taste
- 1/2 teaspoon of dried basil
- 2 tbsps of olive oil
- 1/2 teaspoon of red pepper flakes

INSTRUCTIONS

1. Mix the zucchini with all of the other ingredients.
2. Arrange the zucchini slices in one layer on a baking sheet lined with parchment paper.
3. Place in the oven at 235°F for 90 minutes until they turn crispy and golden brown.
4. The zucchini chips will become crunchy as they cool down. Enjoy your meal!

Nutritional Information: Calories: 48; Fat: 4.2g; Carbs: 2g; Protein: 1.7g

Bell Pepper Boats with Mango Salsa

PREPARATION TIME: 5 MINUTES
COOK TIMING: 0 MINUTES
SERVES: 4

INGREDIENTS

- 1 small shallot, chopped
- 4 bell peppers, seeded and halved
- 1 mango, peeled, pitted, cubed
- 2 tbsps of fresh cilantro, minced
- 1 tbsp of fresh lime juice
- 1 red chile pepper, seeded and chopped

INSTRUCTIONS

1. Mix together the mango, shallot, cilantro, red chili pepper, and lime juice thoroughly.
2. Scoop the blend into the halves of the peppers.
3. Serve immediately and enjoy.

Nutritional Information: Calories: 74; Fat: 1g; Carbs: 17.6g; Protein: 2g

Stuffed Portobellos with Rice and Herbs

PREPARATION TIME: 5 MINUTES
COOK TIMING: 20 MINUTES
SERVES: 6

INGREDIENTS

- 1 cup of cooked brown rice
- 1 red bell pepper, seeded and chopped
- 1 garlic clove, minced
- 3 tbsps of scallions, chopped
- 1/4 cup of raw walnuts, crushed
- 1 tbsp of parsley, minced
- 1 tbsp of cilantro, minced
- 1/2 teaspoon of smoked paprika
- 1 teaspoon of cayenne pepper
- Sea salt and ground black pepper, to taste
- 2 tbsps of olive oil
- 1 tbsp of basil, minced
- 6 portobello mushrooms, stems removed

INSTRUCTIONS

1. Mix together the rice, garlic, walnuts, scallions, pepper, herbs, and spices thoroughly.
2. Evenly distribute the mixture into each mushroom.
3. Drizzle some olive oil over the mushrooms.
4. Place them in the oven preheated to 350°F and bake for 20 minutes until they are tender and fully cooked.
5. Serve and enjoy.

Nutritional Information: Calories: 125; Fat: 7g; Carbs: 13.2g; Protein: 3.6g

NATURAL SWEETS AND DESSERTS

Peanut Butter Date Bites

PREPARATION TIME: 5 MINUTES
COOK TIMING: 0 MINUTES
SERVES: 2

INGREDIENTS

- 8 teaspoons of peanut butter
- 8 fresh dates, pitted and cut into halves
- 1/4 teaspoon of ground cinnamon

INSTRUCTIONS

1. Spread the peanut butter evenly on each half of the dates.
2. Sprinkle a bit of cinnamon on top.
3. Serve immediately.

Nutritional Information: Calories: 143; Fat: 3.9g; Carbs: 26.3g; Protein: 2.6g

Chocolate N'ice Cream

PREPARATION TIME: 5 MINUTES
COOK TIMING: 0 MINUTES
SERVES: 2

INGREDIENTS

- 1 tbsp of chocolate curls
- 2 tbsps of coconut milk
- 1 teaspoon of cocoa powder
- A pinch of grated nutmeg
- 1/8 teaspoon of ground cardamom
- 2 frozen bananas, peeled and sliced
- 1/8 teaspoon of ground cinnamon
- 1 teaspoon of carob powder

INSTRUCTIONS

1. Put all the ingredients in the food processor or a high-speed blender.
2. Blend everything until smooth or until you reach the texture you prefer.
3. Serve immediately, or keep it in the freezer.

Nutritional Information: Calories: 349; Fat: 2.8g; Carbs: 46.1g; Protein: 4.8g

Almond and Chocolate Chip Bars

PREPARATION TIME: 45 MINUTES
COOK TIMING: 0 MINUTES
SERVES: 10

INGREDIENTS

- 1/4 cup of coconut oil, melted
- 1/2 cup of almond butter
- 1/4 cup of agave syrup
- 1 teaspoon of vanilla extract
- 1/4 teaspoon of grated nutmeg
- 1/2 teaspoon of ground cinnamon
- 2 cups of almond flour
- 1/4 cup of agave syrup
- 1 cup of vegan chocolate, cut into chunks
- 1/4 teaspoon of sea salt
- 1 1/3 cups of almonds, ground
- 2 tbsps of cacao powder
- 1/4 cup of flaxseed meal

INSTRUCTIONS

1. In a mixing bowl, thoroughly mix together the almond butter, nutmeg, coconut oil, 1/4 cup of agave syrup, vanilla, salt, and cinnamon.
2. Slowly incorporate the almond flour and flaxseed meal while stirring to mix. Add the chocolate chunks and mix well.
3. In a mixing bowl, mix the almonds, cacao powder, and agave syrup together.
4. Next, spread the ganache over the cake.
5. Place in the freezer for 30 minutes, then cut into bars.
6. Serve chilled, and enjoy!

Nutritional Information: Calories: 295; Fat: 17g; Carbs: 35.2g; Protein: 1.7g

Peanut Butter Oatmeal Bars

PREPARATION TIME: 5 MINUTES
COOK TIMING: 25 MINUTES
SERVES: 10

INGREDIENTS

- 1 teaspoon of pure vanilla extract
- 3/4 cup of coconut sugar
- 1 cup of whole-wheat flour
- 2 tbsps of applesauce
- 1 ¾ cups of old-fashioned oats
- 1 cup of vegan butter
- A pinch of sea salt
- 1 teaspoon of baking soda
- A pinch of grated nutmeg
- 1 cup of oat flour

INSTRUCTIONS

1. Start by preheating your oven to 350°F.
2. Mix together the dry ingredients in a mixing bowl.
3. In another bowl, combine the wet ingredients.
4. Next, gently fold the wet mixture into the dry ingredients until well combined.
5. Pour the batter into a baking pan lined with parchment paper.
6. Place the pan in the oven.
7. Bake for approximately 20 minutes.
8. Enjoy your creation!

Nutritional Information: Calories: 161; Fat: 10.3g; Carbs: 17.5g; Protein: 2.9g

Raw Chocolate Mango Pie

PREPARATION TIME: 15 MINUTES
COOK TIMING: 0 MINUTES
SERVES: 10

INGREDIENTS

- **Avocado layer:**
- 2 tbsps of coconut milk
- 5 tbsps of agave syrup
- 3 ripe avocados, pitted and peeled
- A pinch of sea salt
- 1/3 cup of cocoa powder
- A pinch of ground anise
- 1/2 teaspoon of vanilla paste
- **Crema layer:**
- 1/2 coconut flakes
- 1/3 cup of almond butter
- 2 tbsps of agave syrup
- 1/2 cup of coconut cream
- 1 medium mango, peeled

INSTRUCTIONS

1. In a food processor, combine the avocado layer until it becomes smooth and consistent; set aside.
2. Next, mix the other layer in a bowl. Scoop the layers into a greased baking dish.
3. Place the cake in the freezer for 3 hours. Keep it stored in the freezer.
4. Enjoy your meal!

Nutritional Information: Calories: 196; Fat: 16.8g; Carbs: 14.1g; Protein: 1.8g

Mini Lemon Tarts

PREPARATION TIME: 15 MINUTES
COOK TIMING: 0 MINUTES
SERVES: 9

INGREDIENTS

- 1/2 cup of coconut flakes
- 1 cup of cashews
- 2 tbsps of agave syrup
- 1 cup of dates, pitted
- 3 lemons, freshly squeezed
- 1 cup of coconut cream
- 1/2 teaspoon of anise, ground

INSTRUCTIONS

1. Grease a muffin tray with nonstick cooking spray.
2. Combine cashews, coconut, dates, and anise in a food processor or high-speed blender.
3. Press the mixture into the muffin tin.
4. Next, blend together coconut cream, lemon, and agave syrup. Spoon the cream mixture into the muffin tin.
5. Place in the freezer.
6. Serve and enjoy.

Nutritional Information: Calories: 257; Fat: 16.5g; Carbs: 25.4g; Protein: 4g

Peanut Butter Fudge

PREPARATION TIME: 15 MINUTES
COOK TIMING: 5 MINUTES
SERVES: 10

INGREDIENTS

- 4 tbsps of maple syrup
- 12 ounces of peanut butter, smooth
- 4 tbsps of coconut cream
- Pinch of salt
- 3 tbsps of coconut oil

INSTRUCTIONS

1. Line a baking tray with parchment paper.
2. Gently heat the coconut and maple syrup in a saucepan for around 2 minutes until melted.
3. Add the peanut butter, coconut cream, and salt to the saucepan, mixing thoroughly.
4. Transfer the fudge mixture to the prepared baking dish. Refrigerate for an hour.
5. Cut into pieces, serve, and savor!

Nutritional Information: Calories: 135; Fat: 11.3g; Carbs: 6.2g; Protein: 4.3g

Almond-Date Energy Bites

PREPARATION TIME: 15 MINUTES
COOK TIMING: 0 MINUTES
SERVES: 8 TO 10

INGREDIENTS

- ¼ cup of chia seeds
- 1 cup of dates, pitted
- ¼ cup of cocoa nibs, or non-dairy chocolate chips
- 1 cup of unsweetened shredded coconut
- ¾ cup of ground almonds

INSTRUCTIONS

1. Blend all the ingredients in a food processor until they form a mixture that sticks together, making sure to scrape down the sides as needed to ensure blending. If you don't have a food processor, you can use Medjool dates and mash them instead. For baking dates, soak them first and then attempt to blend them in a blender.
2. Shape the mixture into 24 balls. Place them on a baking sheet lined with parchment or waxed paper. Chill in the refrigerator for 15 minutes or until set.
3. Serve and enjoy.

Nutritional Information: Calories: 152; Fat: 11g; Carbs: 13g; Protein: 3g

Easy Chocolate Squares

PREPARATION TIME: 10 MINUTES
COOK TIMING: 0 MINUTES
SERVES: 10 TO 12

INGREDIENTS

- 1/4 teaspoon of ground cinnamon
- 1 cup of almond butter
- 1/4 cup of coconut oil, melted
- 1 cup of cashew butter
- 1/4 cup of raw cacao powder
- 2 ounces of dark chocolate
- 1/4 teaspoon of ground cloves
- 4 tbsps of agave syrup
- 1 teaspoon of vanilla paste

INSTRUCTIONS

1. Blend all the ingredients in your blender until they are well-mixed and smooth.
2. Transfer the mixture onto a baking sheet lined with parchment paper.
3. Place it in the freezer for an hour to allow it to firm up.
4. Cut it into squares and serve.

Nutritional Information: Calories: 187; Fat: 13.8g; Carbs: 15.1g; Protein: 2.9g

Zesty Orange-Cranberry Energy Bites

PREPARATION TIME: 5 MINUTES
COOK TIMING: 0 MINUTES
SERVES: 4 TO 6

INGREDIENTS

- ½ teaspoon of almond extract, or vanilla extract
- 2 tbsps of almond butter, or cashew or sunflower seed butter
- ¼ cup of ground almonds
- 2 tbsps of maple syrup
- ¼ cup of sesame seeds, toasted
- 1 tbsp of chia seeds
- Zest of 1 orange
- ¾ cup of cooked quinoa
- 1 tbsp of dried cranberries

INSTRUCTIONS

1. In a bowl, mix the nut or seed butter with the syrup until it becomes smooth and creamy.
2. Add the remaining ingredients and ensure that the mixture holds together in a ball.
3. Shape the mixture into 12 balls, then place them on a baking sheet lined with parchment or waxed paper.
4. Allow them to chill in the fridge for 15 minutes to set.

Nutritional Information: Calories: 109; Fat: 7g; Carbs: 11g; Protein: 3g

Tropi-Colada Frozen Pops

PREPARATION TIME: 10 MINUTES
COOK TIMING: 0 MINUTES
SERVES: 6

INGREDIENTS

- 2 cups of chopped fresh pineapple
- ½ cup of unsweetened shredded coconut
- 1 cup of chopped mango, fresh or frozen
- ¾ cup of canned coconut milk

INSTRUCTIONS

1. Blend all the ingredients in a food processor or blender until they are mostly smooth, leaving some pieces for texture.
2. Pour the mixture into ice pop molds, making sure to leave a space at the top for it to expand as it freezes.
3. Place the molds in the freezer until the pops are completely frozen.
4. Serve and enjoy.

Nutritional Information: Calories: 224; Fat: 18g; Carbs: 17g; Protein: 2g

Funky Monkey Sorbet

PREPARATION TIME: 10 MINUTES
COOK TIMING: 0 MINUTES
SERVES: 1

INGREDIENTS

- 1 tbsp of almond butter, or peanut butter, or other seed or nut butter
- ½ Banana chocolate cupcake, crumbled
- 1 frozen banana
- 2 to 3 tbsps of non-dairy milk, or water (only if needed)
- 1 tbsp of walnuts, chopped

INSTRUCTIONS

1. Blend the banana and almond butter in a food processor or blender until smooth. If necessary, add some non-dairy milk to help with blending, but only if necessary to maintain a solid texture.
2. Then mix in the walnuts and cupcake pieces, or simply sprinkle them on top.
3. Enjoy immediately. If the mixture seems soft, chill it in the freezer for a few minutes.

Nutritional Information: Calories: 225; Fat: 11g; Carbs: 31g; Protein: 5g

Mango Coconut Cream Pie

PREPARATION TIME: 15 MINUTES
COOK TIMING: 0 MINUTES
SERVES: 8

INGREDIENTS

For the Crust:
- 1 cup of cashews
- ½ cup of rolled oats
- 1 cup of soft pitted dates

For the Filling:
- 2 large mangos, peeled and chopped, or around 2 cups of frozen chunks
- ½ cup of unsweetened shredded coconut
- 1 cup of canned coconut milk
- ½ cup of water

INSTRUCTIONS

1. Combine all the ingredients for the crust in a food processor and blend until they stick together. If you don't have a food processor, finely chop everything. Substitute half of the cashews with ½ cup of cashew or almond butter. Press the mixture firmly into an 8-inch pie or springform pan.
2. Blend all the filling ingredients in a blender until 1 minute. The mixture should be thick, so you may need to pause and stir occasionally to achieve a smooth consistency.
3. Pour the filling onto the crust, use a rubber spatula to smooth out the top, and place the pie in the freezer for about 30 minutes until it sets.
4. Once frozen, allow it to sit out for 15 minutes before serving after removing it from the freezer to soften slightly.

Nutritional Information: Calories: 427; Fat: 28g; Carbs: 45g; Protein: 8g

Chocolate and Raisin Cookie Bars

PREPARATION TIME: 5 MINUTES
COOK TIMING: 0 MINUTES
SERVES: 2

INGREDIENTS

- 2 cups of almond flour
- 1 cup of agave syrup
- 1 teaspoon of pure vanilla extract
- 1 cup of vegan chocolate, broken into chunks
- 1/4 teaspoon of kosher salt
- 1 teaspoon of baking soda
- 1/2 cup of peanut butter, at room temperature
- 1 cup of raisins

INSTRUCTIONS

1. Mix together the peanut butter, vanilla, agave syrup, and salt in a bowl until well combined.
2. Slowly incorporate the almond flour and baking soda while stirring to blend everything
3. Include the raisins and chocolate chunks into the mixture and stir more.
4. Place in the freezer for around 30 minutes before serving chilled.
5. Serve and enjoy.

Nutritional Information: Calories: 267; Fat: 3g; Carbs: 51.1g; Protein: 2.2g

Lime in the Coconut Chia Pudding

PREPARATION TIME: 10 MINUTES
COOK TIMING: 0 MINUTES
SERVES: 3 TO 4

INGREDIENTS

- 2 teaspoons of matcha green tea powder (optional)
- Zest and juice of 1 lime
- 1 (14-ounce) can of coconut milk
- 2 tbsps of chia seeds, whole or ground
- 1 to 2 dates, or 1 tbsp of coconut sugar, or 1 tbsp of maple syrup

INSTRUCTIONS

1. Mix together all the ingredients using a blender until they reach a smooth consistency.
2. Let it cool in the refrigerator for 20 minutes then present it with your choice of toppings.
3. Serve and enjoy.

Nutritional Information: Calories: 226; Fat: 20g; Carbs: 13g; Protein: 3g

Almond Granola Bars

PREPARATION TIME: 10 MINUTES
COOK TIMING: 20 MINUTES
SERVES: 6 TO 8

INGREDIENTS

- 1 cup of rolled oats
- 1/2 cup of spelt flour
- 1 teaspoon of baking powder
- 1/2 teaspoon of cinnamon
- 1/2 cup of oat flour
- 1/4 teaspoon of freshly grated nutmeg
- 1/2 cup of peanut butter
- 1/8 teaspoon of kosher salt
- 1 cup almond of milk
- 1/2 teaspoon of pure almond extract
- 3 tbsps of agave syrup
- 1/2 cup of applesauce
- 1/2 teaspoon of pure vanilla extract
- 1/2 cup of almonds, slivered
- 1/2 teaspoon of ground cardamom

INSTRUCTIONS

1. Start by preheating your oven to 350°F.
2. In a mixing bowl, thoroughly mix together the flour, baking powder, oats, and spices. In another bowl, combine the wet ingredients.
3. Next, blend the wet mixture into the dry ingredients until well combined.
4. Gently incorporate the slivered almonds.
5. Transfer the batter to a baking pan lined with parchment paper.
6. Place it in the oven. Bake for approximately 20 minutes.
7. Allow it to cool on a wire rack.
8. Slice into bars. Savor each bite!

Nutritional Information: Calories: 147; Fat: 5.9g; Carbs: 21.7g; Protein: 5.2g

Chocolate Dream Balls

PREPARATION TIME: 15 MINUTES
COOK TIMING: 0 MINUTES
SERVES: 8

INGREDIENTS

- 8 fresh dates, pitted and soaked for 15 minutes
- 1 tbsp of coconut oil, at room temperature
- 2 tbsps of tahini, at room temperature
- 1/2 teaspoon of ground cinnamon
- 3 tbsps of cocoa powder
- 1/2 cup of vegan chocolate, broken into chunks

INSTRUCTIONS

1. Combine the cocoa powder, dates, tahini and cinnamon in the bowl of your food processor.
2. Blend until the mixture comes together to form a ball. Use a cookie scoop to shape the mixture into 1-ounce portions.
3. Shape the balls. Place them in the refrigerator for at least 30 minutes.
4. In the meantime, heat the chocolate in the microwave until it melts; then mix in the coconut oil and whisk until combined.
5. Coat the balls with coating. Keep them refrigerated until you are ready to enjoy them. Enjoy your treat!

Nutritional Information: Calories: 107; Fat: 7.2g; Carbs: 10.8g; Protein: 1.8g

Last-Minute Macaroons

PREPARATION TIME: 10 MINUTES
COOK TIMING: 15 MINUTES
SERVES: 10

INGREDIENTS

- 1 teaspoon of ground anise
- 9 ounces of canned coconut milk, sweetened
- 1 teaspoon of vanilla extract
- 3 cups of coconut flakes, sweetened

INSTRUCTIONS

1. Start by preheating your oven to 325°F.
2. Place parchment paper on the baking sheets.
3. Mix all the ingredients together until they are well combined.
4. Use a cookie scoop to place dollops of the dough onto the baking sheets.
5. Bake for around 11 to 12 minutes until they turn golden brown. Enjoy your treat!

Nutritional Information: Calories: 125; Fat: 7.2g; Carbs: 14.3g; Protein: 1.1g

Chocolate Hazelnut Fudge

PREPARATION TIME: 15 MINUTES
COOK TIMING: 0 MINUTES
SERVES: 10

INGREDIENTS

- 1 teaspoon of matcha powder
- 1/4 cup of cocoa powder
- 1 cup of cashew butter
- 1/4 teaspoon of ground cloves
- 1 teaspoon of vanilla extract
- 1/2 cup of hazelnuts, coarsely chopped
- 1 cup of fresh dates, pitted

INSTRUCTIONS

1. Blend all the ingredients together until they are well-mixed and smooth.
2. Transfer the batter onto a baking sheet lined with parchment paper.
3. Put it in the freezer for a minimum of 1 hour to allow it to firm up.
4. Slice into squares and enjoy your treat.

Nutritional Information: Calories: 140; Fat: 11g; Carbs: 4.6g; Protein: 10.6g

Decadent Hazelnut Halvah

PREPARATION TIME: 15 MINUTES
COOK TIMING: 0 MINUTES
SERVES: 8

INGREDIENTS

- 1/2 cup of tahini
- 4 tbsps of agave nectar
- 1/2 cup of almond butter
- 1/2 teaspoon of pure almond extract
- 1/8 teaspoon of freshly grated nutmeg
- 1/2 teaspoon of pure vanilla extract
- 1/8 teaspoon of salt
- 1/2 cup of hazelnuts, chopped
- 1/4 cup of coconut oil, melted

INSTRUCTIONS

1. Prepare a baking pan by lining it with parchment paper.
2. Combine all the ingredients, excluding the hazelnuts, until they are thoroughly mixed.
3. Transfer the batter to the pan lined with parchment paper.
4. Gently press the hazelnuts into the batter. Place the pan in the freezer until you are ready to enjoy.
5. Enjoy your meal!

Nutritional Information: Calories: 169; Fat: 15.5g; Carbs: 6.6g; Protein: 1.9g

Berry Compote with Red Wine

PREPARATION TIME: 5 MINUTES
COOK TIMING: 20 MINUTES
SERVES: 4

INGREDIENTS

- 1 cup of sweet red wine
- A pinch of grated nutmeg
- 1 cup of agave syrup
- 4 cups of mixed berries, fresh or frozen
- 1/2 teaspoon of star anise
- 3 to 4 cloves
- 1 cinnamon stick
- A pinch of sea salt

INSTRUCTIONS

1. Put all the ingredients into a saucepan.
2. Make sure the water covers the ingredients by an inch.
3. Bring it to a boil and then lower the heat to let it simmer.
4. Leave it to simmer for 9 to 11 minutes.
5. Let it cool down completely before enjoying your meal!

Nutritional Information: Calories: 260; Fat: 0.5g; Carbs: 54.1g; Protein: 1.1g

Coconut Cream Pie

PREPARATION TIME: 15 MINUTES
COOK TIMING: 0 MINUTES
SERVES: 8 TO 10

INGREDIENTS

- **Crust:**
- 1 teaspoon of vanilla extract
- 2 cups of walnuts
- 1/4 teaspoon of ground cardamom
- 2 tbsps of coconut oil at room temperature
- 10 fresh dates, pitted
- 1/2 teaspoon of ground cinnamon
- **Filling:**
- 1/3 cup of agave syrup
- 2 medium over-ripe bananas
- 1 cup of full-fat coconut cream, chilled
- 2 frozen bananas
- **Garnish:**
- 3 ounces of vegan dark chocolate, shaved

INSTRUCTIONS

1. In your food processor, mix the crust ingredients until they combine; press the mixture into a baking pan lightly greased with oil.
2. Next, blend the filling layer. Spread the filling over the crust evenly using a spatula.
3. Place the cake in the freezer for 3 hours. Keep it stored in the freezer.
4. Add chocolate curls as a garnish before serving.
5. Enjoy your meal!

Nutritional Information: Calories: 295; Fat: 21.1g; Carbs: 27.1g; Protein: 3.8g

Easy Chocolate Candy

PREPARATION TIME: 5 MINUTES
COOK TIMING: 0 MINUTES
SERVES: 2

INGREDIENTS

- 1/4 teaspoon of ground cinnamon
- 10 ounces of dark chocolate, broken into chunks
- 1/4 cup of cacao powder, unsweetened
- 6 tbsps of coconut milk, warm
- 1/2 teaspoon of vanilla extract
- 1/4 teaspoon of ground anise

INSTRUCTIONS

1. Mix together the chocolate, warm coconut milk, cinnamon, anise, and vanilla until they are fully blended.
2. Scoop out the mixture into 1-ounce portions using a cookie scoop.
3. Shape the portions into balls with your hands. Chill them in the refrigerator for at least 30 minutes.
4. Coat the chocolate balls with cacao powder. Keep them in the fridge until you are ready to enjoy.
5. Enjoy your treat!

Nutritional Information: Calories: 232; Fat: 15.5g; Carbs: 19.6g; Protein: 3.4g

Greek-Style Fruit Compote

PREPARATION TIME: 10 MINUTES
COOK TIMING: 20 MINUTES
SERVES: 4

INGREDIENTS

- 4 apricots, halved and pitted
- 3 peaches, pitted and sliced
- 1 cup of dried figs
- 4 dried apricots
- 1 cup of sweet red wine
- 4 tbsps of agave syrup
- 1 cinnamon stick
- 1 cup of full-fat coconut yogurt
- 3 to 4 cloves
- 1 vanilla bean

INSTRUCTIONS

1. Mix together the fruits, dried fruits, wine, cinnamon, agave syrup, cloves, and vanilla in a saucepan.
2. Ensure the ingredients are covered with water by an inch. Bring it to a boil. Then, lower the heat to let it simmer. Allow it to simmer for 15 minutes while partially covered.
3. Let it cool down completely.
4. Scoop the mixture into bowls.
5. Enjoy with some nicely chilled coconut yogurt.

Nutritional Information: Calories: 294; Fat: 2g; Carbs: 46.8g; Protein: 7.8g

Vanilla Ice Cream

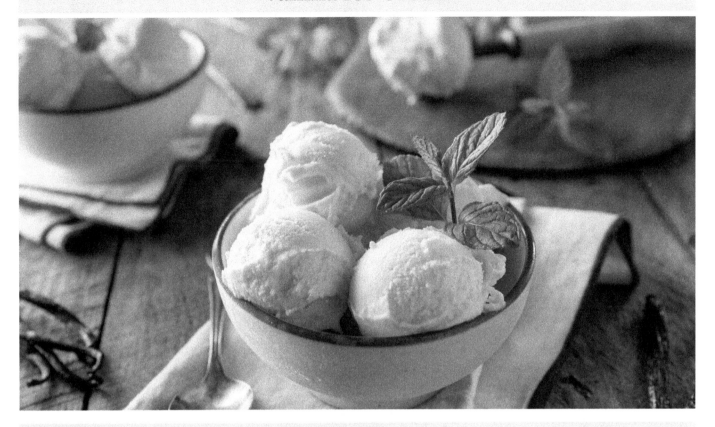

PREPARATION TIME: 5 MINUTES
COOK TIMING: 0 MINUTES
SERVES: 4

INGREDIENTS

- 1 tbsp of pure vanilla extract
- 1/2 cup of raw cashews, soaked overnight and drained
- A pinch of ground anise
- 1 cup of coconut milk
- A pinch of Himalayan salt
- 1/4 cup of agave syrup

INSTRUCTIONS

1. Put all the items into the bowl of your food processor or high-speed blender.
2. Blend the mixture until it becomes creamy, even, and smooth.
3. Chill your ice cream in the freezer for a minimum of 3 hours.
4. Enjoy your treat!

Nutritional Information: Calories: 205; Fat: 9.9g; Carbs: 25.2g; Protein: 4.5g

GLOSSARY

Have you ever come across a recipe and felt puzzled by the meaning of certain terms? Refer to this glossary to familiarize yourself with commonly used cooking terminology found in recipes.

- **Bake:** To cook without covering using dry heat in an oven or oven-like device.
- **Baste:** To add pan drippings or sauces to foods while cooking to enhance taste and prevent them from becoming dry.
- **Batter:** A blend of flour and liquid that has a thin consistency for pouring.
- **Beat:** To swiftly and rapidly blend ingredients, incorporating air, to create an airy and smooth mixture.
- **Blanch:** To partially cook food in boiling water, followed by submerging it in cold water to halt the cooking.
- **Blend:** Mixing two or more ingredients together gently until they are thoroughly combined.
- **Boil:** Heating a liquid on heat until bubbles consistently rise and break on the surface.
- **Braise:** Slowly cooking meat or poultry with a small amount of liquid in a covered pot.
- **Broil:** Cooking food under direct heat on a rack.
- **Caramelize:** Slowly cook a fruit or vegetable until it caramelizes and becomes sweet and brown. This process can also involve cooking sugar slowly to achieve a result or cooking foods like nuts in sugar until they caramelize.
- **Chop:** To chop food into bite-sized pieces.
- **Cream:** To smooth out a fat, such as butter, by beating it with a spoon or mixer. Another method is to combine fat with another ingredient, like blending butter and sugar.
- **Cube:** Cutting food into small pieces, measuring about ½ inch on all sides.
- **Cure:** To preserve fish or meat by drying, salting, or smoking it.
- **Dice:** Cutting the food into ¼ inch pieces all around.
- **Dissolve:** Mix a dry ingredient into a liquid while heating it.
- **Drain:** Strain out all the liquid using a colander, or strainer, or by pressing a lid or plate against the food and tilting the container.
- **Fold:** To Mix the ingredients by swirling in a gentle motion to blend them together then scrape along the bottom of the bowl to incorporate some of the mixture onto the top.
- **Fry:** Cooking in hot oil. Sauté in a small quantity of fat on medium heat or deep fry in hot oil where the food can float freely.
- **Garnish:** Adding a touch of garnish to elevate the appeal and taste of a dish.
- **Grate:** Grating food against the surface to create medium or coarse particles (can also be done by chopping in a blender or food processor).
- **Grease:** Applying a layer of oil or fat to prevent food from adhering to the pan during cooking or baking.
- **Julienne:** Slicing veggies, fruits, or cheese thinly.
- **Knead:** Kneading dough, by pressing, folding and stretching until it becomes smooth typically using the heels of the hands.
- **Marinate:** Marinating food involves soaking it in a flavored liquid to enhance tenderness and taste.
- **Mash:** To mash up food using a fork, spoon, or masher until it becomes smooth.
- **Mince:** Cutting food into small bits.
- **Parboil:** Simmering until partially cooked then typically finishing the cooking process in a sauce.
- **Pare or peel:** To strip off the layer of food by cutting away with a knife or peeler.
- **Pinch:** A small quantity of seasoning added to a dish. An amount that fits between your thumb and forefinger.
- **Pit:** To extract the core or seed from a fruit.
- **Plump:** Soaking dried fruit in liquid until they plump up.
- **Preheat:** Preheating the oven in advance so it's ready when needed (usually takes 5 to 10 minutes).
- **Poach:** Simmering food gently in a small amount of simmering, hot liquid over low heat.
- **Puree:** Reducing the volume of liquid by blending it using a hand or blender.

- **Reduce:** Boiling liquid to reduce its volume.
- **Roast:** Cooking (meat) in an oven using dry heat is known as roasting.
- **Sauté:** Searing food quickly in a small amount of fat, like oil or butter, is called sautéing.
- **Scald:** Heating liquid to below boiling is referred to as scalding.
- **Sear:** Quickly browning food over high heat to enhance flavor and appearance is called searing.
- **Shred:** Cutting or tearing food into long and thin strips.
- **Sift:** Passing dry ingredients through a sifter or strainer to remove lumps or incorporate air is called sifting.
- **Simmer:** To simmer the liquid gently over low heat until it is just about to boil allowing small bubbles to form slowly.
- **Skim:** To skim off any fat or impurities that rise to the surface of a liquid.
- **Slice:** To slice food into thin pieces.
- **Steam:** To steam food on a rack or in a colander inside a covered pot with a small amount of boiling water.
- **Stew:** Slowly simmering food in a small amount of liquid over low heat for an extended period of time.
- **Stir fry:** Cooking food pieces rapidly over high heat with continuous stirring until they reach a tender yet crisp texture.
- **Thaw:** Gradually thawing from a frozen state to become liquid.
- **Toss:** Gently combining ingredients by lifting and mixing them with forks or spoons.
- **Whip:** Whisking vigorously to incorporate air and create a light and fluffy texture, commonly done with egg whites or heavy cream.

MEASUREMENT CONVERSION TABLE

CUP	OUNCES	MILLILITERS	TABLESPOONS
8 cup	64 oz.	1895 ml	128
6 cup	48 oz.	1420 ml	96
5 cup	40 oz.	1180 ml	80
4 cup	32 oz.	960 ml	64
2 cup	16 oz.	480 ml	32
1 cup	8 oz.	240 ml	16
3/4 cup	6 oz.	177 ml	12
2/3 cup	5 oz.	158 ml	11
1/2 cup	4 oz.	118 ml	8
3/8 cup	3 oz.	90 ml	6
1/3 cup	2.5 oz.	79 ml	5.5

1/4 cup	2 oz.	59 ml	4
1/8 cup	1 oz.	30 ml	3
1/16 cup	1/2 oz.	15 ml	1

30-DAY MEAL PLAN

DAY	BREAKFAST	LUNCH	SNACKS	DINNER
1	Simple Avocado Toast	Curried Mango Chickpea Wrap	Carrot Energy Balls	Veggie Curry
2	Oatmeal with Banana and Figs	Loaded Kale Salad	Oven-Baked Kale Chips	Sweet Potato Patties
3	Cheeky Cereal	Classic Lentil Soup with Swiss Chard	Peppery Hummus Dip	Vietnamese Summer Rolls
4	Raspberry and Chia Smoothie Bowl	Roasted Fennel Salad	Traditional Baba Ganoush	Greek-Style Eggplant Skillet
5	Iced Matcha Latte	Cannellini Bean Soup with Kale	Roasted Chickpeas	Pesto and Sun-dried Tomato Quinoa
6	Oatmeal-Free Breakfast	Quinoa and Black Bean Salad	Hummus Avocado Boats	Blackeyed Peas Burritos
7	Plant-Powered Pancakes	Creamy Pumpkin and Toasted Walnut Soup	Baked Zucchini Chips	Falafel Burgers
8	Banana Nut Smoothie	Classic Roasted Pepper Salad	Lettuce Wraps with Hummus and Avocado	Oil-Free Rice-and-Vegetable Stir-Fry
9	Breakfast Scramble	Roasted Beet and Avocado Salad	Bell Pepper Boats with Mango Salsa	Mango-Ginger Chickpea Curry
10	Cinnamon Apple Toast	Moroccan Aubergine Salad	Easy Zucchini Roll-Ups	Rice with Asparagus and Cauliflower

DAY	BREAKFAST	LUNCH	SNACKS	DINNER
11	Chocolate Chia Pudding	Green Lentil Salad	Oven-Roasted Button Mushrooms	Swiss Chard Skillet
12	Oat and Peanut Butter Breakfast Bar	Hearty Winter Quinoa Soup	Stuffed Portobellos with Rice and Herbs	Avocado Bread with Chickpeas
13	Berry Blast Smoothie	Tomato Pumpkin Soup	Aromatic Sautéed Swiss Chard	Chili Sin Carne
14	Classic Tofu Scramble	Chilled Avocado Mint Soup	Sautéed Turnip Greens	Brown Rice with Vegetables and Tofu
15	Goji Breakfast Bowl	Cream of Green Bean Soup	Roasted Garden Vegetables	Barley Pilaf with Wild Mushrooms
16	Mixed Berry and Almond Butter Swirl Bowl	Cauliflower Spinach Soup	Creamy Rosemary Broccoli Mash	Potage au Quinoa
17	Fig Protein Smoothie	Cherry Tomato Salad with Soy Chorizo	Sautéed Zucchini with Herbs	Old-Fashioned Pilaf
18	Everyday Oats with Coconut and Strawberries	Creamy Squash Soup	Herb Cauliflower Mash	Barley with Portobello Mushrooms and Chard
19	Peaches and Cream Oats	Roasted Carrot Soup	Traditional Sautéed Bell Peppers	Traditional Tuscan Bean Stew
20	Frosty Hemp and Blackberry Smoothie Bowl	Rocket Chickpeas Salad	Yukon Gold Mashed Potatoes	Beluga Lentil and Vegetable Mélange
21	Buckwheat Porridge with Apples and Almonds	Classic Cream of Broccoli Soup	Classic Sautéed Bell Peppers	Green Lentil Stew with Collard Greens
22	Tropical Paradise Smoothie	Tarragon Cauli Salad	Easy Braised Green Beans	Classic Italian Minestrone
23	Chocolate Oat Smoothie	Old-Fashioned Green Bean Salad	Braised Kale with Sesame Seeds	Mexican-Style Bean Bowl
24	Raw Morning Pudding	Italian-Style Cremini Mushroom Soup	Sautéed Cauliflower with Sesame Seeds	Chickpea Garden Vegetable Medley

DAY	BREAKFAST	LUNCH	SNACKS	DINNER
25	Peach Crumble Shake	Romaine and Grape Tomato Salad with Avocado and Baby Peas	Easy Braised Green Beans	Old-Fashioned Lentil and Vegetable Stew
26	Banana Cream Pie Chia Pudding	Quinoa and Avocado Salad	Roasted Carrots with Herbs	Brown Lentil Bowl
27	Oatmeal-Banana Pancakes	Red Bean and Corn Salad	Herb Cauliflower Mash	Sushi Bowl
28	Pumpkin Spice Protein Oatmeal	Spring Vegetable Soup	Braised Kale with Sesame Seeds	Sweet Potato Patties
29	Chocolate Quinoa Breakfast Bowl	Kidney Bean and Potato Soup	Classic Sautéed Bell Peppers	Savory Sweet Potato Casserole
30	Baked Banana French Toast with Raspberry Syrup	Creamy Golden Veggie Soup	Creamy Rosemary Broccoli Mash	Olive and White Bean Pasta

CONCLUSION

As we reach the final page of "The Dr. Barbara Cookbook," I want to express my heartfelt gratitude for your invaluable participation in this culinary expedition. Inspired by Barbara O'Neill's wisdom, we've delved into 150 plant-based and natural recipes, each crafted to nourish your body and elevate your soul. From salads to comforting soups and main dishes to delightful desserts, every recipe has been lovingly prepared to support your unique path to well-being.

It is my sincere belief that this cookbook has not only introduced you to a wealth of ingredients but also uncovered the joy of cooking. By integrating these recipes into your routine, I hope you have begun to experience the transformative power of plant-based eating and its profound effects on your health and overall wellness.

With the provided 30-day meal plan, you have a guide leading you towards optimal health and energy. Let every meal serve as a tribute to nourishment and self-love as you foster a bond with your body and the environment around you.

Thank you for allowing me to be a part of your journey towards well-being. Here's to continued progress, vitality, and delightful culinary explorations in the kitchen. Bon appétit!

BOOK 14

Dr Barbara 15-Day Gut Cleanse Plan

UNDERSTANDING GUT HEALTH: THE FOUNDATION OF WELL-BEING

The human gut functions like a city, where trillions of bacteria collaborate intricately to maintain health and balance. Despite its significance, this intricate microbial community often goes unnoticed. Imagine yourself exploring this world teeming with microbes. Each member of this ensemble plays a role in sustaining the gut's delicate harmony. Our microbiome is vital for aspects of being, such as digestion, nutrient absorption, immune system regulation, and even influencing mood and cognition.

Our gut microbiota is a system that evolves due to factors like genetics, diet, environment and lifestyle; it serves as the core of this changing metropolis. Factors like birth method, breastfeeding practices, antibiotic use and dietary choices all influence the composition of these microorganisms. Imbalances in these microbes can lead to health issues; however, some bacteria are beneficial. Promote well-being.

Referred to as the " brain," the gut-brain axis facilitates communication between the system and the central nervous system.

The intricate network of neurons, hormones and microbial metabolites in the gut does not impact digestion. Also influences mood, emotions and cognitive functions. Disruptions in the gut-brain axis have been associated with conditions like anxiety, depression and neurodegenerative diseases.

Beyond its role in responses and infection prevention, the gut microbiota plays a part in modulating the immune system. A balanced gut microbiome promotes tolerance, while imbalances can contribute to auto-immune disorders and chronic inflammation. Recent studies suggest that changes in our gut microbiota can affect inflammation throughout the body, potentially leading to metabolic disorders, heart issues and cancer.

One's dietary choices significantly influence their gut microbiome by altering the composition and function of bacteria present. To promote metabolic health and diversity among microbes, it is recommended to consume a variety of fiber fruits, vegetables and fermented foods. Conversely, diets high in processed foods, sugar and unhealthy fats may contribute to inflammation and imbalances that support bacteria growth.

Probiotics— microbes offering health benefits—and prebiotics— fibers that nourish beneficial gut bacteria—are essential for maintaining optimal gut health.

To boost your digestion and enhance the variety of microbes in your body, try incorporating foods like kimchi, sauerkraut, kefir and yogurt into your diet. Additionally, including foods such as bananas, garlic, onions and leeks can help support the growth of bacteria in your gut, promoting a diverse and thriving microbial community.

Maintaining good gut health isn't about what you eat; factors like activity, sleep patterns, stress levels and environmental exposures also influence it. Regular exercise can positively impact both metabolic health and microbial diversity within the gut. Adequate sleep is essential for a healthy gut-brain connection, as sleep disturbances can disrupt the balance of gut bacteria and lead to inflammation.

External factors like antibiotic use, pollution exposure and household chemicals can also impact gut health by altering the microbiota. While antibiotics are sometimes necessary for treating illnesses, they have the potential to harm gut bacteria along with ones. Environmental pollutants can trigger inflammation and disrupt function when absorbed into the body.

To enhance gut health and overall well-being, it's essential to grasp the interplay between the gut microbiome, diet, lifestyle choices and environmental factors. Building a foundation for health involves adopting a holistic approach that encompasses a diverse diet incorporating probiotic and prebiotic-rich foods, engaging in regular physical activity, getting sufficient rest, managing stress effectively and minimizing exposure to harmful substances. These practices contribute to fostering a gut microbiome.

The well-being of our system, function, mental wellness, metabolism and overall vitality are all influenced by the state of our gut health. This underscores the role that gut health plays in maintaining wellness. By adopting eco behaviors, practicing eating habits, and nurturing a symbiotic relationship with our gut flora, we can unlock the transformative power of gut health to enhance longevity and elevate our quality of life.

WHY A 15-DAY GUT CLEANSE? THE SCIENCE BEHIND SHORT-TERM INTERVENTIONS

During a "gut cleanse," it is recommended to stay hydrated by drinking water to clear out your colon, which is the large intestine.

People often refer to procedures like "colon cleanse," " irrigation," and "colonic hydrotherapy" when discussing this process.

The concept of autointoxication, a theory, forms the basis for this practice. It suggests that removing substances from the system is crucial for maintaining good health.

While there isn't evidence supporting this idea, healthcare providers may recommend a gut cleanse in certain situations.

This article explores the science behind gut cleanses, examining their benefits and risks.

WHAT DOES THE SCIENCE SAY ABOUT GUT CLEANSES?

Having a gut cleanse involves flushing out the intestine with an amount of warm water-based solution, typically, around 60 liters. The process usually takes about half an hour. It is common during this time to have a tube inserted 1.5 inches into your rectum.

In cases undergoing a colon cleanse can be advantageous. For instance, research has shown that a year-long gut cleansing regimen has led to improved gut function and quality of life for individuals dealing with constipation or fecal incontinence.

However, it appears that gut cleanses may not benefit everyone equally, as 43% of participants reported outcomes after 12 months. Previous studies have indicated that gut cleanses could offer relief for conditions like chronic constipation.

Moreover, there is evidence suggesting that a gut cleanse might help alleviate symptoms such as discomfort, diarrhea and constipation in individuals with bowel syndrome (IBS). It's important to note that these studies typically involve individuals with conditions and are conducted under the supervision of experts in the field.

While some people may experience relief from problems through a gut cleanse, it's essential to remember that this approach does not address the underlying causes.

For a period, someone with a colon evacuation may experience temporary relief after emptying it. However, this does not necessarily signify health. It simply offers comfort for a health issue.

The dangers of gut cleanses

There isn't evidence to support the idea that gut cleanses enhance health except for the instances noted earlier. Additionally, there are risks associated with them.

Unwanted gut symptoms

Mild and temporary gastrointestinal issues, such as gas, discomfort and diarrhea, can occur when undergoing gut cleanses. They might also lead to sensitivity or discomfort in the area.

Perforation

During a cleanse of the system, the large intestine is at a heightened risk of perforation. Immediate medical attention becomes crucial under the circumstances.

Gut microbiome disruption

A gut can disrupt the balance of bacteria in your system, potentially harming your digestive health. Studies indicate that bowel cleansing procedures may have an impact on the microbiota. Repeating this process could exacerbate problems. According to experts, while you may feel relief, you might actually be damaging your gut microbiome in the term.

Infection

Due to the nature of gut cleanses harmful bacteria could enter your colon during the process, potentially leading to an infection.

Overview of Dr. Barbara's Holistic Health Philosophy

Dr. Barbara's approach to health considers the well-being of individuals, encompassing their mental, physical and spiritual aspects to enhance overall wellness. By integrating medicine with therapies, Dr. Barbara aims to address the entirety of a person's health issues at their core and foster a state of optimal health. Central to Dr. Barbara's philosophy is the belief in interconnectedness and the importance of achieving balance in all aspects of life.

Mind-Body Connection

Dr. Barbara is well aware of how mental, emotional and spiritual well-being can affect one's health. She emphasizes the importance of maintaining an attitude, managing stress effectively, and developing strength to support overall health.

Nutrition as Medicine

Dr. Barbara believes that a diet centered around plant-based foods is essential for maintaining health. She advises against consuming processed foods, refined carbohydrates and unhealthy fats while recommending an increase in foods like legumes, fruits, vegetables, and whole grains. Dr. Barbara also emphasizes the healing properties of food, suggesting that it can play a role in preventing and treating illnesses while also fueling the body with energy.

Lifestyle Medicine

Dr. Barbara emphasizes the importance of nurturing connections, ensuring rest, handling stress effectively and staying active as key components of a holistic strategy for enhancing health. She encourages the adoption of behaviors that support energy and longevity since she understands that the decisions we make in our lives greatly impact our emotional, mental and physical health.

Holistic Approaches to Healing

She takes an approach to wellness using a range of methods such as care, acupuncture, massage therapy, herbal remedies and practices like tai chi, yoga and meditation. She believes in the body's natural healing capacity. Aims to nurture it through techniques that address the root causes of illness.

Preventive Healthcare

Dr. Barbara emphasizes the importance of detection and treatment of health issues to prevent them from escalating. She recommends screenings, vaccinations and health checkups as preventive measures for maintaining good health. Dr. Barbara encourages individuals to care for their well-being by incorporating strategies that can improve both longevity and overall quality of life.

Environmental Health

Dr. Barbara recognizes the impact of factors on health. Encourages sustainable practices that benefit people and the planet. She promotes eco-lifestyle decisions to preserve resources and protect the environment for future generations, aiming to reduce exposure to pollution, toxins and harmful chemicals.

Patient-Centred Care

Respecting each individual's circumstances, including their values, priorities and health considerations, is an aspect of Dr. Barbara's holistic approach to health. She believes in empowering patients to participate in making decisions about their healthcare and treatment plans and advocating for collaboration between healthcare providers and patients to achieve outcomes.

At the core of Dr. Barbara's health philosophy is the idea of addressing the person—mind, body and spirit. By promoting treatment approaches that target the causes of illness and support overall well-being, she underscores the importance of patient-centered care, nutrition, preventive medicine, mind-body techniques, environmental wellness and lifestyle factors, among other aspects.

BOOK 15

Preparing for Your Gut Cleanse

ASSESSING YOUR CURRENT HEALTH

How to Understand and Record Your Baseline Gut Health

Improving your health and overall well-being starts with getting a grasp of your baseline gut health. Here's a simple guide to help you along the way: 1. Watch for Any Signs of Trouble. Begin by paying attention to how your gut feels and any issues you might be experiencing with digestion. Keep a diary noting any symptoms, like gas, bloating, constipation, diarrhea, indigestion, stomach discomfort and irregular bowel movements. Record the frequency, severity and duration of these symptoms while also observing any patterns or triggers.2. Keep Tabs on Your Diet: To understand how your food choices impact your system, maintain a food journal. Record everything you eat and drink throughout the day including portion sizes and meal timings. Note how different foods make you feel emotionally and whether they worsen or improve your gut issues. Don't forget to mention any sensitivities or intolerances such as gluten or lactose intolerance.

Evaluate Your Lifestyle Factors: Factors like stress levels, quality of sleep, physical activity levels and medication usage all play a role in your health. A person's digestive system and the balance of bacteria in their gut can be influenced by factors like stress, lack of sleep, a sedentary lifestyle and certain medications. It's important to monitor how changes in these aspects may impact your gut health. Reflect on your history. Consider all the information your healthcare provider has shared with you regarding your well, especially concerning any stomach-related issues, autoimmune conditions, allergies or chronic illnesses. Some medical conditions can affect gut health. It may require adjustments to your diet or daily routine. Discuss your health background with your doctor and its implications for your system. Assess the Diversity of Gut Microbiota: Think about undergoing testing to examine the diversity and composition of bacteria in your gut. Specialized laboratories may perform stool analyses or microbiome tests for this purpose. These tests can offer insights into the types and quantities of microbes in your gut, aiding in identifying any dysbiosis or microbial imbalances that could contribute to gastrointestinal issues. Seek Guidance from a Specialist; Consult with a healthcare provider or qualified nutritionist who specializes in gut health to gain insight into your symptoms, choices, lifestyle factors and test results.

Making changes to your diet, taking supplements, adjusting your lifestyle and focusing on treatments to support gut healing and maintain balance could be part of the personalized recommendations they provide. Setting Initial Key Performance Indicators (KPIs): Once you gather all the information about your health, establish baseline metrics to track your progress. Monitoring symptom severity scores, compliance with gut foods in your diet, gut microbiota composition and assessing your quality of life are all metrics to consider. Regularly reassessing these indicators is crucial to monitor changes and gauge the effectiveness of treatments. Defining Improvement Goals: Develop a plan to enhance your health and overall well-being based on the findings from the assessment. Objectives such as reducing symptoms through diet, optimizing gut microbiota diversity, improving absorption, boosting function and promoting general digestive wellness can guide you. Create a plan. Monitor your advancements by breaking down these goals into achievable steps. An effective approach to improving health is understanding and monitoring your baseline gut health. By receiving guidance and taking targeted actions, you can attain gut health and enhance overall well-being. Remember that maintaining gut health involves factors, so it's important to make adjustments and monitor your progress regularly to ensure long-term gut health and well-being.

Symptoms That Indicate Poor Gut Health

If your stomach isn't feeling right, how can you tell? Dr. Diondra Atoyebi, from Piedmont Family Medicine, sheds light on the signs of issues and ways to address them. Why is gut health important? A balanced mix of bacteria in your gut indicates a healthy digestive system. These microbes play roles such as breaking down food, for energy detoxifying the body, defending against germs and boosting the production of serotonin, a neurotransmitter that promotes well-being.

Signs of poor gut health

When there is a shortage of bacteria, harmful bacteria can thrive. Imbalances in bacteria might lead to issues, such as immune system-related conditions like thyroid problems, rheumatoid arthritis and type 1 diabetes. Additionally, digestive system troubles like IBS, constipation, diarrhea, bloating, heartburn, sleep disorders and environmental sensitivities may arise. Cravings for foods, unexplained weakness or fatigue unexplained mood swings, like anxiety and sadness, are also symptoms. Dr. Atoyebi mentions that when people mention these symptoms to him/her/they/them/ he/she/they often inquire about their habits and food choices because these symptoms could be linked to problems if no other medical cause is identified.

Does good gut health impact mood?

Maintaining a gut can greatly affect how you feel emotionally and your overall sense of wellness. Surprisingly, there are connections between gut health and feelings of anxiety, sadness and fatigue. It's common for me to find that individuals experiencing tiredness or low moods tend to consume an amount of processed foods when I review their dietary habits. What you eat can have an impact on how you feel, which in turn influences your state. While not the sole factor, the health of your gut does play a role in managing mood-related issues.

Steps to a healthier digestive system

You can improve your health by limiting the use of antibiotics unless necessary. Antibiotics have the potential to reduce harmful bacteria in your system.

Foods you consume can contain beneficial probiotics for your gut health. Through fermentation, foods like yogurt, sauerkraut, kombucha, kefir and kimchi can introduce bacteria into your diet.

Reduce your intake of processed foods. Dr. Atoyebi suggests reassessing your food choices to align with what your ancestors would recognize as food. Claims of added nutrients in processed foods are often just marketing strategies. Instead, consider reverting to a plant-based diet that has sustained humans for generations.

Include prebiotics in your diet. Prebiotics, abundant in plant-based foods such as fruits, vegetables and whole grains, support the growth of microbes in your gut. Foods like apples, asparagus, bananas, corn, garlic, flaxseeds, onions, leeks, oats, lentils, walnuts and others are examples of options that promote gut health.

Stay hydrated by drinking plenty of water daily. Avoid vitamin supplement drinks as they may not be beneficial for you according to my opinion.

Enhance the taste of water by adding fruit slices.

Browse around the sections at the grocery store.

Around the edges, you can find meats, healthy grains, low-fat dairy products, as well as fresh and frozen vegetables.

FUNDAMENTALS OF GUT CLEANSING

Detox has become synonymous with being and energy in a world filled with detox teas, diets and juice cleanses. It's crucial to distinguish fact from fiction and understand the essence of detox amidst all the marketing hype and celebrity promotions.

What is Detoxification? Separating Fact from Fiction

Eliminating toxins and waste products is crucial for the body's natural detox process, which plays a role in maintaining health for everyone. This process involves getting rid of substances and waste products through organs like the digestive system, skin, lungs, kidneys and liver. When these organs function properly, the body can effectively remove toxins. Maintain its balance.

To stay healthy and full of energy, your body detoxifies itself daily. It's important to focus on making lifestyle changes that support your body's natural detox processes instead of relying on quick fixes or extreme methods. To boost your health and well-being by aiding your body's detoxification mechanisms, make sure to eat meals, stay hydrated, exercise regularly, manage stress levels effectively and prioritize self-care.

Debunking Detox Myths

Detoxification is often misunderstood by individuals, which is unfortunate considering its significant importance. Let's debunk some misconceptions surrounding the process of detox.

Detox Diets Are a Quick Fix

By following diets that focus on cutting calories and eliminating foods, many detox programs promise to help you lose weight fast and improve your well-being. However, these restrictive diets often lead to deficiencies, fatigue and even muscle loss by omitting nutrients. Of making short-term sacrifices for health, it's more beneficial to make sustainable lifestyle changes for long-term well-being.

Detox Teas and Supplements Are Magic Bullets

The assertions promoted by detox teas and pills about their ability to eliminate toxins from your body lack substantiated proof. Consuming detox products may lead to effects such as imbalances in electrolytes and dehydration, often attributed to the presence of chemicals like laxatives and diuretics. It is advisable to maintain a diet with nutrients, have meals, and stay hydrated by drinking an ample amount of water and herbal teas instead of resorting to quick fixes.

Detoxing Requires Extreme Measures

To support your body in detoxifying, you don't have to follow fasting routines or cleansing rituals, as many believe. Instead, focus on incorporating a range of fruits, whole grains, vegetables, lean proteins and good fats into your diet. A key part of living also involves ensuring you get rest, handling stress effectively, and engaging in regular physical activity.

Promoting Gentle Detox Practices

Some methods could potentially support your body's natural detox processes. Excessive detox regimens might end up causing harm rather than offering any real benefits.

1. Hydration

Ensuring your body eliminates toxins and maintaining the health of your kidneys and liver can be supported by staying hydrated. It is recommended to drink 8 to 10 glasses of water each day; for added flavor and detox benefits, consider including slices of lemon or cucumber in your water.

2. Nutrient-Rich Foods

Consume a diet of proteins, diverse fruits and vegetables, nuts, seeds, legumes and whole grains. By incorporating these foods into your meals, you can support your body's natural detoxification process. Maintain well-being due to their high fiber content, antioxidants, vitamins and minerals.

3. Herbal Support

Throughout history, individuals have depended on spices and herbs such as ginger, turmeric, milk thistle and dandelion root to support liver cleansing and maintenance of its health. It's advisable to consult your physician before embarking on a treatment regimen. Experimenting with incorporating these herbs into your cooking or consuming them in the form of teas or supplements could be worth considering.

4. Physical Activity

The body benefits from exercise as it supports its natural detoxification mechanisms, boosts circulation, and enhances drainage. To maintain health and well-being, strive to engage in a workout routine that includes exercises, strength training and flexibility workouts.

5. Stress Management

When long-term stress harmful substances hinder the body's detoxification processes can accumulate. To promote relaxation and harmony, consider engaging in activities such as yoga, deep breathing exercises, meditation, or simply immersing yourself in the world.

The Role of Your Gut Microbiome in Overall Health

The tiny living organisms and germs in your gut help with digesting food and might also support your body's system, heart health and brain function. There are billions of bacteria, viruses and fungi inside you, collectively known as the microbiome. While some bacteria can be harmful, others are essential for keeping your system, heart health, weight and various bodily functions in check. This book guides you through understanding the gut microbiota.

What Is the Gut Microbiome?

Tiny living organisms, commonly referred to as microbes encompass bacteria, viruses, fungi and other types. Your skin and digestive system serve as the residences for these bacteria. Most of the microorganisms dwelling in your gut are concentrated in a region called the cecum within the intestine. This collective population is recognized as the gut microbiome.

While microorganisms are abundant in your body, researchers have primarily focused on bacteria. The quantity of cells within your system surpasses that of cells significantly. In comparison to the 30 trillion cells, your body houses over 40 trillion cells. Hence, you bear a resemblance to a bacterium than a being.

Furthermore, the microbiome inhabiting the gut consists of up to a thousand bacterial species, each playing a crucial role in maintaining your health. While most are beneficial for your well being some may pose risks.

Collectively these microorganisms might weigh between 2–5 pounds (1 2 kg) to the weight of your brain. When combined, they function akin to an organ within your body that's indispensable for your overall health.

The collection of organisms residing in your gut, often referred to as the gut microbiome, is considered a part of your body.

How Does It Affect Your Body?

Throughout history, humans have evolved to live alongside microorganisms, with these tiny beings playing roles in our bodies. The presence of the gut microbiome is essential for our existence. From the moment of birth, when we encounter microbes during passage through the mother's birth canal, the gut microbiome begins to affect our bodies. Recent findings suggest that babies may even encounter some microbes while in the womb. As we grow, the diversity of species in our gut microbiome expands, which is beneficial for our well-being. Interestingly, what we eat influences the diversity of bacteria in our gut. As our microbiome develops it has an impact on our health.

Bifidobacteria are a type of bacteria that initially inhabit a baby's intestines through breastfeeding. These tiny organisms break down growth-promoting carbohydrates found in breast milk.

When beneficial microbes in the gut metabolize fiber, they produce short-chain fatty acids that support gut health. A diet rich in fiber could potentially lower the risk of developing conditions such as cancer, diabetes, heart disease and excess body weight.

Moreover, the gut microbiota plays a role in regulating system function.

The gut microbiota can influence the way your body reacts to infections through its interaction with cells. Recent research has indicated that the gut microbiota plays a role in regulating brain function, potentially impacting the system. Consequently, the gut microbiota can have effects on your health, some of which are more apparent than others. Throughout life, from conception to age, the gut microbiome manages bodily functions such as digestion, immunity and the central nervous system.

The Gut Microbiome May Affect Your Weight

Your stomach houses types of bacteria, most of which play a role in maintaining your overall health. However, an overabundance of bacteria can lead to sickness. When there is an imbalance between bad bacteria in the gut, known as gut dysbiosis, it may contribute to weight gain.

Studies have shown that the gut microbiota of obese and non-identical twins differ significantly, indicating that these differences are not solely due to genetics. Intriguingly, research on mice revealed that those receiving microbiota from their siblings gained weight despite consuming the same diet as the control group.

These findings suggest a link between imbalance and obesity. Fortunately, probiotics can aid in weight loss. Help maintain a balance of gut bacteria. Research suggests that probiotics may have an impact on weight loss, with participants losing more than 2.2 lbs (1 kilogram).

It Affects Gut Health

Irritable bowel syndrome (IBS) and inflammatory bowel disease (IBD) are both conditions affecting the gut that could be linked to the microbiome.

Individuals experiencing bowel syndrome (IBS) might face an imbalance in their gut bacteria, leading to symptoms like bloating, cramps and stomach discomfort. This is because the smelling gases and other byproducts from these microbes can worsen issues.

On the side the microbiome also houses bacteria that can support healthy digestion.

Consuming probiotics and yogurt-containing strains of Bifidobacteria and Lactobacilli could help prevent gut syndrome.

These friendly bacteria may also prevent bacteria from sticking to the intestines.

In fact, some individuals have found relief from IBS symptoms by incorporating probiotics with Bifidobacteria and Lactobacilli into their routine.

The Gut Microbiome May Benefit Heart Health

The bacteria could influence the health of the heart in the gut.

Recent research involving 1,500 individuals suggests that the gut microbiota plays a role in raising levels of "HDL cholesterol and triglycerides.

The presence of bacteria in the gut microbiome producing trimethylamine N oxide (TMAO) has been associated with an increased risk of heart disease.

TMAO is a compound that could lead to blockages in arteries, potentially resulting in heart attacks and strokes.

Certain bacteria found in meat and animal-based foods, such as choline and L carnitine, can be transformed into TMAO within the gut microbiome. This transformation may elevate the risk of issues.

However, specific microbes like Lactobacilli in the gut microbiome have shown a potential to reduce cholesterol levels when taken as probiotics.

A substance created by gut bacteria has been identified as a risk factor for atherosclerosis and cardiovascular disease. On a note probiotics have displayed effectiveness in lowering cholesterol levels and reducing cardiovascular disease risks.

It might aid in regulating blood sugar levels and decreasing diabetes risk

The composition of gut flora also holds the potential for influencing blood sugar control, which could impact the chances of developing type 1 or type 2 diabetes.

33 infants with a family history of type 1 diabetes were involved in the study. Before the onset of type 1 diabetes there was a drop in diversity observed. Additionally, it was found that certain harmful bacterial species experienced an increase in levels prior to the beginning of type 1 diabetes.

In a study, researchers found that individuals may exhibit differences in blood sugar levels even when consuming the same meals. This variation could potentially be attributed to the microorganisms in their systems.

The gut flora plays a role in both the development of type 1 diabetes in children and the regulation of blood sugar levels.

It May Affect Brain Health

The community of microorganisms in the gut could potentially have effects on brain health. Certain types of bacteria might help with the production of neurotransmitters in the brain; for instance, most of the mood-regulating neurotransmitter serotonin is actually produced in the intestines. Additionally, millions of nerves physically connect the intestines to the brain. Consequently, like how it affects these nerve's health, the gut microbiota may also impact brain health.

Studies have shown that the gut microbiome of individuals with health disorders differs from that of those who are healthy. This suggests that the gut microbiota could play a role in well-being. However, whether this is solely due to differences in people's diets and lifestyles remains uncertain.

A few research studies suggest that certain probiotics might help alleviate symptoms of depression and other mental health conditions. Through chemical interactions and communication with neurons that connect to the brain, the gut microbiota may influence brain health.

How Can You Improve Your Gut Microbiome?

Improving the balance of your gut bacteria can be done through methods like;

Having a range of microbes in your gut indicates gut health, and consuming a varied diet can help achieve this. For example, eating fruits, beans and legumes in fiber may support the growth of Bifidobacteria.

Including fermented foods in your diet; Yogurt sauerkraut and kefir are examples of fermented foods that contain bacteria like Lactobacilli and could reduce the species causing stomach issues.

Avoiding sugar substitutes like aspartame can lead to a rise in blood sugar levels by promoting the growth of bacteria such as Enterobacteriaceae in the gut microbiome. It's advisable to limit the intake of these sweeteners.

Consuming meals high in fiber is beneficial for fostering the growth of bacteria in your gut. Rich fruits and vegetables, like apples, bananas, asparagus, oats and artichokes, support this process.

For the development of gut flora, it is recommended to breastfeed for at least six months. Research suggests that individuals breastfed for this duration tend to have levels of Bifidobacteria compared to those who are bottle-fed.

Include grains in your diet. These foods contain fiber and beneficial carbohydrates, like beta-glucan, which the bacteria in your gut can utilize to enhance various aspects of your health, such as weight management, cancer risk reduction and diabetes prevention.

Opting for a vegetarian diet offers health advantages, including reduced cholesterol levels, inflammation and harmful bacteria like E. Coli. One notable benefit is the decrease in food-related illnesses.

Embrace foods in polyphenols; Items such as wine, tea, olive oil, dark chocolate and whole grains are sources of polyphenols. Natural compounds found in plants. The microbiome breaks down these substances to support the growth of bacteria.

Consider using a supplement; Probiotics consist of bacteria that can help restore balance to an imbalanced gut (dysbiosis). By reintroducing bacteria into the gut through "reseeding " probiotics play a role in promoting gut health.

Follow usage guidelines strictly; Antibiotics have the potential to disrupt harmful bacteria within the gut microbiome, leading to issues like antibiotic resistance and weight fluctuations. Only take antibiotics under the instruction of your healthcare provider.

FOODS TO EMBRACE AND AVOID

There isn't an agreed-upon definition for "gut health ". It is commonly thought of as the well-being of the 300–500 microbial species, including bacteria residing in the large intestine. The bacteria in your gut play a role in helping your body digest food. Good gut health is connected to well-being, as 70% of the immune system is situated in the gut. Various autoimmune diseases, disorders, mental health issues, heart conditions and other ailments have been associated with gut health.

Comprehensive Lists of Beneficial and Harmful Foods

Yogurt and whole grains are a couple of examples of foods that can help maintain a balance in your digestive system. Let's discuss some foods that promote gut health, that you should avoid completely, and why probiotics trump prebiotics.

Five Gut Health Foods to Try

In a way, you could say the digestive system acts as the entrance to our body. The intestines are protected by a cell membrane that separates what's inside from what gets absorbed and circulates throughout the body. These cells make up the gut barrier, which consists of not a mucosal layer but the immune system and gut microbiota.

To fend off factors, it's important to have a microbiome.

Keeping your gut necessitates eating a diet that incorporates various types of foods for

- Preserving a Balanced Microbiome in the Gut
- Guarding the gut lining
- Boosting Digestive Health

The following are five meals that are great for your digestive system.

Fiber

Ensuring a variety of bacteria in your gut and lowering the chances of getting sick from germs are two key reasons why consuming enough dietary fiber is essential for gut well-being. Furthermore, having a diet high in fiber could also help with;

- The digestive process
- Nutrient absorption
- Avoiding constipation

Eating a diet of fiber has been linked to a reduced risk of developing type 2 diabetes, heart disease and colon cancer. Conversely, a low-fiber diet may reduce gut bacteria while promoting pathogens. It is recommended to consume between 18 to 38 grams of fiber daily, depending on your information source. Foods high in fiber include grains like barley, buckwheat and brown rice well as fruits and vegetables, nuts and seeds and various beans such as kidney beans, chickpeas and lentils.

Fermented Foods

Foods that have fermentation have had their carbohydrates broken down by microorganisms such as yeast and bacteria. Fermented foods utilize microbes, with common types being Lactobacillus and Bifidobacteria. A diet rich in fermented foods has been associated with increased diversity and potential reductions in inflammation markers. These foods contain probiotics, live bacteria believed to offer health benefits. They can be destroyed by heat. Avoiding heat when cooking allows them to be added at the end or used as a topping. Some examples of fermented foods include culture yogurt refrigerated sauerkraut kombucha tea, Korean kimchi (fermented vegetables), tempeh (a thick soybean dish), yogurt kefir and chilled sourdough miso (made from fermented soybeans).

- Fermented vegetables
- Salted of vinegared
- cheeses (verify if the cultures are live and active on the label)
- Also referred to as fermented cottage cheese or dry curd cottage cheese farmers' cheese
- Beverages with probiotics, like apple cider or beet kvass

Polyphenols

Plants contain substances known as polyphenols, which can be challenging for the stomach to break down. The colon's microbes play a role in breaking them down.

Polyphenols might support gut bacteria. Deter harmful species, but further research is needed to confirm this.

Here are some sources of polyphenols;

- Fruits like blueberries, strawberries, grapes, cherries, apples and pears
- Vegetables such as tomatoes, Brussels sprouts, broccoli, cauliflower and cabbage
- Soy-based food products
- Spices and herbs like turmeric, ginger and red pepper flakes
- fruits, seeds and nuts
- Black tea, green tea, coffee
- Indulgent chocolatey taste
- Sweet chocolate bars

Omega-3 Fatty Acids

Omega 3 fatty acids, a type of fat, are believed to possess inflammatory properties that support gut health and contribute to a diverse microbiota balance. Sources of omega-3 fatty acids include cold-water fish, like albacore, sardines, tuna, mackerel and herring;

- nuts and seeds such as flaxseeds
- walnuts and chia seeds as oils
- like canola and soybean.

Water

To keep your system healthy, it's crucial to stay hydrated. Water plays a role in aiding the absorption of nutrients while digesting meals. Additionally ensuring hydration may lead to a variety of gut bacteria potentially benefiting overall gut health.

Three Gut Health Foods to Avoid or Limit

When considering gut health, it's better to limit or steer clear of items than solely concentrate on the overall diet. A functioning gut necessitates steering clear of foods, which are outlined further below.

Ultra-Processed Foods

Even though most foods undergo processing, it's generally better to enjoy them in their processed state. For example, an entire apple contains more fiber than applesauce or apple juice. Processed meals often contain sugar, salt, and trans fats, which can impact health. Ingredients like emulsifiers and artificial sweeteners are commonly found in meals. While many believe that food additives are harmless, studies suggest they could have effects on the gut microbiota. Ultra-processed foods can be found in places;

- Meats in deli
- A wide variety of cereals
- A variety of snack foods
- Delightful sweets
- Prepared dinners

Greasy Fried Foods

Indulging in dishes, chips, burgers, and similar greasy foods high in saturated fats could lead to challenges in digestion. Potentially trigger gastrointestinal issues like heartburn.

Artificial Sweeteners

Further research is required to validate the assertions. There are signs suggesting that sucralose, aspartame and saccharin, along with other substances, could potentially disturb the intricate equilibrium and diversity of gut bacteria.

Prebiotic Foods for Good Gut Health: An Extra Perk

Although not all foods that are rich in fiber include prebiotics, a large number of foods do.

Raw foods that are rich in prebiotics include:

- Artichokes from Jerusalem
- Fresh Onions Garlic

- Garlic Sprawl
- French bananas
- Radish leaves
- Seaweed food

Additional dietary sources of prebiotics include:
- A family of legumes that includes peas, beans, and lentils
- Oats, barley, wheat, and rye bread are examples of whole grains.
- Various nuts, such as almonds, pistachios, and cashews
- Sweet maple syrup
- Roots of yams and jicama

The Importance of Organic and Whole Foods

It's no wonder that the food we eat can have such an impact on our well-being and health. Our gut is home to 100 million neurons, serotonin receptors than even our brain and over a hundred billion microorganisms in every gram of intestinal content. Scientists are uncovering evidence that the quality of our food, down to how it's grown, the pesticides used and how far it travels before reaching our plate, plays a role in shaping the diverse community of microorganisms in our gut. Having a varied and plentiful array of gut microbes could potentially lift our spirits and hasten recovery from illnesses and medical treatments like antibiotics rev up metabolism and assist in shedding weight. Are you still following along?

Recent research suggests that consuming food could be beneficial for the microbiota. Opting for organic may mean exposure to pesticides that can disrupt gut flora and lead to health issues. Foods grown in soil deemed organic are generally richer in nutrients. The advice to "eat the rainbow" is more important now than before, as dietary variety has significantly dwindled in societies over the past seven decades.

Many individuals believe that incorporating fermented foods into their diet and taking probiotics might promote health.

Eating probiotics, which are foods containing colonies, can boost the number of these colonies in your gut. But that's not all – there are prebiotics, too. Prebiotics are fibers that nourish colonies, supporting their growth and activity.

Natural sources of fiber can be found in a variety of foods, like fruits, vegetables and whole grains. The types of fiber that get lost during processing are abundant in processed and fermented veggies. Not only does this benefit your gut health. It also helps produce "short chain fatty acids," which fuel colon cells. When these fatty acids are absorbed into the bloodstream, they have effects such as improving metabolic health, reducing inflammation, managing insulin and cholesterol levels better and potentially lowering the risk of colon cancer.

Moving on to polyphenols – the P" in the story – they're micronutrients in specific plant-based diets known for their strong antioxidant properties. Conditions like weight loss, diabetes, neurological diseases and cardiovascular issues could see improvements from consuming these foods that also support bacteria in your system.

So what's next? I suggest opting for a diet;

It's no wonder that the food we eat can have such an impact on our well-being and health. Our gut is home to 100 million neurons, serotonin receptors than even our brain and over a hundred billion microorganisms in every gram of intestinal content. Scientists are uncovering evidence that the quality of our food, down to how it's grown, the pesticides used and how far it travels before reaching our plate, plays a role in shaping the diverse community of microorganisms in our gut. Having a varied and plentiful array of gut microbes could potentially lift our spirits and hasten recovery from illnesses and medical treatments like antibiotics rev up metabolism and assist in shedding weight. Are you still following along?

Recent research suggests that consuming food could be beneficial for the microbiota. Opting for organic may mean exposure to pesticides that can disrupt gut flora and lead to health issues. Foods grown in soil deemed organic are generally richer in nutrients. The advice to "eat the rainbow" is more important now than before, as dietary variety has significantly dwindled in societies over the past seven decades.

Many individuals believe that incorporating fermented foods into their diet and taking probiotics might promote health.

Eating probiotics, which are foods containing colonies, can boost the number of these colonies in your gut. But that's not all – there are prebiotics, too. Prebiotics are fibers that nourish colonies, supporting their growth and activity.

Natural sources of fiber can be found in a variety of foods, like fruits, vegetables and whole grains. The types of fiber that get lost during processing are abundant in processed and fermented veggies. Not only does this benefit your gut health. It also helps produce "short chain fatty acids," which fuel colon cells. When these fatty acids are absorbed into the bloodstream, they have effects such as improving metabolic health, reducing inflammation, managing insulin and cholesterol levels better and potentially lowering the risk of colon cancer.

Moving on to polyphenols – the P" in the story – they're micronutrients in specific plant-based diets known for their strong antioxidant properties. Conditions like weight loss, diabetes, neurological diseases and cardiovascular issues could see improvements from consuming these foods that also support bacteria in your system.

BOOK 16

The 15-Day Gut Cleanse Plan

BREAKFAST RECIPES

Berry Chia Pudding

PREPARATION TIME: 5 MINUTES
COOK TIME: 0 MINUTES
SERVINGS: 2

INGREDIENTS

- 1 cup almond milk
- 1/4 cup chia seeds
- 1/2 teaspoon vanilla extract
- Mixed berries

INSTRUCTIONS

1. In a bowl, combine almond milk, chia seeds and vanilla extract. Allow it to rest for 10 minutes until it thickens. Serve the chia pudding garnished with berries.

Nutritional Information (per serving): Calories: 150; Carbs: 15g; Protein: 5g; Fats: 8g

Turmeric Oatmeal

PREPARATION TIME: 5 MINUTES
COOK TIME: 10 MINUTES
SERVINGS: 2

INGREDIENTS

- 1 cup rolled oats
- 2 cups water
- 1 teaspoon turmeric powder
- Pinch of black pepper
- Maple syrup (optional)

INSTRUCTIONS

1. In a saucepan, heat the water until it boils. Put in rolled oats, turmeric and black pepper. Cook for 5 to 7 minutes until the oats are smooth and soft.
2. Add maple syrup for sweetness if you like.

Nutritional Information (per serving): Calories: 150; Carbs: 27g; Protein: 5g; Fats: 2g

Spinach and Mushroom Egg Muffins

PREPARATION TIME: 10 MINUTES
COOK TIME: 20 MINUTES
SERVINGS: 4

INGREDIENTS

- 6 eggs
- 1 cup chopped spinach
- 1/2 cup sliced mushrooms
- Salt and pepper to taste

INSTRUCTIONS

1. Preheat your oven to 350°F (175°C).
2. Prepare a muffin tray by greasing it.
3. In a bowl, beat the eggs. Add some salt and pepper for seasoning. Mix in the chopped spinach and sliced mushrooms.
4. Fill the muffin cups with the mixture. Bake for 15 to 20 minutes until they are cooked through.

Nutritional Information (per serving) Calories: 120; Carbs: 2g; Protein: 10g; Fats: 8g

Coconut Yogurt Parfait

PREPARATION TIME: 5 MINUTES
COOK TIME: 0 MINUTES
SERVINGS: 2

INGREDIENTS

- 1 cup coconut yogurt
- 1/2 cup granola
- Sliced bananas
- Shredded coconut (optional)

INSTRUCTIONS

1. Layer coconut yogurt, granola and sliced bananas in a glass or bowl.
2. Repeat the layering process until you've used all the ingredients.
3. If you like, sprinkle some shredded coconut on top as a finishing touch.

Nutritional Information (per serving) Calories: 250; Carbs: 30g; Protein: 5g; Fats: 10g

Avocado Breakfast Salad

PREPARATION TIME: 10 MINUTES
COOK TIME: 0 MINUTES
SERVINGS: 2

INGREDIENTS

- 1 avocado, diced
- 1 cup cherry tomatoes, halved
- 1/4 cup diced cucumber
- 2 tablespoons chopped cilantro
- Lime juice
- Salt and pepper to taste

INSTRUCTIONS

1. 1. Combine the avocado, cherry tomatoes, diced cucumber and chopped cilantro in a bowl.
2. 2. Drizzle lime juice over the salad. Add salt and pepper to taste.

Nutritional Information (per serving): Calories: 200; Carbs: 12g; Protein: 3g; Fats: 18g

Almond Butter Banana Toast

PREPARATION TIME: 5 MINUTES
COOK TIME: 0 MINUTES
SERVINGS: 2

INGREDIENTS

- 2 slices whole grain bread, toasted
- 2 tablespoons almond butter
- 1 banana, sliced
- Drizzle of honey (optional)

INSTRUCTIONS

1. 1. Spread almonds spread evenly over the toasted bread slices.
2. 2. Arrange sliced bananas on top. Add a drizzle of honey if preferred.

Nutritional Information (per serving): Calories: 250; Carbs: 30g; Protein: 7g; Fats: 12g

Veggie Breakfast Burrito

PREPARATION TIME: 10 MINUTES
COOK TIME: 10 MINUTES
SERVINGS: 2

INGREDIENTS

- 4 whole grain tortillas
- 4 eggs, scrambled
- 1/2 cup black beans, drained and rinsed
- 1/2 cup diced bell peppers
- 1/4 cup diced onion
- Salsa or hot sauce (optional)

INSTRUCTIONS

1. 1. Warm up the tortillas in a pan until they are soft and flexible.
2. 2. Stuff each tortilla with scrambled eggs, beans, chopped bell peppers and onions.
3. 3. Roll up the tortillas. Enjoy them with salsa or hot sauce if you like.

Nutritional Information (per serving): Calories: 300; Carbs: 30g; Protein: 15g; Fats: 12g

Blueberry Buckwheat Pancakes

PREPARATION TIME: 10 MINUTES
COOK TIME: 10 MINUTES
SERVINGS: 2

INGREDIENTS

- 1 cup buckwheat flour
- 1 tablespoon baking powder
- 1 tablespoon maple syrup
- 1/2 cup almond milk
- 1/2 cup fresh blueberries

INSTRUCTIONS

1. 1. In a mixing bowl, combine flour, baking powder, maple syrup and almond milk until the mixture is smooth.
2. 2. Carefully incorporate blueberries. Heat a stick pan over medium heat and pour the batter onto it to create pancakes.
3. 3. Cook until bubbles appear on the surface then. Cook until brown.

Nutritional Information (per serving): Calories: 250; Carbs: 45g; Protein: 8g; Fats: 5g

Greek Yogurt Breakfast Bowl

PREPARATION TIME: 5 MINUTES
COOK TIME: 0 MINUTES
SERVINGS: 1

INGREDIENTS

- 1 cup Greek yogurt
- 1/2 cup granola
- 1/2 cup mixed berries
- Drizzle of honey (optional)

INSTRUCTIONS

1. 1. Layer Greek yogurt, granola and mixed berries in a bowl.
2. 2. Add a drizzle of honey if you like.

Nutritional Information (per serving): Calories: 300; Carbs: 30g; Protein: 20g; Fats: 12g

Tofu Scramble

PREPARATION TIME: 10 MINUTES
COOK TIME: 10 MINUTES
SERVINGS: 2

INGREDIENTS

- 1 tablespoon olive oil
- 1/2 block firm tofu, crumbled
- 1/2 cup diced bell peppers
- 1/4 cup diced onion
- 1/4 teaspoon turmeric powder
- Salt and pepper to taste

INSTRUCTIONS

1. 1. Start by heating some olive oil in a skillet on the heat.
2. 2. Next, add tofu, diced bell peppers and diced onion to the skillet and cook until the vegetables are soft.
3. 3. Finally, season with powder, salt and pepper.

Nutritional Information (per serving): Calories: 150; Carbs: 8g; Protein: 10g; Fats: 8g

LUNCH RECIPES

Quinoa Salad with Lemon Herb Dressing

PREPARATION TIME: 10 MINUTES
COOK TIME: 15 MINUTES
SERVINGS: 4

INGREDIENTS

- 1 cup quinoa
- 2 cups water
- 1 cup cherry tomatoes, halved
- 1 cucumber, diced
- 1/4 cup chopped fresh herbs (such as parsley, basil, or cilantro)
- Juice of 1 lemon
- 2 tablespoons olive oil
- Salt and pepper to taste

INSTRUCTIONS

1. 1. Wash the quinoa with water.
2. 2. Boil water in a saucepan, then add the quinoa cover and let it simmer for 15 minutes.
3. 3. In a bowl, mix the quinoa with cherry tomatoes, cucumber and finely chopped herbs. In a bowl, blend lemon juice, olive oil, salt and pepper.
4. 4. Drizzle this mixture over the salad. Gently mix everything.

Nutritional Information (per serving): Calories: 200; Carbs: 30g; Protein: 6g; Fats: 8g

Veggie Stir-Fry with Tofu

PREPARATION TIME: 10 MINUTES
COOK TIME: 15 MINUTES
SERVINGS: 4

INGREDIENTS

- 1 block tofu, pressed and cubed
- 2 cups mixed vegetables (such as bell peppers, broccoli, carrots)
- 2 tablespoons soy sauce
- 1 tablespoon sesame oil
- 1 clove garlic, minced
- Cooked brown rice or quinoa for serving

INSTRUCTIONS

1. 1. Heat some oil in a skillet on medium heat. Put in the tofu cubes. Cook them until they turn brown from all angles.
2. 2. Then, add a mix of vegetables and minced garlic to the skillet. Stir everything around until the veggies are right. Not soft, not too firm.
3. 3. Pour in some soy sauce. Let it cook for one minute. Finally dish out the stir fry over a bed of rice or quinoa.

Nutritional Information (per serving): Calories: 250; Carbs: 20g; Protein: 15g; Fats: 12g

Lentil Soup

PREPARATION TIME: 10 MINUTES
COOK TIME: 30 MINUTES
SERVINGS: 4

INGREDIENTS

- 1 cup dry lentils, rinsed
- 4 cups vegetable broth
- 1 onion, diced
- 2 carrots, diced
- 2 celery stalks, diced
- 2 cloves garlic, minced
- 1 teaspoon dried thyme
- Salt and pepper to taste

INSTRUCTIONS

1. 1. In a pot, mix lentils, vegetable broth, onion, carrots, celery, garlic and thyme.
2. 2. Let it come to a boil then lower the heat and let it simmer for 25 30 minutes until the lentils and veggies are soft.
3. 3. Add salt and pepper as needed for flavor before serving.

Nutritional Information (per serving): Calories: 200; Carbs: 35g; Protein: 12g; Fats: 2g

Zucchini Noodles with Pesto

PREPARATION TIME: 10 MINUTES
COOK TIME: 10 MINUTES
SERVINGS: 2

INGREDIENTS

- 2 zucchinis large
- 1/4 cup pesto sauce homemade
- halved Cherry tomatoes
- toasted Pine nuts

INSTRUCTIONS

1. 1. Heat the pesto sauce in a skillet on the heat.
2. 2. Toss the zucchini noodles until they are warmed through and evenly coated with the pesto.
3. 3. If preferred, serve the zucchini noodles with halved cherry tomatoes.
4. 4. Toasted pine nuts on top.

Nutritional Information (per serving): Calories: 180; Carbs: 10g; Protein: 5g; Fats: 14g

Greek Quinoa Stuffed Peppers

PREPARATION TIME: 15 MINUTES
COOK TIME: 30 MINUTES
SERVINGS: 4

INGREDIENTS

- 4 bell peppers, halved and seeds removed
- 1 cup cooked quinoa
- 1 cup diced tomatoes
- 1/2 cup diced cucumber
- 1/4 cup chopped kalamata olives
- 1/4 cup crumbled feta cheese
- 1 tablespoon olive oil
- 1 teaspoon dried oregano
- Salt and pepper to taste

INSTRUCTIONS

1. 1. Start by preheating the oven to 375°F (190°C).
2. 2. Next, arrange the bell pepper halves in a baking dish. In a mixing bowl, mix the quinoa, tomatoes, cucumber, olives, feta cheese, olive oil, oregano, salt and pepper.
3. 3. Fill each bell pepper half with the quinoa mixture. Cover them with foil. Bake for 25 minutes. After that time is up, remove the foil.
4. 4. Bake for 5 minutes until they are nicely cooked. Enjoy your delicious stuffed bell peppers!

Nutritional Information (per serving): Calories: 220; Carbs: 30g; Protein: 8g; Fats: 8g

Vegan Lentil Tacos

PREPARATION TIME: 10 MINUTES
COOK TIME: 20 MINUTES
SERVINGS: 4

INGREDIENTS

- 1 cup lentils cooked
- 1 tablespoon oil olive
- 1 diced onion
- 2 cloves garlic, minced
- 1 tablespoon powder chili
- 1 teaspoon cumin ground
- 1/2 teaspoon paprika smoked
- Salt & pepper
- for serving Corn tortillas
- **Toppings:** diced avocado, salsa, shredded lettuce, chopped cilantro

INSTRUCTIONS

1. Start by heating some olive oil in a skillet on the heat.
2. Next, sauté the onions and minced garlic until they become soft. After that, mix in the lentils along with powder, cumin, smoked paprika, salt and pepper.
3. Let it cook for 5 to 7 minutes while stirring occasionally.
4. Meanwhile, warm up some corn tortillas either in a skillet or in the microwave.
5. Finally, assemble your tacos by filling them with the lentil mixture and any desired toppings.

Nutritional Information (per serving): Calories: 200; Carbs: 30g; Protein: 10g; Fats: 6g

Cauliflower Fried Rice

PREPARATION TIME: 10 MINUTES
COOK TIME: 15 MINUTES
SERVINGS: 4

INGREDIENTS

- 1 head cauliflower, grated into rice-like pieces
- 2 tablespoons sesame oil
- 2 cloves garlic, minced
- 1 cup mixed vegetables (such as peas, carrots, corn)
- 2 eggs, beaten (optional)
- 3 tablespoons soy sauce
- 1 teaspoon ginger, grated
- Green onions, chopped (for garnish)

INSTRUCTIONS

1. In a frying pan, warm up some oil on medium heat. Put in the minced garlic and grated cauliflower. Cook for about 5 to 7 minutes until the cauliflower is soft.
2. Move the cauliflower to one side of the pan and pour in beaten eggs on the side. Scramble the eggs until they're fully cooked.
3. Add in a mix of veggies, soy sauce, and grated ginger. Cook for another 3 to 5 minutes until the veggies are heated through.
4. Sprinkle some chopped onions on top before serving.

Nutritional Information (per serving): Calories: 150; Carbs: 10g; Protein: 6g; Fats: 10g

Sweet Potato and Black Bean Salad

PREPARATION TIME: 15 MINUTES
COOK TIME: 20 MINUTES
SERVINGS: 4

INGREDIENTS

- 2 medium sweet potatoes, diced
- 1 can black beans, drained and rinsed
- 1/2 red onion, diced
- 1/4 cup chopped cilantro
- Juice of 1 lime
- 2 tablespoons olive oil
- Salt and pepper to taste

INSTRUCTIONS

1. 1. Preheat your oven to 400°F (200°C). Put the potatoes on a baking sheet and sprinkle them with olive oil. Add some salt and pepper for seasoning. Bake for 20 minutes until they are soft.
2. 2. In a bowl, mix the sweet potatoes, black beans, diced red onion, chopped cilantro, lime juice and a bit of olive oil. Toss everything together until well combined.

Nutritional Information (per serving): Calories: 220; Carbs: 30g; Protein: 8g; Fats: 8g

Mediterranean Chickpea Salad

PREPARATION TIME: 10 MINUTES
COOK TIME: 0 MINUTES
SERVINGS: 4

INGREDIENTS

- 2 cans chickpeas, drained and rinsed
- 1 cup diced cucumber
- 1 cup cherry tomatoes, halved
- 1/4 cup diced red onion
- 1/4 cup chopped fresh parsley
- Juice of 1 lemon
- 2 tablespoons olive oil
- Salt and pepper to taste

INSTRUCTIONS

1. Combine chickpeas, cucumber, cherry tomatoes, red onion and parsley in a bowl.
2. Drizzle some lemon juice and olive oil over the mixture. Add salt and pepper for seasoning, then mix everything.
3. Enjoy it cold or at room temperature.

Nutritional Information (per serving): Calories: 220; Carbs: 30g; Protein: 10g; Fats: 8g

DINNER RECIPES

Quinoa and Black Bean Stuffed Bell Peppers

PREPARATION TIME: 15 MINUTES
COOK TIME: 30 MINUTES
SERVINGS: 4

INGREDIENTS

- 4 bell peppers, halved and seeds removed
- 1 cup cooked quinoa
- 1 can black beans, drained and rinsed
- 1 cup diced tomatoes
- 1/2 cup diced onion
- 1/2 cup shredded cheese (optional)
- 1 teaspoon cumin
- Salt and pepper to taste

INSTRUCTIONS

1. 1. Preheat your oven to 375°F (190°C).
2. 2. Place the bell pepper halves in a baking dish. In a bowl, combine the quinoa, black beans, diced tomatoes, chopped onion, optional shredded cheese, cumin, salt and pepper.
3. 3. Fill each bell pepper half with the quinoa mixture. Cover the baking dish with foil. Bake for 25 minutes.
4. 4. Remove the foil. Bake for 5 minutes until the peppers are soft.

Nutritional Information (per serving): Calories: 250; Carbs: 40g; Protein: 12g; Fats: 5g

Chicken and Vegetable Stir-Fry

PREPARATION TIME: 15 MINUTES
COOK TIME: 15 MINUTES
SERVINGS: 4

INGREDIENTS

- 2 boneless, skinless chicken breasts, thinly sliced
- 2 cups mixed vegetables (such as broccoli, bell peppers, snap peas)
- 2 tablespoons soy sauce
- 1 tablespoon hoisin sauce
- 1 tablespoon sesame oil
- 2 cloves garlic, minced
- Cooked brown rice for serving

INSTRUCTIONS

1. 1. Heat some oil in a skillet or wok on medium-high heat. Throw in some minced garlic and sliced chicken breasts. Cook them until the chicken turns brown and is fully cooked.
2. 2. Drop some veggies into the skillet and stir fry until they are just tender.
3. 3. Mix in soy sauce and hoisin sauce, then cook for another 2 to 3 minutes.
4. 4. Serve the stir fry on top of some cooked rice.

Nutritional Information (per serving): Calories: 300; Carbs: 25g; Protein: 30g; Fats: 8g

Zucchini Noodles with Grilled Shrimp And Pesto

PREPARATION TIME: 10 MINUTES
COOK TIME: 10 MINUTES
SERVINGS: 2

INGREDIENTS

- 2 zucchinis large
- ¼ cup pesto sauce homemade
- 8 peeled & deveined large shrimp
- 1 tablespoon olive oil
- Salt and pepper to taste

INSTRUCTIONS

1. 1. Start by heating some olive oil in a pan or skillet over high heat. Season the shrimp with a bit of salt and pepper, then grill them for 2 to 3 minutes on each side until they are fully cooked.
2. 2. In another skillet, warm up the pesto sauce over heat. Add the zucchini noodles. Mix them well until they are heated through and nicely coated with the pesto.
3. 3. Divide the zucchini noodles between plates and place the grilled shrimp on top.

Nutritional Information (per serving): Calories: 250; Carbs: 10g; Protein: 20g; Fats: 14g

Turkey and Vegetable Skillet

PREPARATION TIME: 10 MINUTES
COOK TIME: 20 MINUTES
SERVINGS: 4

INGREDIENTS

- 1 tablespoon olive oil
- 1 pound ground turkey
- 1 onion, diced
- 2 cloves garlic, minced
- 2 cups mixed vegetables (such as bell peppers, zucchini, and carrots)
- 1 teaspoon Italian seasoning
- Salt and pepper to taste

INSTRUCTIONS

1. Start by heating some olive oil in a skillet on the heat. Put in chopped onions and minced garlic and cook until they become soft.
2. Next, add the ground turkey to the skillet.
3. Cook it until it turns brown. Mix in a variety of vegetables and Italian seasoning, cooking until the vegetables are nice and tender.
4. Finally, season with salt and pepper according to your taste before serving.

Nutritional Information (per serving): Calories: 280; Carbs: 10g; Protein: 25g; Fats: 16g

Salmon and Asparagus Foil Packets

PREPARATION TIME: 10 MINUTES
COOK TIME: 20 MINUTES
SERVINGS: 2

INGREDIENTS

- 2 fillets salmon
- 1 trimmed bunch asparagus
- 2 tablespoons oil olive
- 2 minced cloves garlic
- 1 lemon Juice
- Salt & pepper

INSTRUCTIONS

1. 1. Preheat your oven to 400 degrees Fahrenheit (200 degrees Celsius). Put each piece of salmon on a sheet of aluminum foil.
2. 2. Surround the salmon with asparagus. Pour olive oil over the salmon and asparagus. Sprinkle minced garlic, lemon juice, salt and pepper on top.
3. 3. Fold the foil edges to form a packet and seal it securely. Put the foil packets on a baking sheet.
4. 4. Bake for 15 to 20 minutes until the salmon is cooked through and the asparagus is tender.

Nutritional Information (per serving): Calories: 320; Carbs: 10g; Protein: 25g; Fats: 20g

Vegetarian Lentil Curry

PREPARATION TIME: 10 MINUTES
COOK TIME: 25 MINUTES
SERVINGS: 4

INGREDIENTS

- 1 cup dry lentils, rinsed
- 1 can of coconut milk
- 1 onion, diced
- 2 cloves garlic, minced
- 1 tablespoon curry powder
- 1 teaspoon turmeric
- 1 teaspoon ground cumin
- 2 cups vegetable broth
- Salt and pepper to taste

INSTRUCTIONS

1. Combine lentils, coconut milk, chopped onion, minced garlic, curry powder, turmeric, cumin, vegetable broth, salt and pepper in a pot.
2. Let it boil first and then simmer on the heat for 20 to 25 minutes until the lentils are soft and the curry thickens.
3. Enjoy it over a bed of rice or quinoa.

Nutritional Information (per serving): Calories: 280; Carbs: 35g; Protein: 15g; Fats: 10g

Stuffed Portobello Mushrooms

PREPARATION TIME: 15 MINUTES
COOK TIME: 20 MINUTES
SERVINGS: 2

INGREDIENTS

- 4 large portobello mushrooms, stems removed
- 1 cup cooked quinoa
- 1 cup spinach, chopped
- 1/2 cup diced tomatoes
- 1/4 cup crumbled feta cheese
- 2 tablespoons balsamic glaze
- Salt and pepper to taste

INSTRUCTIONS

1. 1. Preheat your oven to 375°F (190°C).
2. 2. Place the mushrooms on a baking sheet. In a mixing bowl, combine the quinoa, chopped spinach, tomatoes, crumbled feta cheese, salt and pepper.
3. 3. Fill each mushroom with the quinoa mixture. Drizzle some glaze over the stuffed mushrooms.
4. 4. Bake for 15 to 20 minutes until the mushrooms are tender.

Nutritional Information (per serving): Calories: 250; Carbs: 30g; Protein: 12g; Fats: 8g

Vegetable and Tofu Stir-Fry With Peanut Sauce

PREPARATION TIME: 15 MINUTES
COOK TIME: 15 MINUTES
SERVINGS: 4

INGREDIENTS

- 1 block of firm tofu, pressed and cubed
- 2 cups mixed vegetables (such as bell peppers, broccoli, snap peas)
- 2 tablespoons peanut butter
- 2 tablespoons soy sauce
- 1 tablespoon rice vinegar
- 1 tablespoon of honey
- 1 clove garlic, minced
- Cooked brown rice for serving

INSTRUCTIONS

1. In a pan or wok, heat some oil on medium-high heat.
2. Put in the tofu and cook until it's nice and golden on all sides. Add in the veggies. Stir fry until they are just tender and crisp.
3. In a bowl, mix peanut butter, soy sauce, rice vinegar, honey or maple syrup and minced garlic to create the peanut sauce.
4. Drizzle the peanut sauce over the tofu and veggies in the pan, then mix well to coat everything evenly. Serve the stir fry on top of some cooked rice.

Nutritional Information (per serving): Calories: 300; Carbs: 25g; Protein: 18g; Fats: 15g

Miso Glazed Eggplant with Brown Rice

PREPARATION TIME: 10 MINUTES
COOK TIME: 20 MINUTES
SERVINGS: 2

INGREDIENTS

- 2 small eggplants, halved lengthwise
- 2 tablespoons miso paste
- 1 tablespoon soy sauce
- 1 tablespoon rice vinegar
- 1 tablespoon of honey
- 1 clove garlic, minced
- Cooked brown rice for serving
- Green onions, sliced (for garnish)

INSTRUCTIONS

1. 1. Preheat your oven to 400°F (200°C). Place the halves on your baking sheet with the cut side facing up.
2. 2. Combine miso paste, soy sauce, rice vinegar, honey or maple syrup and minced garlic in a bowl to create the glaze.
3. 3. Spread the miso glaze on the side of each half.
4. 4. Bake for 15 to 20 minutes until the eggplant is soft and golden brown.
5. 5. Serve the miso glazed eggplant on top of rice topped with sliced green onions.

Nutritional Information (per serving): Calories: 250; Carbs: 35g; Protein: 5g; Fats: 10g

Lemon Garlic Salmon 2ith Roasted Vegetables

PREPARATION TIME: 10 MINUTES
COOK TIME: 20 MINUTES
SERVINGS: 2

INGREDIENTS

- 2 salmon fillets
- 2 cups mixed vegetables (such as broccoli, bell peppers, and carrots)
- 2 tablespoons olive oil
- 2 cloves garlic, minced
- Juice of 1 lemon
- Salt and pepper to taste

INSTRUCTIONS

1. 1. Preheat your oven to 400°F (200°C).
2. 2. Place the salmon fillets on a baking sheet. In a bowl, mix the vegetables with olive oil, minced garlic, lemon juice, salt and pepper.
3. 3. Spread the vegetables around the salmon on the baking sheet.
4. 4. Bake for 15 to 20 minutes until the salmon is fully cooked and the vegetables are soft.

Nutritional Information (per serving): Calories: 300; Carbs: 10g; Protein: 25g; Fats: 18g

SNACK RECIPES

Avocado and Rice Cake

PREPARATION TIME: 5 MINUTES
COOK TIME: 0 MINUTES
SERVINGS: 1

INGREDIENTS

- 1 rice cake
- 1/2 avocado, mashed
- Sprinkle of sea salt and black pepper
- **Optional toppings:** sliced tomato, cucumber, or radish

INSTRUCTIONS

1. 1. Spread the avocado over the rice cake, then sprinkle with sea salt and black pepper.
2. 2. Feel free to add any toppings you like.

Nutritional Information (per serving): Calories: 120; Carbs: 10g; Protein: 2g; Fats: 9g

Cucumber and Hummus Bites

PREPARATION TIME: 5 MINUTES
COOK TIME: 0 MINUTES
SERVINGS: 2

INGREDIENTS

- 1 cucumber, sliced
- 1/4 cup hummus
- Paprika or chili flakes for garnish (optional)

INSTRUCTIONS

1. 1. Spread some hummus on every cucumber slice, then add a dash of paprika or chili flakes for a burst of flavor.

Nutritional Information (per serving): Calories: 70; Carbs: 8g; Protein: 3g; Fats: 3g

Energy Bites

PREPARATION TIME: 10 MINUTES
CHILL TIME: 30 MINUTES
SERVINGS: 10

INGREDIENTS

- 1 cup rolled oats
- 1/2 cup almond butter
- 1/4 cup honey or maple syrup
- 1/4 cup dark chocolate chips
- 1 tablespoon chia seeds
- 1 teaspoon vanilla extract

INSTRUCTIONS

1. Mix all the ingredients in a bowl until they are thoroughly combined. Shape the mixture into balls. Place them on a baking sheet.
2. Let them chill in the fridge for 30 minutes before serving.

Nutritional Information (per serving, 1 bite): Calories: 120; Carbs: 12g; Protein: 4g; Fats: 7g

Apple Slices with Almond Butter

PREPARATION TIME: 5 MINUTES
COOK TIME: 0 MINUTES
SERVINGS: 1

INGREDIENTS

- 1 apple, sliced
- 2 tablespoons almond butter

INSTRUCTIONS:

1. Spread almond butter on apple slices.

Nutritional Information (per serving): Calories: 200; Carbs: 25g; Protein: 5g; Fats: 10g

Rice Cake with Cottage Cheese And Sliced Strawberries

PREPARATION TIME: 5 MINUTES
COOK TIME: 0 MINUTES
SERVINGS: 1

INGREDIENTS

- 1 rice cake
- 1/4 cup cottage cheese
- 3-4 sliced strawberries
- Drizzle of honey (optional)

INSTRUCTIONS

1. 1. Spread a layer of cottage cheese over the rice cake, then place the sliced strawberries on top.
2. 2. If you like, you can add a drizzle of honey for sweetness.

Nutritional Information (per serving): Calories: 120; Carbs: 20g; Protein: 5g; Fats: 2g

Carrot Sticks with Hummus

PREPARATION TIME: 5 MINUTES
COOK TIME: 0 MINUTES
SERVINGS: 2

INGREDIENTS

- 2 carrots, cut into sticks
- 1/4 cup hummus

INSTRUCTIONS

1. 1. Try serving carrot sticks along with hummus for dipping.

Nutritional Information (per serving): Calories: 70; Carbs: 10g; Protein: 3g; Fats: 3g

Trail Mix

PREPARATION TIME: 5 MINUTES
COOK TIME: 0 MINUTES
SERVINGS: 4

INGREDIENTS

- 1/2 cup almonds
- 1/2 cup cashews
- 1/4 cup pumpkin seeds
- 1/4 cup dried cranberries
- 1/4 cup dark chocolate chips

INSTRUCTIONS

1. 1. Combine all the ingredients in a bowl.

Nutritional Information (per serving): Calories: 180; Carbs: 10g; Protein: 5g; Fats: 14g

Greek Yogurt with Berries

PREPARATION TIME: 5 MINUTES
COOK TIME: 0 MINUTES
SERVINGS: 1

INGREDIENTS

- 1/2 cup Greek yogurt
- 1/4 cup mixed berries (such as blueberries, strawberries, raspberries)
- Drizzle of honey (optional)

INSTRUCTIONS

1. 1. Enjoy a bowl of Greek yogurt with a helping of berries on top.
2. 2. For a touch of sweetness, add a drizzle of honey to taste.

Nutritional Information (per serving): Calories: 120; Carbs: 15g; Protein: 10g; Fats: 2g

Edamame

PREPARATION TIME: 5 MINUTES
COOK TIME: 5 MINUTES
SERVINGS: 2

INGREDIENTS

- 1 cup frozen edamame, thawed
- Sea salt for sprinkling

INSTRUCTIONS

1. Follow the package instructions to steam or boil edamame.
2. Add a sprinkle of sea salt before serving.

Nutritional Information (per serving): Calories: 100; Carbs: 8g; Protein: 9g; Fats: 4g

Rice Cake with Smashed Avocado and Cherry Tomatoes

PREPARATION TIME: 5 MINUTES
COOK TIME: 0 MINUTES
SERVINGS: 1

INGREDIENTS

- 1 rice cake
- 1/2 avocado, smashed
- 1/4 cup cherry tomatoes, halved
- Sprinkle of sea salt and black pepper

INSTRUCTIONS

1. Spread the avocado over the rice cake, then add halved cherry tomatoes on top.
2. Finish by sprinkling sea salt and black pepper.

Nutritional Information (per serving): Calories: 150; Carbs: 15g; Protein: 2g; Fats: 10g

Cottage Cheese with Pineapple

PREPARATION TIME: 5 MINUTES
COOK TIME: 0 MINUTES
SERVINGS: 1

INGREDIENTS

- 1/2 cup cottage cheese
- 1/4 cup pineapple chunks (fresh or canned in juice)

INSTRUCTIONS

1. 1. Serve a dish of cottage cheese with a garnish of pineapple pieces.

Nutritional Information (per serving): Calories: 120; Carbs: 15g; Protein: 14g; Fats: 2g

Almond Butter and Banana Rice Cake

PREPARATION TIME: 5 MINUTES
COOK TIME: 0 MINUTES
SERVINGS: 1

INGREDIENTS

- 1 rice cake
- 1 tablespoon almond butter
- 1/2 banana, sliced

INSTRUCTIONS

1. 1. Spread some almond butter over the rice cake. Then, place slices of banana on top.

Nutritional Information (per serving): Calories: 180; Carbs: 20g; Protein: 4g; Fats: 10g

Stuffed Bell Pepper Halves

PREPARATION TIME: 10 MINUTES
COOK TIME: 0 MINUTES
SERVINGS: 2

INGREDIENTS

- 1 bell pepper, halved and seeds removed
- 1/4 cup hummus
- Sliced cucumber, cherry tomatoes, or other veggies for topping

INSTRUCTIONS

1. Stuff each bell pepper half with hummus.
2. Add a variety of toppings, like sliced cucumbers, cherry tomatoes or any other veggies you prefer.

Nutritional Information (per serving): Calories: 70; Carbs: 10g; Protein: 3g; Fats: 3g

Chia Seed Pudding

PREPARATION TIME: 5 MINUTES
CHILL TIME: 2 HOURS
SERVINGS: 2

INGREDIENTS

- 1/4 cup chia seeds
- 1 cup unsweetened almond milk
- 1 tablespoon maple syrup or honey
- 1/2 teaspoon vanilla extract

INSTRUCTIONS

1. Combine chia seeds, almond milk, maple syrup or honey and vanilla extract in a bowl. Allow it to rest for 5 minutes; stir it to avoid clumping.
2. Place in the refrigerator for a minimum of 2 hours or overnight until it thickens. Enjoy chilled with fruit or nuts sprinkled on top.

Nutritional Information (per serving): Calories: 120; Carbs: 10g; Protein: 4g; Fats: 7g

Turkey and Cheese Roll-Ups

PREPARATION TIME: 5 MINUTES
COOK TIME: 0 MINUTES
SERVINGS: 1

INGREDIENTS

- 2 slices deli turkey breast
- 1 slice cheese (such as cheddar or Swiss)
- Baby spinach leaves

INSTRUCTIONS

1. 1. Place the turkey slices flat. Then, add a slice of cheese to each one.
2. 2. Next, place a few baby spinach leaves on top of the cheese.
3. 3. Roll them up tightly. Use toothpicks to secure if necessary.

Nutritional Information (per serving): Calories: 150; Carbs: 2g; Protein: 18g; Fats: 8g

Caprese Skewers

PREPARATION TIME: 10 MINUTES
COOK TIME: 0 MINUTES
SERVINGS: 2

INGREDIENTS

- Cherry tomatoes
- Fresh mozzarella balls
- Fresh basil leaves
- Balsamic glaze for drizzling

INSTRUCTIONS

1. 1. Skewer cherry tomatoes, mozzarella balls and basil leaves in alternating layers.
2. 2. Before serving, drizzle them with a bit of glaze.

Nutritional Information (per serving): Calories: 100; Carbs: 4g; Protein: 6g; Fats: 7g

Seaweed Snack

PREPARATION TIME: 2 MINUTES
COOK TIME: 0 MINUTES
SERVINGS: 1

INGREDIENTS

- 1 sheet of roasted seaweed
- Sesame seeds for sprinkling (optional)

INSTRUCTIONS

1. 1. Savor the crispy and flavourful roasted seaweed sheets for a snack.
2. 2. Add some seeds for a burst of flavor if you like.

Nutritional Information (per serving): Calories: 20; Carbs: 1g; Protein: 1g; Fats: 1g

Cucumber Slices with Tzatziki

PREPARATION TIME: 5 MINUTES
COOK TIME: 0 MINUTES
SERVINGS: 2

INGREDIENTS

- 1 cucumber, sliced.
- 1/4 cup tzatziki sauce

INSTRUCTIONS

1. 1. Serve some cucumber slices alongside a tzatziki sauce for dipping.

Nutritional Information (per serving): Calories: 40; Carbs: 5g; Protein: 2g; Fats: 2g

Greek Yogurt Parfait

PREPARATION TIME: 5 MINUTES
COOK TIME: 0 MINUTES
SERVINGS: 1

INGREDIENTS

- 1/2 cup Greek yogurt
- 1/4 cup granola
- 1/4 cup mixed berries
- Drizzle of honey (optional)

INSTRUCTIONS

1. 1. Layer Greek yogurt, granola and mixed berries in a glass or bowl, then add a drizzle of honey if you like.

Nutritional Information (per serving): Calories: 200; Carbs: 25g; Protein: 15g; Fats: 6g

Coconut Yogurt with Mango

PREPARATION TIME: 5 MINUTES
COOK TIME: 0 MINUTES
SERVINGS: 1

INGREDIENTS

- 1/2 cup coconut yogurt
- 1/4 cup diced mango
- Toasted coconut flakes for garnish (optional)

INSTRUCTIONS

1. 1. Enjoy some coconut yogurt with chopped mango on top.
2. 2. Sprinkle some toasted coconut flakes for a touch if you like.

Nutritional Information (per serving): Calories: 120; Carbs: 15g; Protein: 3g; Fats: 6g

15-DAY MEAL PLAN

Day 1
- **Breakfast:** BERRY CHIA PUDDING
- **Lunch:** QUINOA SALAD WITH LEMON HERB DRESSING
- **Dinner:** LEMON GARLIC SALMON WITH ROASTED VEGETABLES

Day 2
- **Breakfast:** TURMERIC OATMEAL
- **Lunch:** VEGGIE STIR-FRY WITH TOFU
- **Dinner:** QUINOA AND BLACK BEAN STUFFED BELL PEPPERS

Day 3
- **Breakfast:** SPINACH AND MUSHROOM EGG MUFFINS
- **Lunch:** MEDITERRANEAN CHICKPEA SALAD
- **Dinner:** CHICKEN AND VEGETABLE STIR-FRY

Day 4
- **Breakfast:** COCONUT YOGURT PARFAIT
- **Lunch:** LENTIL SOUP
- **Dinner:** ZUCCHINI NOODLES WITH GRILLED SHRIMP AND PESTO

Day 5
- **Breakfast:** AVOCADO BREAKFAST SALAD
- **Lunch:** GREEK QUINOA STUFFED PEPPERS
- **Dinner:** TURKEY AND VEGETABLE SKILLET

Day 6
- **Breakfast:** ALMOND BUTTER BANANA TOAST
- **Lunch:** VEGAN LENTIL TACOS
- **Dinner:** SALMON AND ASPARAGUS FOIL PACKETS

Day 7
- **Breakfast:** VEGGIE BREAKFAST BURRITO
- **Lunch:** ZUCCHINI NOODLES WITH PESTO
- **Dinner:** VEGETARIAN LENTIL CURRY

Day 8
- **Breakfast:** BLUEBERRY BUCKWHEAT PANCAKES
- **Lunch:** CAULIFLOWER FRIED RICE

- **Dinner:** STUFFED PORTOBELLO MUSHROOMS

Day 9
- **Breakfast:** GREEK YOGURT BREAKFAST BOWL
- **Lunch:** VEGGIE AND HUMMUS WRAP
- **Dinner:** VEGETABLE AND TOFU STIR-FRY WITH PEANUT SAUCE

Day 10
- **Breakfast:** TOFU SCRAMBLE
- **Lunch:** SWEET POTATO AND BLACK BEAN SALAD
- **Dinner:** MISO GLAZED EGGPLANT WITH BROWN RICE

Day 11
- **Breakfast:** BERRY CHIA PUDDING
- **Lunch:** QUINOA SALAD WITH LEMON HERB DRESSING
- **Dinner:** LEMON GARLIC SALMON WITH ROASTED VEGETABLES

Day 12
- **Breakfast:** TURMERIC OATMEAL
- **Lunch:** VEGGIE STIR-FRY WITH TOFU
- **Dinner:** QUINOA AND BLACK BEAN STUFFED BELL PEPPERS

Day 13
- **Breakfast:** SPINACH AND MUSHROOM EGG MUFFINS
- **Lunch:** MEDITERRANEAN CHICKPEA SALAD
- **Dinner:** CHICKEN AND VEGETABLE STIR-FRY

Day 14
- **Breakfast:** COCONUT YOGURT PARFAIT
- **Lunch:** LENTIL SOUP
- **Dinner:** ZUCCHINI NOODLES WITH GRILLED SHRIMP AND PESTO

Day 15
- **Breakfast:** AVOCADO BREAKFAST SALAD
- **Lunch:** GREEK QUINOA STUFFED PEPPERS
- **Dinner:** TURKEY AND VEGETABLE SKILLET

BOOK 17

Supplements for Enhancing Gut Health

DIETARY SUPPLEMENTS

Certain dietary supplements and vitamins are known to enhance wellness, as supported by research findings and expert advice. Before determining the dosage of a supplement and assessing interactions with medications, it is advisable to consult with a healthcare professional.

Probiotics

Probiotics, which are microorganisms, can change the bacteria in the gut. Dr. Amy Lee, the officer at a weight loss clinic in Southern California called Lindora, mentions that having a good mix and variety of probiotics is important for maintaining a healthy gut.

Natural sources of probiotics include Greek yogurt, kombucha, kimchi and other fermented foods. Additionally, there are powders, pills and tablets with these ingredients that you can take well.

Prebiotics

Prebiotics are a type of fiber that cannot be digested by the system but can be utilized as food by probiotic bacteria in the gut. According to Dr. Lee, many fruits and vegetables contain prebiotics, which are rich in fiber. "For benefits from probiotics, incorporating prebiotics through fruits and vegetables is recommended," says Dr. Lee. Prebiotics can also be obtained through supplements and combined with probiotics; they are not limited to food sources.

Apple Cider Vinegar

Apple cider vinegar, often made by fermenting apple juice, is commonly referred to as ACV. According to Dr. Lee it contains pectin, a substance. Unpasteurized ACV that includes "the mother" may also contain bacteria that support the digestive system's microbiome.

However, there is currently no clinical research linking ACV to specific benefits for digestive health.

Psyllium Husk

Dr. Rao suggests that incorporating fiber into your meals is typically the choice. However, she mentions that using psyllium husk or another fiber supplement could be beneficial for those who do not get fiber daily.

When mixed with water, psyllium husk creates a gel substance that can help move waste materials through the intestines and, in some situations, ease constipation. Moreover, psyllium husk assists, in adding bulk to stools, which could help with diarrhea relief.

Vitamin D

Dr. Rao pointed out that vitamin D insufficiency is quite common among individuals with skin tones and those living in regions like the northeastern United States with limited sunlight exposure. If your blood levels are significantly low, a healthcare provider might suggest taking vitamin D supplements. A recent study review from 2020 emphasized the inflammatory and balance-regulating properties of vitamin D on the digestive system. However, more research is needed to confirm this connection since some of the studies cited in the review involved animal subjects than participants.

Vitamin C

The human body obtains its dose of vitamin C from food or supplements. As it dissolves in water, it eliminates any surplus instead of storing it. Interestingly, vitamin C has the potential to boost feelings of fullness by promoting the production of short-chain fatty acids, which could play a role in connecting the gut to the brain and strengthening the barrier.

You can easily find vitamin C in form as well as in cruciferous vegetables like broccoli and citrus fruits such as oranges.

Butyrate

Dr. Paulvin suggests that butyrate, a type of short-chain fatty acid, supports the growth of cells in the colon by supplying them with nutrients. Butyrate can be obtained through supplements. Produced naturally when beneficial bacteria in the gut digest fiber. However, human clinical trials have shown results regarding the effectiveness of supplementation.

Glutamine

Glutamine, an amino acid that may not be essential for survival, could potentially benefit the system. A review published in Food Science & Human Wellness in 2021 suggests that glutamine could support gut flora, reduce responses, and enhance mucosal wall integrity.

Additionally a clinical trial published in the Gut journal in 2019 examined the impact of glutamine supplementation on symptoms of bowel syndrome (IBS) like bloating and stomach discomfort. The study indicated that glutamine was more effective than a placebo in easing these symptoms. However, it is important to note that further validation through randomized studies is necessary to confirm these findings.

Ginger

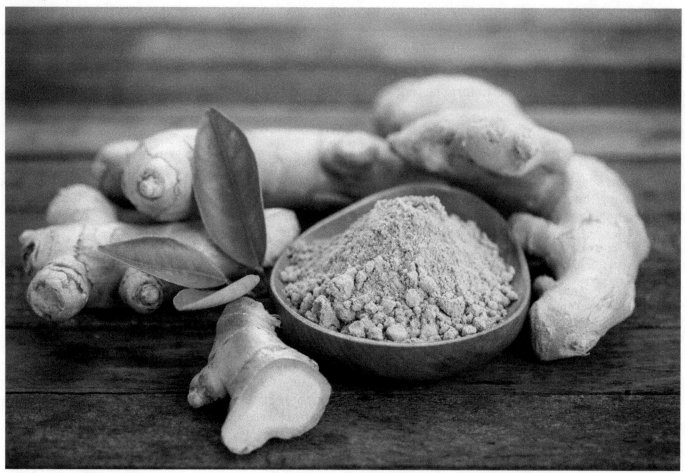

The anti-inflammatory and antioxidant properties of ginger may stem from its roots. A study published in Frontiers in Microbiology in 2020 suggests that drinking ginger juice for a period could have effects on the stomach microbiota. Over two weeks, 123 healthy individuals participated in the experiment, comparing the impacts of ginger juice to a sodium chloride placebo. Researchers concluded that those who consumed ginger had gut microbiomes.

However, further research is needed to explore the potential of ginger as a supplement for health, especially through long-term studies.

Curcumin

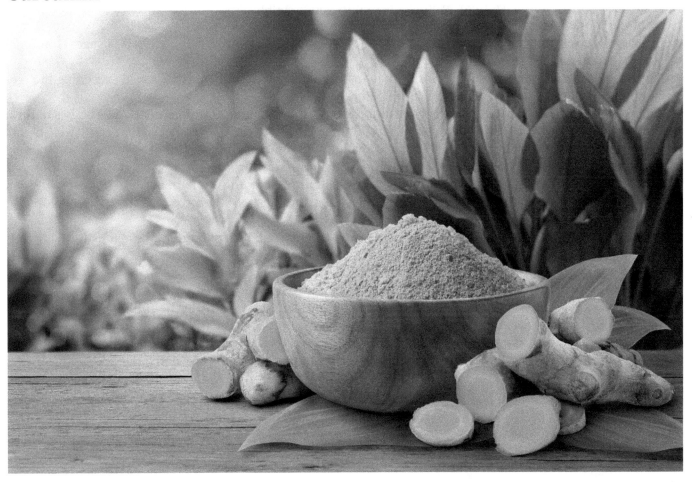

Turmeric contains a compound called curcumin, known for its inflammatory and antioxidant properties. Further research is needed as certain studies suggest that curcumin might benefit the population of gut bacteria, as mentioned in a publication by Nutrients magazine. However, there are conflicting results from studies conducted on individuals.

Health professionals emphasize that lifestyle changes such as diet and physical activity play a role in maintaining gut health. While some supplements could potentially enhance gut flora based on findings, it's essential to consult with a healthcare provider before adding any supplements to your routine.

SAFE USAGE OF SUPPLEMENTS DURING YOUR CLEANSE

Before incorporating any supplements to aid in your system while undertaking a cleanse, it's important to exercise caution and consult with your doctor, especially if you have any existing health issues or are currently taking medication. Here are some general guidelines for using supplements during a gut cleanse;

- Consult a healthcare professional. It is crucial to seek advice from a medical professional before starting any new supplement regimen. They can provide recommendations based on your history and current medications.

- **Choose brands:** When purchasing supplements, opt for brands that adhere to Good Manufacturing Practices (GMP) and have their products tested by independent laboratories. By doing you can ensure that the product you're using is both safe and effective.
- Start to Assess your body's response to new supplements by beginning with a small dosage. Gradually increase the dosage as necessary.
- Review labels. Carefully read labels for dosage instructions and ingredient lists. Avoid exceeding the recommended dosage unless advised by your doctor.
- Stay hydrated; Maintain hydration throughout the day after consuming supplements. The body's natural detoxification processes can benefit from maintaining hydration, which is essential for overall well-being.
- Always be vigilant for any reactions. If you are using supplements, be mindful of any reactions you may experience. Stop using them and seek attention if any adverse effects occur.
- Consider what works best for you. Individuals respond differently to supplements, and not everyone can tolerate them. Take into account your age, gender, diet and lifestyle when creating a regimen tailored to meet your health goals.
- **Prioritize whole foods:** While supplements can be beneficial, they should not be a substitute for consuming meals. In general, promoting gut health can be achieved by incorporating a diet of fruits, vegetables, whole grains, lean proteins and healthy fats.
- Use caution with supplements as some may interact negatively with prescription medications or lead to undesired side effects. Conduct research. Consult your healthcare provider before taking any herbs to ensure they are safe for you.
- Pay attention to your physical well-being; Monitor how you feel during the gut cleanse process and while using vitamins. To maintain your well being it's important to listen to your body and adapt your habits accordingly.

BOOK 18

Mind–Body Practices to Enhance Your Cleanse

INCORPORATING YOGA AND MEDITATION

Many individuals believe that maintaining a rounded diet and incorporating probiotics are crucial for ensuring gut health. However, these are not the factors to consider. Interestingly, engaging in activities like yoga and meditation could also positively impact your system. Recent studies suggest that these traditional practices can greatly benefit gut health in addition to their established reputation for enhancing well-being. Therefore, consider integrating yoga and meditation into your routine to support a system!

Sympathetic Vs. Parasympathetic Nervous System

It's no secret that stress can really mess with your stomach; I mean, we've all had those moments, right? When you're stressed out, your body goes into fight or flight mode, thanks to the system. This can lead to blood flow in your gut, slowing down digestion.

If you try yoga and meditation, it might just do the trick! Studies suggest that doing these activities could help you chill out and trigger your system, which helps your body relax and get into a restful state. The parasympathetic nervous system is like a friend to your gut health because it helps you unwind deeply, which is super good for digestion.

One cool thing about activating the system is that it can slow down your heart rate, sending more blood to your intestines for some much-needed oxygen and nutrients.

Your ability to digest and absorb nutrients from food relies on kicking up the production of enzymes.

Relaxing those muscles could ease constipation and bloating.

You want to make sure those digestive hormones, like gastrin and cholecystokinin (CCK), are doing their job properly.

Your gut lining stays healthy when you give it some love by promoting cell growth and repair. Engaging in meditation and practicing mindfulness, though not a cure could potentially. Prevent stress, an aspect of everyday life.

Meditation And Gut Health

One effective method to reduce stress and promote the body's relaxation is through practicing meditation. By engaging the system and reducing stress levels, one may achieve a more stable gut microbiota and decreased inflammation, leading to an improved gut-brain connection.

A recent study focused on the impact of meditation on the structure of the gut microbiome. The research compared the gut flora of monks who practiced meditation regularly with a control group that did not meditate. The results were fascinating! They revealed that consistent deep meditation practice positively influenced the composition and health of the gut microbiota.

When engaging in meditation.

- Choose an environment (such as an organized space)
- Put away distractions like your phone and TV and simply be present
- Focus closely on each breath and how your body responds
- Let go of worries or judgments about your thoughts

Understanding these practices can help bring peace not only to your mind but also to your stomach during future meditation sessions.

Yoga And Gut Health

By incorporating yoga sessions and practicing breathing exercises, you're essentially signaling to your body's system that everything is okay. It's time to unwind. Yoga offers health perks, such as enhancing digestion, muscle tone and flexibility. The twists and forward bends in yoga poses also provide the bonus of massaging organs and encouraging the release of digestive enzymes. This can help promote bowel movements and facilitate food passage through the digestive system.

Moreover, the controlled breathing techniques used in yoga, known as pranayama, can stimulate waves that move food through the intestines. Employing breathing is an effective approach. To achieve this stance, place your hands facing upwards with one on your abdomen. Inhale through your nostrils, allowing the breath to fill your abdomen before reaching your chest. This technique helps regulate your breath to originate from your diaphragm rather than your chest. It's efficient, simple and effective!

It's essential to listen to your body's limits during yoga practice and not push yourself hard. Following a teacher's guidance is crucial for ensuring a yoga experience.

Enhance the functioning of your system by incorporating three practices: mastering your breath control, focusing on the present moment and reducing stress and anxiety levels. Show some care to your stomach to ensure it operates optimally by putting yourself. Therefore, lay out your yoga mat. Show some love to your area!

THE ROLE OF SLEEP AND HOW TO IMPROVE IT

If you've ever struggled to get some shut-eye or woke up feeling not hungry, you understand the significance of a night's sleep for your digestion. Ensuring you get sleep and keep your system in good shape is essential for overall health. Surprisingly, the bond between these two aspects may play a role well.

Often, when we attempt to drift off to dreamland, our minds are preoccupied with thoughts. It's important not to forget about the microbiota during this process.

What is the microbiome?

The microbiome encompasses a range of organisms, including bacteria, fungi, viruses and other microorganisms that reside in our bodies. These tiny inhabitants play a role in influencing aspects of our well-being, such as our system, emotions, digestion, energy levels and sleep patterns. Each person possesses their microbiome composition. While it primarily forms during pregnancy and early childhood, it continues to evolve throughout life due to factors like diet, environmental toxins, medications and other influences. Just as every town within a state has its population mix, parts of the body—like the mouth, skin and gut—harbor their specific bacterial communities.

What does the gut have to do with sleep?

Recent studies have highlighted the connection between the gut and the brain, showcasing how our instincts, often referred to as "gut feelings," can influence our actions. The communication pathway known as the gut-brain axis facilitates the transmission of signals between these two body systems through the system.

It's not surprising that there is a correlation between gut health and sleep patterns, considering the relationship between the brain's cortex and sleep functions as well as its connection with stomach processes.

Dr. Amy Burkhart, a nutritionist and physician, points out that our gut microbiome. Comprising all microorganisms in our system. Possesses its distinct genetic makeup. Traditionally, human DNA has been considered the blueprint for functions. However recent findings suggest that bacteria in our gut could also impact processes. Given that DNA outweighs human genetic material in our bodies, microbes' influence on health could be extensive and significant. How these gut microbes affect sleep is one illustration of their impact.

Good sleep helps the gut

The significance of maintaining digestion has drawn attention to the importance of gut health. It's not without reason. Many serious diseases are associated with gut issues, such as bowel conditions like Crohn's disease and ulcerative colitis. Health risks also include cancer, diabetes, liver problems and heart conditions.

Various factors play a role in how sleep quality can affect gut health negatively. Research suggests that two days of sleep can disturb the balance of gut bacteria. Short sleep duration is linked to inflammation and stress hormone levels.

Unhealthy sleep patterns that disrupt rest can also have an impact on your system. Since both systems are interconnected, anything that disturbs sleep can harm gut health. According to Burkhart, factors that are harmful to gut health include stress, lack of activity, excessive sugar intake, consumption of processed foods and alcohol exposure to light before bedtime and drinking coffee late in the day.

Recognizing this connection emphasizes the importance of being mindful of our sleeping habits for our well-being. Making changes such as following a routine and spending time could significantly improve both your digestive health and the quality of your sleep.

A healthy gut helps with sleep

A balanced microbiome could potentially enhance the quality and duration of sleep, as getting a good night's rest can positively impact the gut. According to Soni, studies have indicated that a diverse microbiome is linked to sleep efficiency and longer durations of sleep. Nourishing the gut microorganisms properly may lead to sleep disturbances and an uplifted mood.

Maintaining a system can help regulate our internal clock effectively. Burkhart mentioned that research from the University of Missouri highlights the role of the gut microbiome in governing sleep patterns. The gut microbes play a role in enhancing one's sleep quality by influencing rhythms.

How to improve both gut health and sleep

Improving your digestion and ensuring a night's sleep are influenced by the habits you might already be working on changing. Here are some examples.

- Eat foods. Burkhart mentions that eating a diet in foods low in processed foods and sugars can have a positive impact on the gut microbiome. Soni suggests including a variety of plant-based foods like fruits, nuts, seeds, and vegetables as pre and probiotic meals.
- Increase your protein intake. Recent research indicates that consuming protein could enhance sleep quality.
- Stay active throughout the day. Regular exercise can benefit both your system and your sleep quality. Aim for 30 minutes of physical activity daily.
- Manage stress levels. Burkhart recommends establishing a routine to reduce stress, whether it's spending time in nature doing breathing exercises, reading, writing or practicing meditation. Lowering stress levels is linked to sleep and a healthier microbiota balance.
- Stay hydrated. The positive effects of water on health and sleep are well documented.

Don't worry much if you slip up on your diet or sleep – our bodies are resilient. Use this as a health guide. Tweak it to suit your lifestyle for overall well-being.

COMMON CHALLENGES AND HOW TO OVERCOME THEM

Dealing with Detox Symptoms

Various factors such as well-being, diet, lifestyle, and the specific detox plan being followed can lead to varying detox symptoms among individuals. For some, detox can be quite demanding, while others may experience symptoms. Here are some common challenges and remedies for dealing with detox symptoms;

1. Headaches and fatigue:

Symptoms of detox may manifest as headaches and fatigue when the body adapts to alterations in diet, hydration and the elimination of toxins. These symptoms could stem from factors like lack of fluids withdrawal, from caffeine or the release of built-up toxins.

Triumph over it: Remember to drink plenty of water throughout the day to stay hydrated. For a hydrating option consider sipping on teas or infused water. If you're looking to reduce your caffeine intake it's best to cut to minimize any withdrawal discomfort. Ensuring you get sleep can also support your body's detoxification efforts.

2. Digestive issues

When going through a detox process, some individuals may encounter issues like gas, bloating, constipation or diarrhea. These symptoms often arise as your body adjusts to a diet and eliminates toxins.

Victory awaits: Incorporate fiber into your diet by consuming a variety of vegetables, whole grains, legumes and fruits. Yogurt sauerkraut, kefir and kimchi are examples of foods with probiotics that can support digestion and enhance gut health. Stay hydrated by drinking an amount of water to facilitate bowel movements, and consider incorporating gentle physical activity or movement to aid in digestion.

3. Flu-like symptoms

Sometimes, when going through a detox process, you might feel flu symptoms such as chills, body aches and a general feeling of being unwell. Your body may react this way as it adapts to a diet and lifestyle, working to rid itself of toxins.

Triumph over it: Make sure to include a variety of foods with vitamins, minerals and antioxidants, such as garlic, berries, citrus fruits and leafy greens to support your system. Consider taking immune boosting supplements, like Vitamin C, zinc and echinacea, after consulting with your doctor before starting any regimen.

4. Mood swings and irritability

Sometimes, detoxification might impact emotional and mental health, causing irritation, mood swings, anxiety, or sadness. Possible causes of these shifts include variations in hormone levels, disruptions in neurotransmitter balance, or even mental health issues.

Triumph over it: Engaging in breathing, practicing yoga, meditation and mindfulness are ways to reduce stress and achieve emotional balance. Pursue activities that bring you joy and fulfillment, such as taking a stroll in the park, bonding with loved ones or nurturing a hobby. If you encounter challenges while undergoing detoxification, seeking guidance from a counselor or therapist could be beneficial.

5. Skin issues

When the body is detoxifying, it might show signs like acne, skin rashes or increased sweating. These issues are likely to improve as the detox process goes on.

Triumph over it: Taking care of your skin, eating foods in antioxidants and essential fatty acids and staying well hydrated are key practices to maintain healthy skin. To support the body's natural detoxification mechanisms, consider detox methods such as using a sauna or dry brushing.

6. Cravings and food withdrawal

When going through a detox process, certain individuals may experience cravings and withdrawal symptoms due to the need to eliminate foods and food groups from their diet.

Triumph over it: To help balance your blood sugar and reduce cravings, focus on eating rich meals. Plan your meals and snacks with a mix of carbohydrates, proteins and fats to keep you satisfied and energized if you're craving comfort foods. Want to stick to your detox goals, look for alternatives to satisfy those cravings.

Social and environmental challenges

It can be challenging to stick to a detox plan when you're out, at restaurants, social gatherings or the workplace where unhealthy food and temptations are around.

Triumph over it: Engage the people around you by discussing your detox goals and dietary preferences with them. Kickstart your detox journey by preparing meals in advance or bringing snacks to social events. During your detox process, it can be beneficial to have a network, whether it is through face-to-face interactions or online connections.

To overcome detox symptoms and challenges, it's important to stay determined, reflect on your progress and adapt your approach when needed. Listen to your body, prioritize self-care and don't hesitate to seek advice from trusted individuals or healthcare professionals if you encounter any issues while detoxing.

Adjusting the Cleanse to Fit Your Lifestyle and Needs

To have an effective detox that lasts it's important to customize it according to your needs and lifestyle. If you're looking to personalize a cleanse based on what works for you, consider these suggestions;

- Adjust the duration; of strictly adhering to a pre-set cleanse schedule think about tailoring the duration to suit your goals and requirements. Opt for a cleanse if you're pressed for time but still want to rid your body of toxins. Conversely, if you're aiming for a detox due to dietary concerns, consider extending the cleanse period.
- If you discover that a particular diet plan is too stringent or impractical for your preferences, consider tweaking it to better align with your tastes and nutritional needs. Then, following an elimination diet, perhaps focus on cutting out specific food groups like processed foods, sugar or dairy.
- **Be flexible:** Allow yourself some flexibility within the guidelines of the cleanse to accommodate social events, special occasions and unexpected situations. Aim for moderation while staying true to the core principles of the cleanse; view it as an opportunity for balance rather than an all-or-nothing scenario.
- Of focusing on counting calories or eliminating certain foods, consider prioritizing the consumption of whole nutrient rich meals. Opt for fruits and vegetables, lean proteins, whole grains and healthy fats to nourish your body and support its detoxification processes.
- Adjust your supplement intake based on your needs, health goals and existing health conditions. Consult with your healthcare provider to determine the supplements for you and the appropriate dosages if you are taking supplements.
- Pay attention to your well-being by monitoring your energy levels, digestion, emotions and overall health during the cleanse. Make adjustments based on what you observe. Always prioritize self-care. Trust your instincts.
- Take an approach to maintain emotional well-being throughout the cleanse by incorporating mindfulness practices such as journaling, deep breathing exercises or meditation into your daily routine. These practices can help alleviate stress, enhance self-awareness and promote balance and clarity.
- Stay adequately hydrated by drinking plenty of water throughout the day to support hydration levels in your body and aid, in its natural detoxification processes.

- To add some flavor and stay hydrated, consider trying infused water, herbal teas or beverages rich in electrolytes.
- **Seek support:** If you're looking for someone to encourage you and keep you on track. Offer advice during your cleanse: reach out to friends, family or online acquaintances. Sharing your experiences and challenges with others can help you stay motivated and committed to your goals.
- Be kind to yourself; a cleanse is not about perfection or strict rules; it's about enhancing your health and well-being. Treat yourself with care, celebrate your achievements, and remember that it's okay to adjust along the way to fit your needs and lifestyle.

FAQS AND EXPERT ANSWERS

Responses to the Most Commonly Asked Questions

The term "gut health" is frequently mentioned. What does it mean, and why is the digestive system important for our overall health? What factors impact your gut health? How can you improve it? We'll delve into questions like these and more. Let's explore together to gain expertise in well-being.

1. What does gut health mean?
To maintain health, it begins with the balance of microbes, in your gut. Ensuring a community of potentially harmful bacteria and yeast in your digestive system is crucial for overall gut well-being.

2. Is gut health key to overall health?
I totally agree with that. It's important to note that your digestive system works well when your gut microbiota, made up of the microbes in your tract, is healthy.
- digestive tract
- immune system
- the skin
- cardiovascular system
- endocrine system
- skeletal system
- the brain

That's quite a bit of information! The digestive system houses two-thirds of the system. Interestingly, it's responsible for generating 95% of the body's serotonin, often referred to as the "feel good" hormone. It's essential to maintain gut flora for well-being; without it, one cannot truly be healthy on their own.

3. Which gut health tips actually work?
There are recommendations for keeping your system in good shape, but since each person's digestive system is different, the trick is to try different approaches until you find what suits you best. The top priorities for improving your gut health naturally include consuming foods and embracing lifestyle habits such as;
- **eating fiber-rich & probiotic-packed food** – think lentils, beans, yogurts, whole grains, tempeh and kefir.
- **Supplements** – like live-friendly bacteria, turmeric & apple cider vinegar.

- **Frequent exercise** – Regular physical activity plays a role in maintaining your mental well-being. Engaging in exercise offers advantages for your digestive system, emotions and overall health, leading to a healthier gut.
- **Limit your alcohol intake** – Have you ever experienced a stomach after a night of drinking? Alcohol can affect the bacteria in your gut microbiome, leading to symptoms like bloating, flatulence and diarrhea.
- **Reduce stress levels** – Feeling uneasy, bloating, and irregularity in bowel movements could indicate problems linked to stress.

4. Which foods improve gut health?

Explore further about the 18 foods for promoting gut health!. If you're curious, here's a quick look at some of our good foods for your digestive system;

- chia seeds
- black beans
- oats
- almonds
- garlic
- avocado
- lentils

Plus more!

5. What are the symptoms of an unhealthy gut?

It might come as a surprise to learn that quite a few people exhibit symptoms of issues. Signs that your digestive system may require some attention include;

- constipation
- bloating
- cramps/stomach pain
- diarrhoea
- heartburn

6. What are the signs of a healthy gut?

Here are six common signs of a functioning system;

- Regular and comfortable bowel movements
- Normal levels of gas and bloating consistent energy
- Sharp mental focus, regular digestion
- Effective stress management techniques and healthy eating habits

7. How can I detox my stomach?

The concept of a stomach cleanse is to rid your intestines of toxins and waste material. To enhance the health of your system, try the following suggestions;

- Stay well hydrated.
- Include plenty of fiber foods in your diet.
- Explore options like teas herbal teas, fresh juices, water with honey lemon or smoothies.
- Enjoy some ginger, or consider taking a ginger supplement.
- Add starches to your meals.
- Ponder fasting as a potential approach.

8. How does gut health affect mental health?

There have been terms suggested to describe the connection between the brain and the digestive system, such as the mind-gut connection, the brain-gut axis and the gut-brain link. Feelings of anxiety or stress can sometimes be linked to stomach problems like loss of appetite, bloating or stomach cramps. Research has shown that certain gastrointestinal conditions like bowel syndrome (IBS) and celiac disease are connected to feelings of anxiety and depression. If you're dealing with anxiety or depression along with symptoms, it's crucial to consult a doctor for proper treatment.

9. Why can gut health affect your skin?

A problematic digestive system can impact your health, leading to effects on your skin. Maintaining a balance of gut bacteria is crucial for skin well-being. If your digestive system is not working at its best, you may experience skin problems.

- Rosacea
- Psoriasis
- Redness & Inflammation
- Acne vulgaris
- Dry skin

Seek advice from a skin specialist. Try out some of the mentioned methods to enhance your well-being.

10. Can the heat cause bloating?

Summer is a time of year for many. Did you realize that the heat can sometimes lead to feeling gassy? This happens because the harmful bacteria in our stomachs may multiply in response to temperatures.

If you're experiencing gas due to the heat, here are some ways to help alleviate it;

- It might be tempting to stay indoors during the weather. Keep in mind that your digestive system functions less effectively when you're sedentary.
- Stay hydrated by drinking plenty of water.
- Avoid beverages.
- Ensure you get a night's sleep—lack of sleep can trigger cravings for processed foods, which may worsen bloating in high temperatures.

With any luck you now have solutions to your questions about gut health. Are ready to move toward achieving and sustaining gut health. However, it's always advisable to consult with your doctor if you have concerns about your well-being.

BOOK 19

Beyond the Cleanse

TRANSITIONING TO A LONG-TERM GUT HEALTH PLAN

How to Safely Conclude Your Cleanse

It's just as important to end a cleanse as it's to start one. Here are some tips to finish your cleanse safely without putting your health at risk;

1. **Gradually reintroduce foods:** After a period of eliminating or restricting foods it's best to ease into your regular meals gradually to help your body adjust and avoid stomach issues. If you find that some foods are hard to digest, consider starting with vegetables, lean proteins and whole grains before reintroducing the challenging items once your body gets used to them again.
2. **Pay attention to how you feel:** Be attentive to how your body responds when you start eating. Monitor any shifts in your health indicators, digestion, emotions or overall well-being. If you experience any effects or unease consider eliminating the food temporarily and reintroducing it later on at your own pace.
3. **Continue with healthy habits:** Maintaining a diet, staying hydrated, staying active, managing stress effectively and getting rest are all beneficial routines that you should uphold beyond the cleansing period. These habits will continue to contribute to your health and wellness even once the detox phase is over.
4. **Monitor portion sizes:** Getting back to your eating habits involves being mindful of how much you eat. Overloading your system by consuming amounts of food or eating too quickly, especially if it's a heavy or processed meal, can lead to discomfort. Pay attention to your body's hunger and fullness cues. Aim to eat in moderation.
5. **Reassess your goals:** Reassess your health and wellness goals based on your cleansing journey. Acknowledge your achievements. Identify areas for improvement and personal growth. Consider leveraging the insights gained from the cleanse to set objectives or aspirations.
6. **Stay hydrated:** Making sure you drink an amount of water every day should be your focus. It's essential for functions like detoxification, maintaining proper hydration levels and overall health and well-being.
7. **Be patient:** Give your body time to adjust to your eating routine and feel the complete benefits of the detox. It's normal to feel a bit different in terms of energy, digestion and mood as you go through this transition period. Trust that your body will find its balance if you give it the time it needs.
8. **Seek professional guidance if needed:** Contact a healthcare professional, such as a functional medicine practitioner or registered dietitian, if you have concerns about completing your cleanse or are experiencing persistent symptoms. They can offer tailored advice and support to help you navigate the cleanse period successfully.

By adhering to these recommendations, you can conclude your cleanse and transition back to a diet with assurance, which will also benefit your well-being in the long term.

STRATEGIES FOR MAINTAINING GUT HEALTH POST-CLEANSE

How can you ensure that the benefits of detox are as long, as possible now that you are aware of the incredible processes happening in your body? Here are some beneficial habits to help you maintain your well-being in the run!

Follow a Plant-Based Diet

Now is the perfect time to consider switching to a plant-based diet if you haven't already done so before starting our detox program. Not a plant-based diet supports detoxification. It also enhances overall well-being and promotes longevity.

Plant-based foods are easier for the body to digest and absorb compared to animal-derived foods. Along with assisting in natural detox processes, the rich assortment of phytonutrients and antioxidants in these foods helps combat damage caused by radicals.

Moreover, choosing plant based diets can significantly reduce your intake of pollutants initially. Many animal products contain hormones and other harmful substances that can negatively impact your health and potentially accumulate in your body tissues.

Stay Hydrated and Start Your Day with Lemon Water

It's crucial to keep up with your fluid intake post-detox to support your body's natural detox processes and help with weight loss. Making sure you drink plenty of water daily should be a priority especially since many people tend to forget. A simple, effective way to boost your body's detoxification and maintain the benefits of your detox is, by starting your day with a glass of lemon water. Drinking water in the morning helps flush out toxins accumulated overnight during fasting, while the lemon further enhances the detox benefits by stimulating the liver's enzymes.

Take Care of Your Gut

After completing a detox program in Thailand, it's crucial to remember the importance of maintaining a system for your overall well-being. A balanced digestive tract not only impacts your mood and hormone levels positively but also plays a role in supporting your immune system.

Once you've detoxed, it's vital to promote the growth of bacteria to sustain their effects. Along with incorporating consuming fermented foods, sticking to a plant based diet is essential.

The role of these bacteria, which also support your liver function, cannot be overstated. Some excellent rich foods to include in your diet are kombucha, sauerkraut, tempeh and kimchi.

Drink Your Greens

To enhance the effectiveness of your detox and support your body's natural cleansing process, consider incorporating juice or a smoothie made from leafy greens into your routine. This is a way to boost your intake of phytonutrients, antioxidants, minerals and vitamins. Be cautious with fruits due to their high sugar content, as they can lead to spikes in blood sugar and insulin levels despite being sugars. Opt for vegetables like arugula, kale, spinach, dandelion greens, herbs, cucumbers and arugula for health benefits. For added flavor, squeeze some lemon or lime juice into your drink. These fruits do not aid in detoxification. Also helps maintain stable blood sugar levels.

Exercise Daily

To maintain mental health, it's important to engage in daily exercise. Not does this support digestion and circulation. It also helps prolong the detoxifying effects on the body.

Prioritize Healthy Sleep

Everyone needs to prioritize getting a night's sleep. Sleep allows your body to heal and recharge. To support your body's rhythm and keep serotonin levels in check, try going to bed around 10 PM or no later than 11 PM.

Wrapping It Up: Foods to Avoid After Your Detox

After completing detox, it is recommended to steer off sugar, gluten, nonfermented dairy and processed foods. Especially those that are fried or overly processed. By avoiding these items post-detox, you can prolong the benefits of your cleanse. Maintain a feeling. Many people opt to cut out alcohol and caffeine.

It's important to remember that everyone is unique, so what works for one person may not work for another. If certain foods don't agree with you, it's best to limit or avoid them; always listen to your body.

It's crucial to be mindful of hydrogenated oils and artificial additives in processed foods for the sake of your health. Keeping these substances off your plate is a choice for well-being.

BUILDING A HOLISTIC LIFESTYLE

Integrating Nutritional Changes into Everyday Life

Usually, when people think of "detox," they imagine getting rid of toxins to boost their health. What about well-being? With many environmental factors affecting our state, isn't it time for a mental cleanse? It's no good having a body if your mind isn't in place. I've created this mental detox plan to help us stay sane in today's world.

Feed yourself on mental peace.

Trying to seek approval from others, engaging in actions and behaving merely to conform can have detrimental effects on our well-being. These harmful substances accumulate in our bodies over time gradually causing damage.

Of subjecting your body to these toxins, prioritize activities that bring you happiness and peace of mind. Shift your focus from meeting the expectations of others to fulfilling your needs and aspirations. Use your time to engage in activities that truly resonate with you. Opt for experiences that nurture tranquility and satisfaction rather than just going through the motions.

Reduce stress intake

Living a stressful life is an aspiration that may not be entirely achievable. However, there are ways to reduce the burden of stress in your life. Factors such as a demanding job, health issues or aimless relationships can contribute to this type of pressure.

Stress can have effects on your mental and emotional well-being. The key to managing stress effectively is to identify and address its root causes. Additionally, finding ways to minimize its impact can be beneficial if complete elimination is not feasible. For instance, practicing mindfulness or incorporating meditation into your routine could prove helpful.

Become a minimalist

When we want to impress people we barely know, we often splurge on things we can't afford and don't actually need. This ongoing debate really speaks to the challenges of our era. We get caught up in trying to be the " one" in our circles, so we end up buying things that serve no real purpose.

Have you ever thought about all the stuff you've accumulated? From gadgets to clothes, shoes and accessories, our possessions pile up without much thought. Each item adds to the clutter that clouds our minds and calls for a decluttering of our lives.

Take good care of your health.

A sound body is essential for a mind. Yet the health advantages of the sedentary lifestyle embraced by millennials are debatable. Physical activity has dwindled in both work settings and homes due to progress. Job satisfaction has waned with escalating work demands.

With everyone lacking the time to prioritize their well-being, overall quality of life has further declined. We opt to drive distances for groceries, indulge in foods, spend extended hours seated while tackling projects and consume alcohol excessively. The detrimental impact on our lives is evident. Making adjustments to these routines will enhance our well-being.

There are ways to uphold our health, such as embracing a lifestyle and engaging in regular exercise. Furthermore, your happiness will be naturally catered to.

Stay hydrated with positive thoughts!

Having a mindset is like nourishing your mind and body with hydration to how water and other bodily fluids support our physical well-being. Negative thoughts, such as engaging in office rumors, criticizing a colleague who didn't help you with a task and blaming management for not approving your time off, can cloud our thinking. Hinder our productivity.

That's why it's crucial to feed our minds with positivity. Surround yourself with optimism and supportive individuals. Eliminate anything that brings negativity into your life—whether it's people or circumstances.

Change the way you think about change!

When someone mentions "change," it often catches people off guard. How do you typically react when asked to adjust your behavior? Do you not give them a look?

The real challenge with change is our resistance to it than the change itself, as Gautam Buddha once pointed out. It's important to acknowledge that if you stick to the ways for too long, you might miss out on opportunities for growth and development. Embrace change as a tool for advancement. To truly savor life, it's essential to evolve and reinvent yourself.

Engaging in a detox diet can significantly enhance your health and well-being. Here are some of my suggestions on how to start one. With the new year underway, now is the time to set goals for achieving things you've never done before.

Give this detox regimen a try for a week. Let me know how it goes.

SUSTAINING MENTAL AND PHYSICAL WELL-BEING

To maintain a happy mind and body, it's important to engage in activities that bring you joy. Here are some suggestions to support your well-being in both aspects;

Physical Well-being:

1. **Regular Exercise:** Strive for 30 minutes of physical activity most days of the week and integrate exer-

cise into your daily schedule. To establish a long-term exercise routine opt, for activities you enjoy such, as walking, jogging, biking, swimming or practicing yoga.

2. **Balanced Diet:** Make sure to include variety vegetables and fruits, lean proteins whole grains and good fats in the meals regularly. To stay healthy, avoid sugar, processed foods and unhealthy fats while focusing on eating whole foods.
3. **Adequate Sleep:** Ensure you aim for seven to eight hours of sleep each night. Create a bedtime to help you drift off peacefully, limit screen time before hitting the hay, and transform your bedroom into a comfortable sanctuary.
4. **Hydration:** Be sure to stay hydrated throughout the day by drinking plenty of water. Try to have around 8 to 10 glasses of water daily, adjusting based on how active you are, the weather and your overall health.
5. **Stress Management:** To unwind and ease stress, consider incorporating relaxation techniques such as breathing, mindfulness, meditation or progressive muscle relaxation into your routine. Make sure to schedule downtime for hobbies and activities that bring you joy and help you recharge regularly.

Mental Well-being:

Engaging in activities expressing gratitude, journaling or exploring outlets are all ways to practice self-care and enhance your mental and emotional well-being. It's essential to prioritize your needs and carve out time for activities that bring you joy and fulfillment.

Building relationships with individuals in your life, whether they are friends, family members, or neighbors, can foster a sense of community and belonging. Regular communication, shared interests and meaningful interactions with loved ones contribute to nurturing connections.

To enhance health, reduce stress levels, and stay present in the moment, incorporating mindfulness practices like meditation is highly recommended. Techniques such as breathing exercises, body scans and guided meditation sessions can help cultivate awareness in your routine.

Continuously seeking opportunities for growth and lifelong learning can engage your mind. Challenge you to expand beyond your comfort zone. Whether through reading books, attending workshops or classes, or exploring hobbies, striving to broaden your knowledge base and explore interests is beneficial.

If you are grappling with mental health challenges, like heightened stress levels, anxiety issues or feelings of depression, it is crucial to seek support.

To receive support in overcoming challenges and enhancing your wellness, consider consulting with a health professional like a therapist, counselor or psychologist. To sustain a harmonious way of life that enhances your well-being and joy, make it a priority to focus on both your physical and mental health by integrating these strategies into your daily routine. While navigating the highs and lows of life, keep in mind that self-care and self-kindness play roles in maintaining your well-being.Top of Form

CONCLUSION

"Summing up the 'Dr. Barbara Inspired 15-Day Gut Cleanse offers a roadmap to improve gut health and overall well-being that can be followed during the cleanse period. This guide enables individuals to boost their gut health and enhance their wellness. It presents readers with a cleansing regimen designed to reset and rejuvenate the system throughout the entire book content. Moreover, the book furnishes a plethora of information backed by studies and practical advice for real-life scenarios.

Highlighting the connection between gut health and various aspects of our mental well-being, Dr. Barbara underscores the vital role that the gut plays in maintaining optimal health by underscoring its significance. Through her blend of knowledge and compassionate insight into topics like microbiota, digestion and dietary selections, she adeptly makes subjects accessible to individuals from diverse backgrounds.

This guide offers a straightforward cleansing program for anyone looking to embark on a journey toward gut health. The author lays out the regimen over fifteen days."

This book offers a guide to meal planning, delicious recipes and strategies for overcoming challenges, equipping readers with the knowledge and tools needed to embark on this transformative journey. The "Dr. Barbara Inspired 15-Day Gut Cleanse" goes beyond recommending foods; it also includes stress management techniques, mindfulness activities and lifestyle adjustments aimed at enhancing well-being. The ultimate purpose of the cleanse is to boost wellness. Dr. Barbara shows her audience how to reclaim their vitality by guiding them through addressing gut imbalances and forming habits. By following the crafted cleansing program outlined in this book, readers are taking a step toward improving their gut health—a truly groundbreaking achievement. Through modifications, lifestyle changes and personalized supplements, individuals can rebalance their gut flora, alleviate discomforts and revitalize their energy levels using various effective approaches.

If you're seeking ways to enhance your system health, reduce pain, and overall improve your quality of life, this book is an option for you. It serves as a guide to help individuals enhance their well-being with "Dr. Barbara Inspired 15 Day Gut Cleanse" standing out as one helpful resource. Dr. Barbara's expertise, compassion and dedication to sharing knowledge make this book a standout choice for anyone looking to prioritize their health.

BOOK 20

430 Extra Remedies

SPECIAL GIFT FOR OUR READERS

Unlock 430 Extra Natural Remedy Recipes!

Thank you for reading Dr. Barbara's Encyclopedia of Natural Remedies. As a token of our appreciation, we're excited to offer you an exclusive bonus

430 ADDITIONAL RECIPES FOR NATURAL REMEDIES

Scan the QR code below to access this treasure trove of natural health wisdom. Enhance your well-being with even more powerful and effective remedies.